Living With a
Below-Knee
Amputation

*A Unique Insight From
a Prosthetist/Amputee*

Living With a
Below-Knee
Amputation

*A Unique Insight From
a Prosthetist/Amputee*

Richard Lee Riley, CP, BS

CEO and Founder Prosthetic Consulting Technologies

Washoe Valley, Nevada

Nancy,
I hope you find some
helpful information in the
book!

Richard Lee Riley
— Rick

Note to Reader

This book was written as a source of information, inspiration, and guidance for anyone who has, works with, or knows someone who has an amputation. The book contains content of an explicit nature. The opinions expressed by the author are not those of the publisher.

ISBN-10: 1-55642-692-5
ISBN-13: 978-1-55642-692-6

Copyright © 2005

This book was originally published by SLACK Incorporated.

The work SLACK Incorporated publishes is peer reviewed. Prior to publication, recognized leaders in the field, educators, and clinicians provide important feedback on the concept and content that we publish. We welcome feedback on this work.

Printed in the United States of America.

Library of Congress Cataloging-in-Publication Data
Riley, Richard, 1954-
    Living with a below-knee amputation : a unique insight from an prosthetist/amputee / Richard Riley.
        p. ; cm.
    Includes bibliographical references and index.
    ISBN 1-55642-692-5 (alk. paper)
    1. Amputees--Rehabilitation. 2. Amputees--United States--Biography. 3. Leg--Amputation. 4. Artificial legs. 5. Riley, Richard, 1954- 6. Prosthetists--United States--Biography.
    [DNLM: 1. Amputees--Personal Narratives. 2. Amputation--Personal Narratives. 3. Artificial Limbs-
-Personal Narratives. 4. Leg--Personal Narratives.] I. Title.

RD756.4.R54 2005
617.5'8--dc22

                                                    2005000332

For more information on this book, contact:

Amputee Prosthetics
220 N. Hwy 395, #303
Washoe Valley, NV 89704
775-849-0958
www.amputeeprosthetist.com
office@amputeeprosthetist.com

Last digit is print number: 10   9   8   7   6   5   4   3   2   1

Contents

Acknowledgments

The knowledge in this book has been accumulated over the past 30 years of my life as an amputee. I learned most of it through listening to other professionals and amputees, as well as through my relationships with my employees. Most everything that I have talked about in this book has already been said before by more esteemed and learned persons. I just hope that I made reading about it a little more fun.

I want to thank all of the authors of all of the other books about amputation. Especially those authors who are also amputees. Their candor and selfless communications give so much for other amputees. In particular I wish to thank Ellen Winchell, author of *Coping With Limb Loss,* for her quote on the stages of grieving.

This work would not have been possible had I not had the advice and support of my colleagues around the world who shared their knowledge with me. I am not much of a scholar, but I love to listen to the advice of other professionals. Their unselfish sharing of information is the core of what makes us professionals.

I have to thank all of the amputees that I have had the pleasure to work with during my years as a prosthetist. I used bits and pieces of all of you in my stories, drawing on your experiences to tell the tale of the amputee. I got so much from the opportunity to be a part of my clients' lives that I could never repay it.

I wish to thank all of the companies that sent me photos for the book. Their contributions made the book easier to read and gave life to the project. A special thanks is given to Silipos and Ossur for their outstanding photos. Other companies that contributed to the book were Alps South, Freedom Innovations, Otto Bock Orthopedic, Artech, Endolite, FLO-TECH, Rampro, Ohio Willow Wood, Hanger Specialty Prosthetics of Reno, and College Park Industries. A special thanks to the people at the Amputee Coalition of America who supported my project and provided most of the books I used.

None of the photos would have made it into the book had it not been for my friend Dale Horkey. He took many of the photos and helped me prepare them for the publisher. Along the way I leaned on Nick, Dave, Katryn, Dick, Karen, Jerome, Chris, Mark, Steve, John, Doug, Jimmy, Kevin, Bill, Marty, Don, Treat, Sally, Jay, and Peter as well as all the other friends who lent their support. My good friend, Bob Guerrero who did all of the drawings, added a certain beauty to the project.

The publisher and editors at SLACK Incorporated deserve all of the credit for making this a legible document. Without their support, the book would never have been written. A special thanks to Carrie Kotlar, who supported me during the year and a half it took to write it.

I owe everything to my family, especially to my lovely wife Jill. She and my two boys, Jeff and John, have put up with the long days locked away with my computer. They had to live with me throughout the process, and their love and understanding allowed me to complete this book.

I am truly grateful to have had the privilege of knowing so many dynamic and interesting people in my life. I feel that my friendships and my family are the most wonderful gifts that a man can have. Thanks.

About the Author

Richard Lee Riley, CP, BS has been an amputee for 30 years and a prosthetist for over 22 years. His experiences in life from the perspective of the prosthetist/amputee provide a unique insight into life as an amputee. As he turns 50, he can look back over a life filled with rich and rewarding experiences. He has a degree in education from Miami University of Ohio and has taught elementary school in Mexico and Egypt. He bicycled the Alps and went on safari in Kenya. He built a house and decided to change careers. Eight years after the motorcycle accident that resulted in his amputation, he became a prosthetist and got married.

He attended Northwestern University's Prosthetic Program and founded an Atlanta-based handicapped sports association. He became an avid sportsman and began skiing, both downhill and cross-country. In 1983, he became a member of the U.S. Disabled Nordic team for the next 6 years. Rick took a job with a prosthetics firm in New Hampshire and he and his wife moved north. He competed in two Olympics and one World Championship, as well as the U.S. National Biathlon Championships.

Richard and his wife divorced and he headed west to Nevada. He started a business from scratch in Reno and eventually moved outside of town into nearby Washoe Valley. His business grew and he remarried and began a family. Rick's business flourished as he hired mostly amputees to work for him. In 2000, he sold his business and moved with his wife and two sons to Spain for a year.

He now lives with his family in their home in Washoe Valley where he writes and provides consulting services. He is a member of Rotary International and continues to remain active in the prosthetics industry.

Introduction

I lost my leg over 30 years ago in a motorcycle accident. I became a prosthetist after 8 years as a prosthetic client and eventually had my own practice outside of Reno, Nev for 12 years. After selling my practice, I felt that there was a lot of knowledge of living with an amputation that needed to be put into the hands of amputees. I have attempted to write a multidisciplinary book, one that will be interesting to the amputee as well as the professional. The format for the book utilizes stories at the beginning of each chapter, beginning with my personal story, to describe each phase of the experience. I have changed the names of all amputees in the stories to protect the innocent or guilty, depending upon your point of view. Most of the stories are compilations of several amputees, but all of them are true with a little embellishment from me. The end of each chapter contains reference and technical information that seeks to inform the reader of options and terminology, giving him or her enough background to be knowledgeable. **The personal preferences and prosthetic recommendations are not meant to be interpreted as "gospel," but as guidelines based on my experience.**

As I prepared to put my story into words, I read as much of the literature as I could find about amputees. There were some excellent books about physical therapy written for professionals, great reference material relating to amputation surgery, books on the lives of inspiring amputees, and superb material on the psychology of recovery. There were specific books on upper extremity amputees and on sexuality, but nothing specifically for the below-knee amputee, who make up nearly 70% of the prosthetic wearers. I found only one thing missing as I read all of these great books. There seemed to be a real lack of a sense of humor in the relation of the experience of being an amputee. Do not misunderstand me. I am not saying that losing your leg is a funny thing; it is tragic and painful, but the experience can also contain some humor. I relate some stories in a humorous way because throughout my experience as an amputee, I always found some parts of it funny. My experience as a prosthetist showed me that people who could find the humor in their tragedy often returned to a nearly normal life much quicker than those who were mired in their grief.

This book is for amputees, their relatives, and friends as well as physical therapists, rehabilitation professionals, surgeons, and any other person who needs to know about the below-knee amputee. Following the stories, there are charts and explanations of concepts in an outline format for easy reference. Diagrams and pictures are used to illustrate techniques and components with the emphasis on ease of access rather than a deluge of information. My hope is that after reading this book you will have a working knowledge of the prosthetic process, the phases of rehabilitation, and an empathy for the challenges faced by the amputee, not to mention a chuckle or two.

Much of the information in this book is based on the work of the numerous other authors of books relating to amputation. I have credited where I have quoted other authors directly and included all of the reference books that I utilized. I want to thank all of the friends and colleagues who generously shared their stories and knowledge with me over the years. The experience has been rewarding and enlightening.

CHAPTER 1

Amputation

Stories

My Experience

It was a Tuesday afternoon, hot and sultry as most August afternoons in Georgia. It was 1974, and I was returning from my day job as the recreation director of a children's home, hoping to catch a catnap before I started my night job. The staccato whine of the tiny engine on my Honda 100 stabbed through the afternoon heat as I turned onto the road behind my parent's house. Ahead was the construction zone I went through earlier in the day. I came to a stop as the lazy flagman glanced in my direction.

"Is it OK for me to go?" I yelled through my helmet.

His only response was a nod and quick wave of the flag, indicating that I could pass. As I accelerated, I saw that a front-end loader was in my lane ahead of me, apparently going toward the line of vehicles parked up ahead. The Honda was hardly an acceleration machine; however, I quickly overtook the front-end loader whose top speed is 13 kilometers (8 miles) per hour. As I pulled up behind, I saw that the flagman at the far end of the construction zone was holding traffic, so I eased out to pass. Just as I came up beside the loader, I caught a movement of the driver's left arm and instinctively I throttled down. I was too late. The huge extended blade of the loader whipped in front of me as the driver made a sudden unsignaled left turn. I swerved on my bike to avoid the blade, but the front corner of the blade caught my front tire and catapulted me from the bike. As I was flying through the air, time slowed to a crawl. Because I was a wrestler and a rugby player, I knew how to land. After flying 10 meters (30 feet), I balled myself up and rolled six or eight times. As I was rolling across the red Georgia clay, I was trying to discern if I was injured but I felt no pain. When my tumble ended, I popped to my feet and found that I was having difficulty balancing on my right foot. I looked down and lifted my foot. It separated from my shin with only a shred of Achilles tendon holding it to my body.

I screamed through the face shield of my helmet. I ripped the helmet from my head and for a split second I had a choice: I could pass out and not have this experience or I could keep my wits about me and deal with it. I decided to deal with it and there was an almost audible click in my brain and all the fuzziness that came with excruciating pain cleared from my mind. All of a sudden I knew exactly what to do. I directed the people at the accident scene to call an ambulance and help me cover the severed leg. A Georgia State Trooper arrived after about 20 minutes and was very persistent about the details of the accident; and even though he really irritated me at the time, my focus on his questions certainly helped me to cope. After 40 minutes, the paramedics arrived and decided to take me to Dekalb General Hospital, which was at least a 30-minute drive from where we were in Conyers. Unfortunately, the ambulance got stuck in rush hour traffic and it took over an hour to make the drive. By the time I got to the emergency room, it had been over 2 hours since my leg had been cut off. I had not received anything for the pain, nor had I gone into shock. Pain and me got to know each other really well that afternoon.

My mom arrived in the operating room to find me lying on the metal gurney. The operating room surgeon came in and lifted the towel covering the barely attached foot and we all agreed that the leg had to come off. It was really tragic for me that my mom had to see the gore but a parent had to give permission because I was not 21 years old. My fondest memory of the otherwise bleak experience was the shot of morphine I received just before going into surgery. The pain, which was probably akin to having someone hold a blowtorch to an open wound, was getting tough to take. It had been almost 3 hours since the accident when the nurse finally gave me the shot in the upper arm. I could feel the pain like a crimson hot volcano erupting from my right leg, but the morphine started to leave a delicious lack of sensation as it traveled down my torso. The pain and the morphine battled in my thigh for a few moments. As the morphine triumphed, I let out a sigh and broke a smile, no more pain.

I woke up in the hospital room and I had the sensation of having a truck parked on my foot. I still had the effect of the morphine working so I didn't experience the searing agonies that would become an all too familiar part of my days. I had a large plaster cast on my stump that extended up my thigh; there was a belt around my waist and a plastic tube coming out of the side of the cast. My feelings immediately after surgery were more in gratitude of being alive than deep grief for my leg. My dad arrived the next day, having been away on business, and was a great comfort to me. I also saw my sister, Jan, and brother, Bill, for the first time. I attempted to be upbeat because I knew they would be freaked by the thought of what it was like to have your leg cut off.

What was it like to have my leg cut off? It was not as bad as I had imagined it to be. Not that I had ever given it much thought. I was a pretty normal kid and just never thought that I would become an amputee. Surprise! Sometimes God has other plans.

The days passed in a fog. My girlfriend Jane arrived from Ohio within a couple of days but I really don't remember a lot about her being there, which did not do much for the relationship. I was getting pain shots every 3 hours and I distinctly recall how the pain would start getting really bad about 2 hours after each shot. I could take it for a half an hour more but then I started badgering the nurses, usually with little success.

I was wheeled down to the operating room on day 3. I had just been given a pain shot so I was just enjoying the ride, not really cognizant of what was going on. When I arrived, my surgeon, Dr. Johnson, was there along with a new person, Grant Rice, my prosthetist. Dr. Johnson, a Korean War surgeon, began to explain what they were going to do. I was still a pretty happy kind of guy from the pain shot so when he said that Grant was going to cut off the cast and remove the drain, I didn't have any serious trepidation. The first clue that I better pay attention was when the prosthetist turned on the cast cutter. I had used a chain saw before and this sound was nearly as scary. I looked down and tried to sit up a little when I realized that I was strapped down to the gurney. I got that, "Oh no" feeling as Grant started to cut the cast off of my leg. It looked as if he was taking a circular saw to my leg. He had to stop and demonstrate to me that the saw actually just vibrates back and forth and would not cut the skin. I later learned that it could cut the skin and also leave burns if not used properly and skillfully. Fortunately for me, Grant knew what he was doing and he soon had the cast off. Doc Johnson briskly removed all the bandages and then grabbed my stump and lifted it up to look at the incision. This was my first glimpse of my stump; it was pretty weird to not see a foot down there. It had a big smiley-faced wound that was stitched up and the skin was all yellow from the Betadine. The sides stuck out like the corners of a ravioli and there were little patches of dried blood stuck to the sutures. It did not upset me as much as I imagined that it would; maybe having experienced the trauma prepared my mind.

Doc Johnson, with his best military sensitivity style, reached down and grabbed my stump. I jumped at his gruff handling of my poor leg. He then reached behind my knee and found the drain tube. The next thing I knew he had taken hold of the tube with a pair of forceps and jerked really hard on the tube, which went through my stump and came out the other side. It unfortunately had healed into part of my body and did not yield easily. The second time he jerked on the drain tube, it came free but this time I was ready. The pain was so excruciating I let out my fiercest growl and kicked for all I was worth with my left leg, which was not strapped down. Thanks to his prior wartime experiences Doc Johnson ducked, but Grant did not and I kicked him right in the face with my best roundhouse. Little did I know that I would later work for him and consider him to be one of the driving forces in my move to become a prosthetist. After Grant recovered from the assault, he reapplied the postoperative cast but this time he attached a device at the bottom of the cast that would allow a rubber foot to be worn. The foot had no toes and was dirty but it would allow me to stand up and walk around. The cast came up over my knee and had an opening where my kneecap poked through. Attached to the top was a strap that looked like an inverted Y, which hooked to a belt that was around my waist. By the next day I was able to stand up on crutches and hobble around with my rubber foot touching the ground. It really hurt but it felt so good to be standing again that I could suffer through the pain.

The next week was a period of weaning me off of the morphine and oxycodone by giving me less and less of the drugs. The pain would get pretty bad sometimes, but I knew that the really good drugs were going to have to go if I was going to have any kind of normal life. I had been in the hospital for over a week and the only physical therapy I had was to learn how to utilize crutches and go up and down steps. No one at the hospital had ever seen a postoperative cast before so they weren't quite sure what to do with me. I only had one really bad day at the hospital. I had been there for about a week and had had several roommates. As long as I had someone to talk to I was OK but on day eight my roommate left and I was alone. It was also a rainy day and I found myself feeling sorry for myself and asking those answerless questions of "Why me?" and "What is going to happen to me?" My father found an amputee that worked in his office and brought him in to see me. I was mostly shocked by the fact that I couldn't tell he was an amputee; he looked just like another businessman. He showed me his prosthesis, which was made of shiny plastic and was held on by a belt that went over his knee.

I don't know what I expected a prosthesis would be like because I had really never thought about it. My father kept encouraging me to learn to walk with one crutch because he knew a man who lost a leg in WWII and that's how he got around for the rest of his life. I tried to get information from anyone who seemed knowledgeable: the nurses, the physical therapist, my surgeon, and, whenever I saw him, the prosthetist. Some people told me that it would just suck onto my leg but most people didn't have much information about what a prosthetic leg was like. The prosthetist, Grant, came in after 10 days and changed my cast. The doctor was there and I got to look at my stump again. It was smaller than before and I could see that the suture line, which was across the front, was healing nicely. They reapplied the cast and I asked a bunch of questions. Of course, since they always gave me pain medication prior to the cast removal, I couldn't remember much of what Grant told me.

There were two other amputees in the hospital with me. One was an above-knee amputee, about my age, who had also been in a motorcycle accident; the other was a man in his thirties who had lost his leg below the knee in an auto accident. I hung out with these guys a lot because they shared my dilemma, although they were as clueless as I as to what was going to happen next. Both of them were fixated on the money they were going to get when their lawsuit came through; the cars they were going to buy and the thought of never having to work again sustained them. I had already contacted an attorney friend of mine in Ohio, where I used to live and where I was attending college. He was researching good attorneys for me in the Atlanta area so I wasn't really focusing too much on the legal side of things. In my gut I felt that these two guys were on the wrong track. I was young and still had a life to live and could not imagine not working.

Finally, after 13 days in the hospital, Doc Johnson came in one morning and said that I could go home. Hallelujah!! Still feeling a little in the dark about what I should be doing, I asked him point blank, "What should I do?" His reply, as he patronizingly patted my shoulder, was, "Son, do what you can." In retrospect, that was probably not the best instruction that he could give to a 20-year-old rugby player who had a dangerously high pain threshold.

I was discharged on a Sunday afternoon and was so glad to get back to my parents' home. There were some visitors, a couple of old friends from my high school in Medina, Ohio that stopped by briefly to say hello and share their condolences. This encounter, which went fairly well, was my first attempt at the humor strategy. I made jokes about my leg and I found that it put my friends at ease with what must have been an uncomfortable situation. From then on, whenever I was faced with new people, I would make some type of joke. If I could get the other party to smile, I knew that they would be able to see me, Rick Riley, instead of the poor guy who had his leg cut off. I figured out that anyone coming to see me had the same thought going on in his or her mind: how it would feel to be in a similar circumstance? If you had asked me prior to amputation what it would be like, I may have replied that I would rather die. But when it does happen to you, you don't want to die. There may be times when it crosses your mind but as long as there is life, there is hope. The best way to cut through the other person's dread at seeing you in this debilitating condition is to make them smile or laugh. Once humor is introduced you are no longer the tragic amputee but a person again and people can relate to you in a normal way.

Other Experiences

My story of amputation is not typical by any means. In fact, amputation by accident or trauma accounts for only about 22% of the total. Most amputations are the result of diseases that can be broken down into three categories: circulatory, cancer, and infection. Disease accounts for nearly 75% of all amputations and congenital birth defects are 3%. Every source that I checked had slightly different statistics, but this is close. I would like to relate the experiences of two other amputee's to illustrate other causes of amputation.

Fred

Fred was 73 years old when he started to notice that his right foot was numb all the time. He had been diagnosed with diabetes 2 years earlier and had pretty much stuck to the diet and taken his medication. His blood sugar was in the normal range most of the time, except for the times when he had a few drinks with his buddies at the local tavern. He maintained an active lifestyle by walking and working in the garden. He also volunteered at the local VA hospital once a week to hang out and provide company to older vets who were bedridden or incapacitated. He felt an obligation because he served in WWII in the Pacific theater. He had been in the Marines and had taken part in the landings at both Okinawa and Iwo Jima and had seen a lot of his buddies die or get maimed. He had a lot of close calls, yet was never wounded himself. He considered himself lucky to be alive and with all of his limbs. There wasn't a day that went by that he didn't give thanks for his blessings.

When his foot started to feel numb he didn't think much about it. After all, he was getting old and it didn't hurt or cause him to lose balance. It was about the same time that his wife of 45 years became ill. The doctors diagnosed her with inoperable cancer and she went downhill rapidly. Fred was heartbroken. He spent his days with her in the hospital and his nights were sleepless and terrifying. It had never occurred to him that Alice would die before him; she was 10 years younger than him. Fred had thought that living through the hell that was Iwo Jima would be the worst thing that could ever happen to him, but he was wrong; watching his wife die slowly ate at his soul like nothing he had ever experienced. He quit eating, and when he did eat it was generally at the hospital cafeteria or a fast food place on the way home from the hospital. His hygiene suffered, he had never done the laundry before, and he was too despondent to take good care of himself. He would often skip his medication and he lost track of whether he was taking his pills on time. Alice died on a Tuesday morning and after taking care of the necessary arrangements he went home and slept for an entire day. His son arrived from overseas on a Thursday and they both attended the memorial service the following day. They had never been very close and Fred's son didn't know what to do for his dad, didn't know what to say. He did notice how empty the refrigerator was and how dirty his dad's clothes were so he did what he could to tidy up and get his dad to eat better.

Saturday night they both were tired but had rented a movie, Midway, Fred's favorite war movie. Fred collapsed onto the couch and propped his feet on the coffee table. As he took his shoes off, his son commented on how bad Fred's feet smelled. It was only then that Fred noticed the dried blood on the sock of his right foot. He slipped off the sock and was shocked to see that his second toe was almost black and that there was an abrasion on the toe from a too long and poorly cut toenail. His son said that they better go to the doctor first thing on Monday and Fred reluctantly agreed. All day Sunday Fred tried to get his mind off of his loss but to no avail. He was depressed and just could not see a way out of the hole that his life had become.

Monday morning came and Fred's son dragged his father to the doctor's office. When the doctor saw the toe and took one whiff of the sock, he immediately called the local hospital. Fred was taken to surgery the same day for the removal of the toe. He lay despondent in his bed and although his son tried to cheer him up, nothing seemed to help. They discharged Fred after a week and he went home to a house that only depressed him more. Memories of Alice were all around him. His son had to return to his job and so Fred was left all alone in his house with his memories. His lifestyle deteriorated rapidly, he quit taking his medicine, and he wouldn't go out with the friends who called. He started to drink more and sleep late into the day. Several months went by and the wife of an old drinking buddy stopped by one afternoon. Her name was Sally and she had been widowed for the last 2 years since her husband had died from leukemia.

Sally entered the house and knew that Fred was in trouble. It was 3:00 in the afternoon, he was still in his bathrobe and slippers, and it looked like he hadn't shaved in 3 days. She remembered how fit and handsome he had been just a year ago when she saw him at the mall and to see him now you wouldn't recognize him. Sally started coming by every day to have coffee with him and to help him get back into life. She needed something to do and Fred had always been a good man. She managed to get him to take off his slippers one day so she could wash them and that's when she noticed that there was another black toe on his foot and an oozing wound on his heel. When asked how long the wound had been there, Fred replied that he had just noticed it a couple of days ago but that it didn't hurt. Sally had been a registered nurse for 20 years and knew this was not good. She hustled Fred to the emergency room and his physician was called. After a brief examination, the physician said there was a serious infection in the foot and that it might have to come off. Fred was not shocked by the news. He had seen amputations on the battlefield but thought that it was ironic that he had lived through 2 years of combat in the Pacific only to lose his leg to infection 40 years later.

For the next month, Fred and Sally went to physical therapy where there was a wound care facility four times a week. The nurses cleaned and dressed the wound each time. He got to spend hours with his foot inside a hyperbaric chamber and was on so many antibiotics that it made him nauseous. After a month, the infection had spread and the doctor said that the foot would have to come off. Fred had never been to a prosthetic shop before and on the advice of his physician he went to one that had been recommended by his physical therapist. The prosthetist was friendly and explained about prostheses and how they function. He explained the process that occurs immediately after amputation and how they would proceed once his wound had healed.

The day came and Sally was with him throughout the whole procedure. When he woke in the recovery room he was groggy but happy to see Sally's smiling but concerned face looking down at him. His leg hurt with a dull throb but it wasn't as bad as he thought it would be. The stump was wrapped in multiple layers of gauze and bandages and it really hurt to move it around or to have someone touch it. Still, he felt better than he had felt in a long time; Sally was beginning to stir feelings in him that he thought would never surface again. Fred found that each day he actually felt stronger and more positive. On the second day, a physical therapist came in and started to work with him on some stretching and exercises. They were painful, but he did them anyway. Sally was there to encourage him and he could not believe how much he looked forward to seeing her every day. If he didn't know better, he would say he was falling in love. On the third day, the doctor took off all of the bandages and gauze and Fred got to see his stump for the first time. It was really strange to look down and not see the leg that had been part of his body for the last 73 years. His stump was swollen; the stitches were sticking out of the wound, which was red and puffy; yellowish Betadine stained the skin; and there were small flakes of skin around the amputation site. The physical therapist was there and she instructed Fred to reach down and gently massage his skin. Sally offered to help, but the physical therapist said that it was very important for Fred to massage himself, as it would improve his proprioception and help retrain his brain to give accurate feedback. She explained that Fred's brain still thought that there was a foot down there and it would take time and retraining to get the brain to integrate this new body part. On the fourth day, the surgeon came in and said that Fred was ready to be discharged from the hospital. The stitches needed to stay in for another couple of weeks depending on how well the healing progressed; he would receive better rehabilitation in a rehab hospital. Fred felt good about things. He had already learned a lot about how to care for his stump from the in-hospital physical therapy staff (eg, not to sit with his leg hanging down, how to work to keep his knee straight, and how to massage his skin to improve the circulation in his stump). He kept the compression bandage on his leg at all times because the physical therapist had told him that it would improve the circulation and because it felt better with slight pressure on it. She had explained that the body was still pumping all of the blood to the foot that it always had but that his plumbing was now all screwed up. His body's ability to return the blood and fluid being pumped down there was severed and he needed to do everything he could to help it get out. This meant that he should keep his leg elevated as much as possible so that gravity pulled the blood and fluid away from the end of his leg. The compression bandage had to be wrapped tight at the end and looser as it came up toward his knee; this would assist the body in removing the swelling that was the result of amputation.

Fred left the hospital on the fourth day after amputation and was transferred to a local rehabilitation hospital where he would spend the next 2 weeks while his wound healed. Sally came and visited every day and he found that he looked forward to her visits more each time. Amputation had not been easy. It was painful and depressing, but Fred had discovered that life did not have to end because he lost his leg. He didn't know what would lay ahead for Sally and him but he was ready to try.

Laura

Laura was born in 1910 on a farm in Washington near the city of Tacoma. Her father was a farmer who raised wheat, corn, hay, and oats, and Laura was the apple of his eye. She often accompanied him into the fields to watch him work and to pick the abundant wildflowers that grew in their hayfields.

One day it was nearly noon and Laura's father, Bruce, was looking forward to the noon meal. He was hungry and had been mowing hay since 6:00 that morning. The old McCormick combine had seen better days and tended to veer to the right if you didn't constantly correct the line. It was tiring work and he looked forward to the big meal that his wife would shortly have ready. He thought he had smelled an apple pie in the oven earlier when he was working near the house and he and Laura had exchanged looks of anticipation. He looked up to see Laura picking flowers off to his left where she was nowhere near the combine with its slashing razor sharp blades.

Laura was bent over picking a group of blue flowers that were all clumped together at the bottom of a little mound of dirt. She was so happy. In 3 weeks she would have her fifth birthday and her daddy told her he would take her to the fair in Tacoma that had a circus, rides, and cotton candy. She was picking flowers for the kitchen table for her mother and was thinking about how good the apple pie that she and her dad had smelled earlier would taste. She then noticed something moving near the mound of dirt. She came closer and saw a small hill of dirt start to come out of the mound. Being only a little taller than the hay gave her a good look at the ground and she could see the little hill of dirt start to move across the ground. How could the ground move, she thought to herself as the little hill crawled through the grass. She started to follow the little hill as it moved. Sometimes she lost it in the taller hay but if she looked carefully, she could always see where it went. Laura looked up to see where her daddy was because she wanted to ask him what could cause the ground to move like that. However, he was way down at the end of the field and the combine made so much noise that he would not be able to hear her anyway. Suddenly, she heard a little rustling sound and saw the ground start to move off again. She followed the moving dirt with intense concentration as it snaked through the hay. When she had followed it for a while, the little hill stopped at another pile of dirt in the hayfield. There on the hill were the same pretty blue flowers that she had picked before. As she knelt down to pick them, she thought how pretty they would look on the kitchen table.

"The damn combine has drifted again, the row will be crooked, and it will take at least two more rows to straighten back out," thought Bruce as he sped along the field. He concentrated on the machine, trying to keep the row straight, and didn't see Laura kneeling by the little pile of dirt. The slicing blades caught both of her tiny feet and severed them in a microsecond. All he heard was the high pitched shriek that only his little girl could make and as he looked to the left, he could just make out something crawling through the grass. He raced to her and found both of her legs neatly cut just above the feet. His horror was unimaginable as he scooped her into his arms and ran toward the house. He was shouting when he got to the farmyard but his wife had already come out of the house, sensing that something was wrong. He gave Laura, who had gone into shock, to his wife who took her into the kitchen. Bruce, in a near state of panic, started running down the lane that led to the county road but the nearest doctor was 7 miles away. He should have rode the horse but it would have taken too long to catch her and saddle her, so he just started running. As he approached the county road, a buggy was coming toward him and to his surprise it was the town doctor who was on his way to the McMullen farm down the road. Bruce breathlessly explained what had happened to Laura and they both took off back to the farm.

There they found Laura deep in shock and cradled in her mother's arms. They cleared off the kitchen table and the doctor performed the amputations right in the kitchen. He stayed with her throughout the night as she drifted in and out of consciousness, giving her what he could for the pain. By the next morning her fever had stabilized and he felt that she would actually survive what in those days should have been a deadly accident. She did recover and was fit with prostheses 6 months later. They were heavy wooden legs with huge metal knee joints and leather thigh lacers that were held on by a belt that went around her waist. She had always been a head- strong little girl but no one could believe how well she got around on those wooden legs. She enjoyed childhood even though her legs were constantly in need of repair and their appearance was less than ladylike.

Laura went on to graduate from high school with honors and to live a long and incredibly productive life. She was a stage performer and singer, an entrepreneur, a newspaperwoman, not to mention mother of four boys and wife to three men. She said she always had trouble with men. I got to work with her as her prosthetist when she was already in her seventies. When I first met her, she was still ballroom dancing two nights a week. All she ever wore were 3-inch high heels, which were a challenge for a woman with two feet let alone a woman with none. She was such a positive person with whom to work, full of life and always ready to help counsel new amputees, but don't ask her to be tactful, she spoke her mind. She was much more likely to say, "Get off your butt and get back into life!" then use gentleness. It was only when her back gave out in her late seventies that she started to slow down, but until then she maintained herself immaculately.

In my private practice I often hosted teaching seminars for my staff as well as other prosthetists in the local area. On one such occasion I was using Laura as my model to demonstrate a new cosmetic covering technique. She was supposed to be at my facility at 10:00 in the morning to begin the seminar. Eleven-thirty came and still no Laura. I called her house and no answer. Finally, at a quarter to twelve she pulled up in her little car. I went out into the parking lot to greet her and ask her what happened. Had I gotten the time wrong with her or something? She apologized for being late and blushed, which is something that Laura never did. "It took a while to get Charlie out the door this morning," she explained. "Who's Charlie?" I asked, expecting her to tell me about some dog or something. "He's my latest boyfriend," was her embarrassed reply.

Laura passed away in 2001 after having lived as full a life as any human. She is a shining example of courage and determination against insurmountable odds. I always felt extremely privileged to have the opportunity to work with her and to become her friend.

Amputation Surgery

The Decision to Amputate

There was not much of a choice in my case. The encounter with the blade of the front-end loader had severed my leg, leaving the Achilles tendon still attached and there was little hope of reattachment. I thought that I could feel my toes, but I later learned that the nerves would continue to send feedback to the brain long after they had been cut. I will deal with this type of sensation later in this chapter (see p. 33). I was, however, conscious throughout the discussions between the surgeon and my mother, who unfortunately was required to consent to the obvious decision. I think back on the moment when the surgeon came into the room, lifted up the sheet that was covering my slightly attached foot, shook his head, and said, "It's got to come off." I cringed at the thought but looked up at him, nodded my head, and said, "OK." I felt clear in my head although there was enormous pain. I regretted that this was happening to me but I continued to surprise myself at my "matter of fact" thinking. In retrospect, I have always considered myself lucky to lose my leg quickly without a lot of time to consider the ramifications.

Unfortunately, this is not typically the case with most amputations. Because most amputations are due to disease, there is time to ponder life as an amputee. In my capacity as an prosthetist/amputee, I had numerous opportunities to consult with persons who were trying to make the decision to undergo amputation. Most people go through hell with the decision. The easiest ones are the ones that are in tremendous pain and the removal of the foot diminishes that pain. Still, there is no easy decision here. You become quite attached to your body, and amputation is something that is pretty much irrevocable. Putting legs back on is not one of your viable options and although it may happen someday, it is definitely worthwhile to explore what life today as an amputee may be like.

Early in my career, I fielded a call from a woman who had been watching a medical show on TV about the reattachment of frog legs. She asked if we could do this at our facility. I replied that yes, we could attach a frog leg to her but it would only come in handy for swimming. She hung up. So much for my tact. I have tried everything to regrow my leg but with no success. I really thought that holding my stump up to the television when the TV preacher was healing things might work but all I got was a static lint collection. **The point is that once you cut off a part of your body, chances are it is gone for good.**

Most amputation scenarios involve a diabetic foot that loses sensation and starts to get sores from blisters or abrasions. The sore does not heal and an infection sets up in the foot or toe. The infection is often confined to a toe and the surgeon opts to remove just one or two toes. Removal of toes will generally not have a dramatic impact on stability unless one of them is the big toe. The big toe provides stability and control for the foot during the push off phases of gait; when you have lost it, you have lost a significant function of the foot. A good fitting prosthesis with an energy storing foot can often provide more function than a foot without a big toe. Most people don't know that and, after all, it is part of their body that the doctors are talking about. It is tough, especially when people allow surgeons to whittle away at them by removing one toe, then another, then the forefoot. Eventually most of these persons end up as below-knee amputees (Figures 1-1 and 1-2), but have had to endure multiple amputations. From someone who has been through one, it is not that much fun so make the first one count.

I am not a physician, but I saw a lot of results from our medical care system and you need to be aware of its weaknesses. Medical professionals are under extreme pressure to make a profit and to avoid liability issues; therefore, it is dangerous for them to always tell you what they truly think because they have to consider the legal results of their recommendation. There are many excellent medical professionals that operate within the system and it is worth your time and effort to seek them out. It is not always easy to get second opinions or to see the best people due to constraints placed by your insurance company or agency. Often times, your best advice may come from a nurse or physical therapist, so be open to the opinions of others. The decision to remove part of your body is also a spiritual one. Consult a religious person of your faith and keep in mind that your life is more important than your foot. With a good prosthesis, you will be able to live a life surprisingly similar to the one you have now.

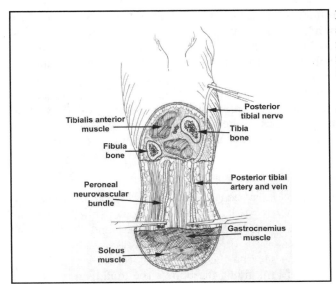

Figure 1-1. A below the knee amputation showing the bones, muscles, nerves, and major arteries/veins. (Illustration by Robert Guerrero, 2004.)

Tibialis anterior muscle

Posterior tibial nerve

Tibia bone

Fibula bone

Peroneal neurovascular bundle

Posterior tibial artery and vein

Gastrocnemius muscle

Soleus muscle

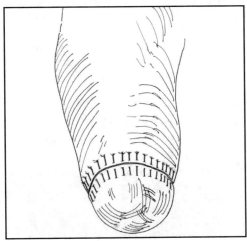

Figure 1-2. A closed transtibial amputation. (Illustration by Robert Guerrero, 2004.)

I strongly advise seeking out other amputees to consult about their lifestyle now versus before amputation. A great place to find these people is in your local amputee support group (see Chapter 12). Licensed counselors, especially ones with experience in disability issues, or ultimately another amputee are excellent sources of comfort and understanding.

I do have some advice for people facing this decision. Don't let a surgeon whittle away at your body by removing toe after toe and then the forefoot. If you have to lose your big toe, you may be functionally better off as a below-knee amputee and you are not likely to have to have surgery again. If you have an injury or infection to your foot and the surgeon gives you an option of grafting skin or muscle onto your foot to save it, you may be better off as a below-knee amputee. These scenarios were so familiar in my practice where someone has undergone multiple amputations or revision surgeries to try to save a foot that even under the best of circumstances would not have more than 50% function. I have counseled numerous persons who were living with a dysfunctional foot for years. If you have a wound that won't heal or there is damage to the foot and you cannot walk without a limp, then you are a candidate for amputation. The problems that are created because of years spent on crutches can be far worse than amputation; plus, the entire focus of your life is trying to heal instead of getting on with your life. The thing about amputation is that once it is over you can start to get your life back. Yes, it hurts but it does get better. Chronic pain saps the life out of anyone and is not only rough on you but everyone who cares about you as well.

Amputation Surgery

Like I said, I'm not a surgeon, but I have seen the results of thousands of amputations and have a pretty good idea of what works the best. I have consulted in dozens of amputations, attended dozens more postoperative procedures, and I have some observations regarding optimal outcomes.

In my particular case, Doc Johnson severed the bone 12 centimeters (4.5 inches) below the knee and beveled it at the front, giving the bone a rounded frontal tip. The muscles were cut smoothly and the skin from my calf was brought around to the front and stitched to the skin of my shin. Since my muscles were not attached to anything but left to float, they quickly began to atrophy. Eventually, after 5 years, my stump shrank to skin and bone with no muscle tissue evident below my knee. This has created some real problems such as neuromas, which could have been prevented with a little muscle covering. Still, I can get into a lot of trouble with a relatively short bony stump.

Today, amputation surgery is a 2- or 3-day stay in the hospital with a quick transfer to a rehabilitation center. In 1974, I was in the hospital for 13 days and they told me that I was out in record time. If you are having elective surgery, then I highly recommend that you talk to your surgeon about the type of amputation he or she will perform and what his or her philosophy of amputation entails. If it is an emergency amputation, then you get the luck of the draw and whatever surgeon happens to be on call, anywhere from ole' Doc Johnson to Marcus Welby.

Bone

The basic anatomy of the below-knee leg is that there are two bones that go from the knee to the ankle: the tibia, which is your shin bone, and the fibula, which is smaller and runs down the outside of your leg. The length of the optimal below-knee limb is subject to some controversy; however, my experience is that 15 to 20 centimeters (6 to 8 inches) below the knee gives the amputee the best weight-bearing surface. Of course, this depends on the height of the individual. From an anatomical view, the optimal place on the tibia is just before the bone reaches its narrowest point.

The tibia should be beveled smooth in the front, creating a rounded appearance and to a lesser degree in the back to eliminate any sharp edges that could surface later. If the bone is left too long, then the stump tends to be sharp and pointy at the end and the added leverage of a longer residual limb is mitigated by discomfort and more limited prosthetic options.

Osteomyoplastic Reconstructive Technique for Primary and Secondary Amputations (Ertl Procedure)

by Jan Ertl, MD

Introduction

Lower extremity amputation is a surgical procedure that dates to prehistory and is one of the oldest surgical procedures described. Neolithic man is known to have survived traumatic, ritualistic, punitive, and therapeutic amputation. Plato and Hypocrites have described therapeutic amputation techniques.

The treatment of severe lower extremity trauma and peripheral vascular disease has made great advances in the modern surgical era. Revascularization, internal fixation of fractures, microvascular techniques, and free tissue procedures have improved and have favorably enhanced the patient's outcome. Failure of these techniques in the lower extremities may result in factors that can lead to amputation surgery. Sometimes all efforts are pursued to salvage and maintain the extremity but amputation is the only alternative to return the patient to his or her family and an active lifestyle. Amputation is then viewed as a failure by both the surgeon and the patient, who then pictures him- or herself as incomplete by societal standards. In many regions of the world, these advanced surgical techniques are unavailable, or even too costly, and amputation remains the primary form of treatment.

When compared to the prosthetic industry, amputation techniques have changed little over the years and are usually performed by the most junior member of the surgical team. In contrast, prosthetists have made significant advances in accommodating the amputated extremity, at times attempting to improve on less than optimal surgical results. In spite of a well-performed amputation and a well-fitted prosthesis, some patients have persistent symptoms of residual extremity pain, swelling, sense of instability, and decreased length of prosthetic wear. These patients pose a challenging situation from a surgical reconstructive perspective. The effects of previous surgery, altered anatomy, muscle and bone atrophy, aerobic deconditioning, and maintenance of residual limb length create additional difficulties when considering surgical reconstruction.

The osteomyoplastic lower extremity amputation procedure was described by Professor Janos V. Ertl, MD, in 1939. This encompassed the sum of his experiences from the Post War eras, operating on an estimated 13,000 amputees.[1,2] The principles of the surgical technique were not only limited to the amputation field but had their origins in the field of reconstructive surgery. The procedure arose from the observation that the periosteum had regenerative potential in bony injuries. Ertl first applied this principle to procedures utilizing osteoperiosteal grafts to the mandible and the skull during World War I.[1,2] As this was a trench war, many soldiers survived with injuries to their face and cranium. Ertl reconstructed these osseous defects with flexible, free osteoperiosteal grafts harvested from the tibia. As the potential for these grafts to regenerate an osseous structure was realized, the grafts were then applied to a wider use, including the spine, long bones, and amputations. Along with osseous reconstruction in amputations, particular attention was also applied to the handling of the soft tissues. Neuromuscular isolation, high ligation of the nerves, myoplasty, and smooth skin closure provided the patient with a cylindrical residual extremity with end-bearing capabilities. Ertl believed that this returned the residual extremity to as normal an anatomic, physiologic, and biologic state as possible. Within the literature, this has been referred to as the Ertl procedure. This procedure is applied to both primary and secondary diaphyseal amputations of the femur, tibia, humerus, metatarsals, and digits.

Our experience with this procedure has been positive and offers the surgeon an option when presented with difficult surgical primary and reconstructive amputee symptoms.

Description of Transtibial Procedure

Informed consent is obtained from all patients. In very short residual extremities, the possibility of knee disarticulation or above the knee amputation is also discussed. Attempts are made to maintain the knee and residual extremity in these patients.

The patient is positioned supine, a bump under the hip may be utilized to control rotation of the limb, and a tourniquet is applied. Use of a tourniquet in vascular patients is used on a discretionary basis. After prepping and draping of the extremity, the previous incisions are identified and utilized. There has been no difference in wound healing between anterior-posterior, oblique, or medial-lateral incisions. Following incision, dissection is carried down to the muscular layer. Frequently, the residual extremity has no distal bony muscular coverage since the musculature was either poorly secured or allowed to retract. Dissection is then carried more proximal with the anterior, lateral, and posterior compartments being identified and isolated. If a long posterior muscle flap was utilized for anterior coverage in the primary amputation, care should be taken to preserve the length of this posterior muscle compartment. During isolation of the muscle compartments, care should be taken to maintain fascial attachments to the musculature for later myoplastic reconstruction. Following isolation of the muscle compartments, the main neurovascular structures are identified, released from scar tissue, and separated. This should include the tibial nerve, artery, and vein; the superficial and deep peroneal nerves; the peroneal nerve (both superficial and deep), artery, and vein; the sural nerve, and the saphenous nerve and vein. Palpation of neuromas may aide in localizing neurovascular bundles as these have commonly been ligated in unison. Once separated, the identified nerve should be transected as high as possible and allowed to retract into the soft tissue bed. The artery and nerve are separated and ligated in a separate fashion.

Once soft tissue dissection is complete, attention is turned to the osseous structures. The periosteum is incised from anterior to posterior on the fibula and tibia. Utilizing a 45-degree angled chisel, an osteoperiosteal flap is elevated medially and laterally, maintaining the proximal attachment. Small cortical fragments are left attached to the periosteum. Once the osteoperiosteal flaps are created, any exposed cortical bone that remains is resected to the same level, facilitating the suturing of the osteoperiosteal flaps. This requires no more than 1.5 to 2 cm of bone to be resected. The medial tibial flap is sutured to the lateral fibular flap and the lateral tibial flap is sutured to the medial fibular flap, resulting in a tube-like structure. Occasionally it is necessary to split the fibula longitudinally creating medial and lateral periosteal-cortical flaps, which are used and secured in the same fashion as above. Care should be taken not to abduct the fibula too much as this will place stress on the proximal tibiofibular joint.

In short or very short residual extremities, free osteoperiosteal grafts are harvested from the proximal tibia, contralateral extremity, or iliac crest to maintain bony length. This may also be performed on any length of residual extremity. We have utilized free osteoperiosteal grafts in primary amputations harvested from the removed limb without difficulty and complete synostosis formation.

Some short transtibial extremities exhibit an abduction of the fibula (abducted fibula) secondary to the pull of the biceps femoris muscle. This may lead to a lateral pressure point and prosthetic difficulties. The fibula is reduced into an adducted position and a lag screw is placed into the proximal tibiofibular joint, stabilizing this dynamic deformity with or without an arthrodesis of this joint.

The mobilized musculature is then brought distally covering the osteoperiosteal bridge and a myoplasty is completed suturing the posterior musculature to the anterior and lateral musculature. (If there is a length discrepancy, then a myodesis can be done). However, the goal is to provide soft tissue coverage to the distal aspect of the residual extremity. Following the completion of the myoplasty, the skin is mobilized over the underlying myoplasty. Care is given to reapproximate the skin in a symmetric fashion, leaving neither dog-ears nor crevices. Drains are placed for hematoma decompression. After sterile dressings are applied, the extremity is placed in a plaster splint in extension. The splint is removed between 2 and 7 days. A temporary total contact end-bearing prosthesis is begun in 5 to 8 weeks. Physical therapy is also instituted for education on transfers, desensitization of the residual extremity, aerobic conditioning, and upper body strengthening.

In primary amputations, the same technique is utilized. Primary amputations are approached in a similar fashion. Care is given to ensure sufficient skin coverage for the greater muscle bulk.

Results: Transtibial

Between January 1980 and January 1995, 3 surgeons performed transtibial osteomyoplastic lower extremity amputation reconstructions in 164 patients. There were 7 bilateral amputees treated in stages. Twelve patients were deceased from unrelated causes and 9 patients were lost to follow-up. A total of 143 patients with 150 osteomyoplastic reconstructions, with a minimum of 2-year follow-up, were available for review. The average follow-up was 9 years with a range of 2 to 15 years. There were 109 males and 41 females with an average age at the time of reconstruction of 48.5 years. Age ranged from 12 to 88 years of age. There were 72 right and 78 left lower extremities involved. The initial causes of amputation were traumatic in 63.3% (95), peripheral vascular disease in 27.3% (41), infection in 7.3% (11), and tumor in 2% (3). The average time to surgical reconstruction after primary amputation was 9.5 years, with a range of 2 months to 47 years.

The overall results when using the 30-point scale (Table 1) for these patients revealed a 73.3% (n = 110) excellent result, 18.7% (n = 28) good result, 5.3% (n = 8) fair result, and 2.7% (n = 4) poor result. The 4 poor results were in dysvascular patients as there was continued pain in spite of improvements in all other categories. When questioned with overall satisfaction, 97.3% of the patients felt their final result improved the residual extremity function and also improved their perceived quality of life.

Table-1

Pain	Points
a) no pain	5
b) slight pain/no compromise with activities	4
c) mild pain with normal activity	3
d) pain with standing in prosthesis	2
e) pain w/out prosthesis	1
Function	**Points**
a) unlimited walking ability	5
b) 6-12 blocks	4
c) 2-5 blocks	3
d) 1-2 blocks	2
e) indoors only or wheelchair assistance	1
Stability	**Points**
a) no weakness/no limitations	5
b) difficulty with uneven terrain	4
c) difficulty with stairs/inclines	3
d) extremity weakness	2
e) thigh lacer/walking aids	1
Swelling	**Points**
a) none/minimal/no socket compromise	5
b) with walking 6-12 blocks	4
c) with walking 2-5 blocks	3
d) with walking 1-2 blocks	2
e) with indoor walking	1
Hours of prosthetic wear	**Points**
a) 14-18 hours	5
b) 10-13 hours	4
c) 6-9 hours	3
d) 3-5 hours	2
e) 1-2 hours	1
Radiographs	**Points**
a) full synostosis	5
b) up to 75%	4
c) up to 50%	3
d) up to 25%	2
e) no synostosis	1
Total	30

(continued)

Table-1 (continued)	
Grading system	Excellent: 25 to 30
	Good: 20 to 24
	Fair: 15 to 19
	Poor: <15

Description of Procedure: Transfemoral

The patient is informed of the surgical risks and complications. All attempts are made to maintain residual extremity length to spare the cost of increased energy expenditure. A diagrammatic transverse section at the appropriate transfemoral level is helpful during surgery. In secondary reconstructive cases, the previous operative report should be reviewed and attention directed toward the treatment of the muscles and nerves, which may assist in the exposure and dissection.

The extremity is prepared in standard fashion. A tourniquet may not always be feasible and a sterile tourniquet may be used. A bump is placed under the hip of the involved extremity to assist with rotational control. The previous incisions are identified and utilized.

Dissection is carried to the muscular layer. The muscles are often retracted and atrophic, necessitating proximal dissection and muscle identification. The adductors, abductors, quadriceps, and hamstrings are isolated in their respective groups. The fascial envelope or more often scar tissue attachments are maintained for subsequent myoplasty. The neurovascular structures are identified, released from scar, and separately isolated. It is important to separate the nerve from the artery as the neurovascular structures have often been ligated together. This avoids pulsatile irritation of the nerve. The sciatic nerve may be identified by palpation of its neuroma, which may reach sizes up to 4 cm. The nerve trunk is mobilized by blunt dissection, distracted and transected at a higher level, allowing retraction into soft tissue surroundings. If a tourniquet has been used, it may be released to evaluate bleeding. The vascular structures are often friable and need to be handled carefully to avoid proximal retraction. The artery and associated veins are separately ligated to avoid arteriovenous connections.

Attention is directed toward the distal residual femur. All exostosis are removed and the periosteum is incised anterior to posterior. Utilizing a 45-degree angled chisel, medial and lateral osteoperiosteal flaps are elevated, maintaining their proximal attachments. Elevation of the flaps is aided by rotating the chisel 180 degrees, lifting and maintaining the osteoperiosteal attachments. The femur is transected at the level of the osteoperiosteal flaps with minimal femur necessitating removal. The medial and lateral flaps are sutured together and circumferential periosteal sutures are placed, occluding the end of the open medullary canal. An alternative method is to prepare a longer medial- or lateral-based osteoperiosteal flap, securing it to the opposing and circumferential periosteum, achieving medullary coverage.

The myoplasty is performed by suturing the antagonistic muscle groups to each other and anchoring them into the periosteum, covering the osteoplasty. The adductors are sutured first to the abductor group or anchored to the lateral femoral periosteum.

The abductors are imbricated over the adductor attachment and additionally secured to the periosteum anterior and posterior. The flexors are sutured to the extensor group and the underlying adductor/abductor groups, centralizing the distal femur in a muscular envelope.

The skin is fashioned to the underlying myoplasty in a symmetric fashion avoiding dog-ears and invaginations of the incision. A smooth contour is the goal allowing for a better limb/prosthetic limb interface. Penrose drains are placed prior to completion of the closure.

Postoperatively, the residual extremity is placed in an compression wrap hip spica or a bulky plaster splint, depending on the length. Sutures are removed at 2 to 3 weeks depending on wound healing. Temporary total contact end bearing prosthetic fitting is coordinated with the patient's prosthetist, between 5 and 8 weeks postoperative. Physical therapy is initiated for transfers, desensitization, range of motion, aerobic conditioning, and upper body strengthening.

Primary amputations are approached in a similar fashion. Care is given to ensure sufficient skin to coverage for the greater muscle bulk.

Results: Transfemoral

Between January 1980 and January 1995, 3 surgeons performed transfemoral osteomyoplastic lower extremity amputation reconstructions in 93 patients. There were 2 bilateral amputees. Thirteen patients were deceased from unrelated causes and 6 patients were lost to follow-up. A total of 72 patients with 74 transfemoral osteomyoplastic amputation reconstructions with a minimum 2 year follow-up were available for review. The average postoperative follow-up was 9.8 years with a range from 2 to 15 years. There were 40 males and 32 females with an average age at operation of 57.4 years. Age ranged from 29 to 79 years. There were 37 right and 37 left lower extremities involved.

The initial causes of amputation were traumatic in 60% (43), peripheral vascular disease in 30% (22), infection 4% (3), and tumor 6% (4). The average time to surgical reconstruction after primary amputation was 13.3 years, with a range of 10 months to 40 years.

The final overall results using the 30-point rating system demonstrated 70% (n = 52) excellent, 20% (n = 15) good, 4% (n = 3) fair, and 6% (n = 4) poor. The 4 poor results occurred in 3 patients, one bilateral amputee, with peripheral vascular disease as there was continued pain in spite of improvements in other categories. When questioned about their overall satisfaction, 95.8% of these patients felt their final result improved the residual extremity function and also improved their perceived quality of life.

Description of Procedure: Transmetatarsal

Use of a tourniquet in vascular patients is used on a discretionary basis. The extremity is prepared in standard fashion. The skin incision is made as distal as feasible and dorsal and plantar flaps created. The flexor and extensor muscle groups are elevated as one musculofascial flap.

The vessels are isolated and ligated and the digital nerves separated, distracted, and ligated at a more proximal level.

Osteoperiosteal flaps are elevated from the first and fifth metatarsals as described above. The metatarsals are equally transected at the level of the osteoperiosteal elevation. The osteoperiosteal flaps are sutured end to end and to each metatarsal, covering (closing) the exposed diaphysis. The flexor and extensor groups are sutured to each other through the fascial attachments, forming the myoplasty.

If used, the tourniquet is released and bleeding controlled. The skin is contoured to the underlying myoplasty, achieving a smooth transition. Penrose drains are placed for hematoma decompression. Sterile dressings and a well-padded posterior splint are applied.

The splint is removed between 2 and 7 days. Physical therapy is also instituted for education on transfers, desensitization of the residual extremity, aerobic conditioning, and upper body strengthening. Full weight bearing is initiated between 4 and 6 weeks or pending wound healing.

Transhumeral

Sterile upper extremity preparation is completed in standard fashion. A sterile tourniquet may be used on a discretionary basis. Previous incisions are utilized and anterior-posterior or medial-lateral flaps elevated. The muscles are separated into anterior and posterior groups. Depending on the amputation level, the median, ulnar, and radial nerves and their extensions are isolated, distracted, and proximally ligated. The brachial artery is separated from its veins and separately ligated. Similar to the transfemoral amputation, osteoperiosteal flaps are created and sutured over the exposed medullary canal. If used, the tourniquet is released and bleeding controlled. The myoplasty is fashioned by suturing the flexor and extensor myofascial groups together and into the underlying periosteum. The skin is contoured to the myoplasty in similar fashion as above. A bulky soft tissue dressing is applied. Prosthetic management is begun between 4 and 6 weeks postoperative.

Discussion

Conventional amputations can create multiple difficulties within the amputee. Loon[3,4] described 2o categories that amputee patients can fall into. The first is those directly related to the amputation and include pain, circulatory disturbance, local osteopenia, and muscle atrophy. The second category consists of those problems related when an attempt is made to restore function by the attachment of prosthesis to the residual extremity. From clinical observations involving amputees and Loon's descriptions, the extremity then becomes a passive, inactive participant in function and the constellation of symptoms is referred to here as the inactive residual extremity syndrome.

Numerous physiologic effects of conventional amputation contribute to the inactive residual extremity syndrome and have been elucidated in both animal and human studies. Conventional amputation procedures leave the intramedullary canal open. Non-traumatized bone exhibits an intramedullary pressure gradient of approximately 65 mmHg.[5] The increased venous pressure is necessary to maintain a centrifugal venous drainage in a rigid tubular bone. This medullary pressure appears to be important in extremity venous drainage[6] and in osteocyte nutrition.[7] When the medullary canal is left open, the normal venous pressure is lost and is measured as 0 mmHg; there is a slowing of dye material on contrast venogram; and dilated, tortuous intramedullary sinuses are also observed.[3,4] With closure of the canal with osteoperiosteal flaps, these conditions reverse themselves as shown on postoperative venograms and in the transtibial amputee additionally stabilizes the fibula, creating a broader surface area to load and accept a prosthesis.[3,4,8-12] Maturation of the bony bridge can allow complete end weight bearing of the residual extremity.

Muscle and soft tissue blood flow is essential for primary healing and future function. Many amputations are performed without restoring the length-tension relationship of the musculature. Subsequently, the muscle can undergo atrophy, fatty degeneration occurs, circulation slows, venous stasis arises as the muscles do not aide in pumping venous blood, and the result can be chronic edema. Shortly following amputation, there occurs a hypervascularity and tortuousity of the vessels.[13] However, this hypervascularity decreases within 1 to 2 weeks following the amputation. The soft tissue then becomes hypovascular but the tortuous vessels remain.[8-11] These similar angiographic findings were seen in patients with vessel occlusion and peripheral vascular disease, indicating pathologic circulation.[13-16] Arteriovenous malformations can also be seen at the distal portion of the stump, creating a shunt in the extremity.

Myoplasty in the transtibial level reapproximates the flexors to the extensors over the bony bridge. For transfemoral amputations, the adductors are attached to the abductors and the flexors to the extensors, centralizing the residual femur and securing the muscles to bone via the periosteum. This restores muscle tension and provides soft tissue covering over the distal osseous structures. Angiographic studies after myoplasty have shown an improvement in circulation on arterial supply and venous drainage.[8] Vasculature changes that are seen with inactivity and immobilization are also reversed with myoplasty.[11] Medhat has also shown that terminal circulation in vascular patients is improved with myoplasty.[17] In relation to function of the residual extremity, a more rhythmic and phasic activity is seen on EMG studies as opposed to an irregular pattern without myoplasty.[18]

With the resultant physiologic changes within the residual extremity, edema can result, which can alter the size and shape of the residual extremity.[3,4] This is believed to result from the relative inactivity of the extremity when myoplasty is not performed. With the resultant volume changes, the patient has difficulty fitting into the prosthetic socket, limiting ambulation, and can result in chronic skin changes. Continuing the cascade of changes, inactivity and the inability to load the bone will lead to atrophy of the muscle and local osteopenia/osteoporosis, poor venous return, loss of the pumping action of muscle, and fatty degeneration. Size and shape of the residual extremity are maintained with osteomyoplastic reconstruction.

Pain is the most frequent and often the most disabling symptom for the amputee and often is the most common reason for seeking medical intervention. The genesis of pain may be phantom sensations, circulatory disturbances, local skin changes, exostosis, bone necrosis, and neuroma formation. Combining medullar closure, high neuroma resection, myoplasty, and meticulous skin closure, pain has been seen to decrease in the majority of patients treated. Four patients within our study group continued to experience pain. These were all in dysvascular patients. Although experiencing an improvement in all other categories that were rated, including length of prosthetic wear, these patients most likely exhibited symptoms that were most likely continued vascular claudication.

Stability of the residual extremity is difficult to objectively measure. The clinician is usually reliant on the patient and his or her ability to function while the prosthesis is in place. The functional gains experienced by these patients were related to the decrease of pain and their ability to remain stable within their socket following reconstruction. As their function improved, patients appeared to become more confident in push off, increasing their overall walking distance. Although 4 vascular patients did not improve on their pain scale, they did show improvement in their ambulatory potential. We postulate that pain may be from persistent vascular claudication.

The efforts of the osteomyoplastic procedure are directed at creating a functional and active residual extremity based on reestablishing a physiologic environment. The resultant residual extremity will afford the amputee with a stronger and more durable limb with improved stability and proprioception. We have utilized free osteoperiosteal grafts to form our bone bridge in short residual limbs in order to maintain length and achieve the desired results. In longer residual limbs, minimal length is removed, in contrast to what has been described.[20-22] In addition, the overlying myoplasty will contribute to the total length of the extremity. The surgeon should not hesitate to sacrifice length when an increase in function can be achieved.[3] This technique has successfully been applied to both primary and secondary amputations.

The difficulty with assessing these patients' final result is that the final outcome involves variables that may affect the results (eg, socket design, prosthetic componentry and the use of different prosthetists with varying experience).

The osteomyoplastic lower extremity amputation reconstruction is technically challenging with a somewhat greater operative time than conventional techniques. It may be used for traumatic and vascular amputations with high success and high patient satisfaction. This procedure offers the surgical community with a dynamic procedure for both primary and secondary reconstructions in lower limb amputation surgery.

References

1. Ertl J. *Regeneration: Ihre Anwedung in der Chirurgie.* Leipzig: Verlag von Johann Ambrosius Barth;1939.

2. Ertl JP, Barrack R, Alexander AH, VanBuecken KP. Triplane fracture of the distal tibial epiphysis. Long-term follow-up. *J Bone Joint Surg.* 1988;70A:967.

3. Loon HE. Biological and Biomechanical Principles in Amputation Surgery. Prosthetics International. Proceedings of the Second International Prosthetics course. Copenhagen: 1962.

4. Loon HE. Below the knee amputations. Artificial limbs. *National Academy of the Sciences-National Research Council.* 1963;6(2):86.

5. Ascenzi A. Physiologic relationship and pathological interferences between bone tissue and marrow. In: Bourne GH, ed. *The Biochemistry and Physiology of Bone.* New York: Academic Press; YEAR:4, 403-444.

6. Lopez-Curto JA, Bassingwaighte JB, Kelly PJ. Anatomy of the microvasculature of the tibia: diaphysis of the adult dog. *J Bone Joint Surg.* 1980;62A:1362-1369.

7. Sturmer KM. Measurement of intramedullary pressure in an animal experiment and propositions to reduce pressure increase. *Injury.* 1993;24(3):S7.

8. Hansen-Leth C, Reiman I. Amputations with and without myoplasty on rabbits with special reference to the vascularization. *Acta Orthop Scand.* 1972;43:68-77.

9. Hansen-Leth C. Muscle blood flow after amputations with special reference to the influence of osseous plugging of the medullary cavity. *Acta Orthop Scand*. 1976;47:613-618.

10. Hansen-Leth C. Muscle blood flow after amputations with special reference to the amputation level. *Acta Orthop Scand*. 1977;48:10-14.

11. Hansen-Leth C. The vascularization in the amputation stumps of rabbits. A microangiographic study. *Acta Orthop Scand*. 1979;50:399-406.

12. Langhagel J. Angiographische Untersuchung der Stumpfdurchblutung bei Beinamputierten. Arbeit und Gesundheit. Stuttgart: Georg Thieme Verlag; 1968.

13. Leriche R. Traitement de certaines ulcerations spontanees des moignons par la sympathectomie priarterielle. *Press Med*. 1950.

14. Erikson U, Hulth A. Circulation of amputations stumps. Arteriographic and temperature studies. *Acta Orthop Scand*. 1962;32:159.

15. Erikson U. Circulation in traumatic amputation stumps. An angiographic and physiologic investigation. *Acta Radiol Suppl*. 1965;238.

16. Erikson U, Olerud S. Healing of amputation stumps, with special reference to vascularity and bone. *Acta Orthop Scan*. 1966;37:20.

17. Medhat MA. Rehabilitation of the vascular amputee. *Orthopaedic Review*. 1983;12(2).

18. Condie DN. Electromyography of the lower limb amputee. Medicine and Sport, Vol 8. Biomechanics 3: 482-488, Karger, Basle, 1973.

19. Bowker JH, Goldberg B, Poonekar PD. Transtibial amputation. *Atlas of Limb Prosthetics. Surgical, Prosthetic, and Rehabilitation Principles*. St. Louis, MO: Mosby; 1992: 18, 429.

20. Smith D. Amputations and prosthetics. *OKU*. 1993;4:23, 267.

21. Smith DG, Fergason JR. Transtibial amputations. *Clin Orth*. 1999;361:108-115.

22. Goldberg VM, Heiple KG, Ratnoff OD, Kurczynski E, Arvan G. Total knee arthroplasty in classic hemophilia. *J Bone Joint Surg*. 1981;63A:695.

23. Hughes SL, Weber H, Willenegger H, Kuner EH. Evaluation of ankle fractures. Nonoperative and operative treatment. *Clin Orthop*. 1979;138:111-119.

Muscle

There are many muscles below the knee that need to be dealt with. You may already be familiar with the major ones. The gastrocnemius and soleus are the 2 big ones that make up your calf muscle, and the anterior tibialis that runs along the front of your leg.

Underlying the muscle is the fascia, a tissue that separates the muscle from the bone and allows the muscle to contract and expand without sticking to the bone. In my case, the muscles were just guillotined, left to atrophy. After 5 years, they eventually shrank to the cellular fibers, leaving no muscle covering whatsoever. When you look at my stump it is skin and bone with no muscle at all. Many stumps that I saw, especially amputations prior to the 1980s, reflected this type of surgery.

Today, the standard procedure is to perform myodesis (the reattachment of the muscle to the bone) and myoplasty (the reattachment of the muscle to other muscles). These procedures give the muscles something to pull against so that they can remain active and will not shrink away to nothing. This can be a great advantage later on as it gives the bones padding and there is better circulation in the residual limb because of the increased muscle mass.

Generally, the surgeon leaves the gastrocnemius and soleus longer than in a guillotine amputation and then brings the two large muscle bellies around to the front where the inner one is sewn to the bone and the outer one is sewn to the front muscle, the anterior tibialis. When these two muscles are intact and have some function, they will provide a far better cushion to the bone than a prosthesis can provide. When this is combined with the Ertl bone bridge, it creates the optimal weight-bearing surface. You will not be able to tell what has been done when you first see your stump because it will be so swollen, but these things can make a huge difference later on in your amputation lifestyle.

Nerves and Fascia

There are many nerves that run to the foot and innervate your leg. The bulk of these run behind the knee and then branch from there to the front of the leg and down to the foot.

When a nerve is severed, it will do what every other tissue in the body does—it will cap itself off and heal with a layer of scar tissue. Unlike other systems in the body, nerves cannot remove scar tissue once it has been laid down. If the nerve continues to be irritated, it will continue to lay down scar tissue. When the scar tissue builds up into a ganglion or ball of nerve tissue, it is called a neuroma. I have had 2 neuromas cut out of my leg and they are no fun. The pain is very invasive and has a distinct sensation.

The surgeon generally will find the major nerves and grab them with a pair of forceps; he or she then pulls the nerve as far out as possible and snips it, letting it retract back into the stump. This works great as long as there is a large muscle mass covering the nerve, the way our bodies were designed. The problem occurs when the muscles atrophy to the point where the nerve becomes exposed beneath the skin and allows pressure or irritation to occur, setting up a cycle of the nerve continually laying down more scar tissue. Since the nerve can't remove the scar tissue, it builds up into a painful ball of nerves that can create unbearable pain. The key to avoiding neuromas is to have a decent amount of muscle covering the bone so that the nerves do not get exposed beneath the skin.

The fascia is the connective tissue that separates the muscles from the bones and from each other. It allows the muscles to move in relation to the bone and in relation to one another. Great care needs to be taken to preserve the fascia to make sure that there is covering over the bone so that the muscle does not scar down to the bone. When this happens it is called an adhesion and is most likely to occur right at the tip of the stump where the muscle can heal to the end of the bone. Since there is no way to ensure that there won't be some fascia damage, the best way to prevent adhesions is with aggressive therapy.

Skin

The final covering of the residual limb is the skin. The surgeon will leave extra skin at the back of the stump to bring around to the front. The skin on the calf of your leg is generally better vascularized and flexible than the skin that covers your shin so it is better to create a good covering for your limb. The most important thing to keep in mind is that the skin will be your first line of defense against infection or damage and it needs to be in good shape.

I have seen many revisions take place because the limb was left long in order to provide more leverage but without viable skin the leverage cannot have the desired effect. A shorter residual limb with good skin covering will lead to a smoother recovery than a stump covered with marginal skin. When you first see your stump, the skin will be yellowish from the Betadine and there will be redness and puffiness at the incision. This will diminish over the course of the next couple of weeks and you should experience a healing of the suture line.

Circulation

The body is still pumping all of the blood and fluid that it previously sent to the foot but it has no way of getting the blood and fluid back out. The plumbing is incomplete there is no return system that can take up the slack. There are still small blood vessels called capillaries that will return the blood to the body but they are very small and were not designed to carry the entire blood flow. Over time they will expand to some degree but will never be able to completely compensate. The more muscle tissue that you have below your knee the better your circulation will be due to the increased number of capillaries that you will have.

This has a major impact on healing and infection. If you are on oral antibiotics than they depend on the blood system to deliver them to the effected area. If you have poor circulation in the affected area than the antibiotics can't get to where they need to be to help fight infection. It is important to help the body as much as possible to improve the circulation through massage and utilizing gravity to your advantage. This will be covered thoroughly in the rehabilitation section.

Syme's Amputation

To remove the foot at the ankle joint is called a Syme's amputation (Figure 1-3), or an ankle disarticulation, and is an option when the disease or damage is confined to the foot. The foot is removed at the joint where the tibia and fibula meet the top of the ankle and then the heel pad of the foot is brought up and sewn in place as the bottom of the stump. The end of the fibula pokes out longer than the end of the tibia and needs to be shaved back so that it does not create a pressure point. This type of amputation makes for a really good weight-bearing surface because the heel pad is preserved, and the heel pad is one of the few skin surfaces on the body that was designed to bear weight. The disadvantage of the Syme's amputation is that it creates a stump that is quite a bit bigger on the end than it is further up the shank of your leg so that fitting a prosthesis is much trickier. There are also less prosthetic options for the

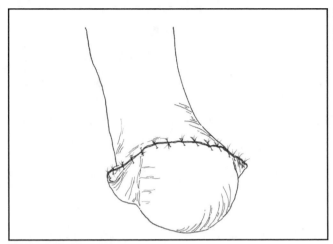

Figure 1-3. A closed Syme's amputation. (Illustration by Robert Guerrero, 2004.)

Syme's amputee, but these have been minimized over the last few years so that this is less of a problem than in the past. The main problem with a Syme's prosthesis is cosmetic. It just isn't possible to make a leg that looks shapely when you have this large distal end of the residual limb to try to work around. If cosmesis is not a problem, circulation is viable to the ankle, and the heel pad is well vascularized, then I believe that the Syme's amputation offers an excellent functional amputation. It is especially useful because after awhile most Syme's amputees can actually weight bear on the end of their stumps, which means late night trips to the bathroom don't require crutches or hopping. If this is one of your options, then careful consideration needs to be taken to make sure you understand the pros and cons of this level of amputation.

Partial Foot Amputations

Many of my clients went through partial foot amputations (Figure 1-4) to eliminate infected toes or forefoot tissue. In many of those cases, the person ended up as a below-knee amputee later on in his or her life. Functionally, these amputees did not have to wear a prosthesis but rather utilized a shoe filler, which as the name implies, filled in the shoe and, in some cases, also provided some push off in the form of an energy storing plate. The problem with this level of amputation is that the foot does not have any large muscle groups that can provide cushion or padding to the exposed bones in the front. Therefore, the bones are left with a thin covering of skin, optimally the skin that covers the ball of the foot, that at least has some end-bearing capacity. If the amputation is due to poor circulation, this is a set up for further problems because healing is a difficult if not impossible outcome. The cut end of the foot ends up having to take the brunt of the forces and there are no anatomical features that can compensate for the lack of push off. A below-knee amputee is often more functional than a partial foot amputee and his or her chances of healing in a vascular compromise situation are greatly enhanced.

Figure 1-4. A closed partial foot amputation. (Illustration by Robert Guerrero, 2004.)

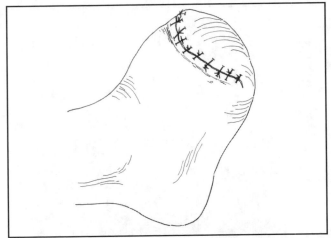

Bilateral Amputations

The only thing worse than losing one leg is losing both. However, there are unique circumstances to the bilateral amputee and although rehabilitation can take longer, the prognosis for function can be very positive. In my private practice, we worked with a large number of bilateral amputees and they were able to perform quite well on prostheses after they developed a sense of balance to accommodate the loss. All of the same postamputation procedures should be followed but more care should be taken to instruct the amputee in the use of wheelchairs because they will not be able to use crutches when there are leg problems. I will discuss prosthetic options in the next chapter.

After Amputation

Immediate Postoperative Prostheses

The immediate postoperative prosthesis was developed in Poland and brought to the United States in the early 1970s by Dr. Ernest Burgess who introduced the technique to American surgeons. The original procedure began in the operating room when a rigid plaster dressing was applied to the residual limb immediately after the amputation surgery. If the patient is projected to be active, then an attachment platform is placed onto the bottom of the rigid plaster cast that can receive a prosthetic foot. The rigid plaster cast is positioned on the stump to allow partial weight bearing and pads are placed over the bony areas so that as the residual limb shrinks inside the cast, there will be minimal pressure on the suture line. The purpose of the postoperative device is to contain the immense swelling that occurs during amputation and to protect the residual limb from impact. Secondarily, the prosthetic foot can be used to get the patient ambulatory from the first day or two on crutches or a walker as well as give the amputee a visual boost to see a foot at the end of the leg.

The "postop," as it is called, can be a very effective device if it is monitored carefully. In a perfect scenario, the cast minimizes edema (swelling) and allows the amputation wound to heal in a clean, protected environment. The amputee can experience an accelerated rehabilitation by early partial weight bearing on the residual limb and developing balance with crutches or a walker. In my experience, postops lost favor in the 1980s due to a high incidence of failure in the healing of the amputation site. The main problem with the system is the inability of the amputee or attending medical professional to monitor the healing process at the end of the stump. When there is a rigid plaster cast around the residual limb, it is very difficult to tell when something is going wrong. Much depends upon the feedback from the amputee. Below are the warning signs.

Warning Signs of Postoperative Procedures

1. If the patient complains of unbearable pain in the residual limb, then the postop needs to be removed to check on the amputation sight.
2. If the patient has a high fever, then it could indicate infection at the wound site and the cast needs to be removed.
3. Generally, there is a hole cut in the cast to allow the knee cap (patella) to be exposed. If you can smell a strong odor from the patellar hole, then the cast needs to be removed and the amputation site checked for infection.

The real problem here is that all of these warning signs come too late and the damage is already done. The patient will have to undergo a longer rehabilitation than normal due to damage to the incision. Because most of the feedback depends on the amputee's sensation, there can be a lot of discrepancy in the accuracy of information. If the amputation is the result of peripheral vascular disease, then the level of sensation at the stump may be severely compromised; they may not be able to feel when something is not right. In addition to poor sensation, there is always the factor of this being a novel experience for the patient. How is it supposed to feel? You have to figure that it is going to hurt, after all you did get your leg cut off, but how much is normal and when is the pain an indication of something going wrong? Certainly, when you get a funky smell coming from the cast it is past the point where effective measures can be taken to correct the problem. In the worst case scenarios, revision surgery is necessary.

Postoperative Solutions

There have been some encouraging improvements in postoperative technology in the past 10 years. This has come in the form of removable systems that allow monitoring of the residual limb while still providing all of the advantages of the traditional postop. Two systems that I am familiar with are the FLO-TECH (Trumansburg, NY) (Figure 1-5) and the Aircast postoperative systems (Summit, NJ), which are both commercially available. The FLO-TECH system uses a thermoplastic prefabricated system of shells that are fit to the patient immediately following surgery and are secured by a waist belt and Velcro straps (Velcro Industries, BV) that allow for some adjustment as the tissue shrinks. These shells can then be fit into an ambulating pylon system that allows for ambulation with crutches or walker. The Aircast system utilizes

Figure 1-5. A removable postoperative device. (Courtesy of FLO-TECH.)

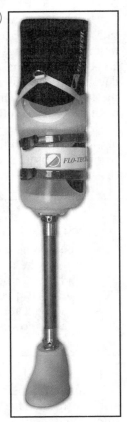

inflatable air bladders to maintain a constant pressure as the residual limb shrinks and also comes with an attachable foot to aid in ambulation. Both of these systems work well if applied properly and monitored regularly. By the same token, they can both fail if they are not carefully monitored.

Because the length of stay in the hospital is only 3 to 4 days on average for the amputee, there is a large gap in the continual monitoring of postoperative devices. If the patient is lucky enough to be placed directly into a rehabilitation center, then there is generally excellent follow-up care; however, there is also a gap in education of therapists and nurses in the management of amputees with postoperative devices. In my private practice, we spent a great deal of time teaching postop management to nurses and physical therapists. Another problem with the system in general is the lack of education on the part of the surgeon to have the postop applied directly after amputation while the patient is still under general anesthesia. My experience was that patients who got their postoperative devices applied during surgery had better tolerance of the device than patients who received their systems the next day. Once the swelling has occurred, the rigid container was normally too painful to tolerate and our success rate dropped dramatically. My personal opinion is that a properly applied and aggressively monitored postoperative device is part of the optimal amputation procedure; however, if all circumstances are not positive, then they can often create more problems than they are worth.

Care of the Residual Limb While the Stitches Are Intact

The surgeon may decide to leave the stitches in your stump for as long as 3 weeks, depending on how well you are healing. The suture line will be tender and sore so keep away from it in any massaging or desensitization that you work on. Gentle rubbing behind the knee and on the front of the knee will feel good and help lessen the skin sensitivity. If you are not in a postoperative device or cast, then you should keep your stump wrapped at all times. This is one of the most critical things you can do because the gentle pressure of the compression bandage wrap or shrinker sock will limit swelling and begin to assist the body in the removal of all excess fluid that has built up in your stump after amputation. It is equally important to keep your stump elevated when you are sitting or in bed. A pillow will keep it elevated and help prevent contractures.

Contractures occur when muscles shorten due to disuse, such as when you lose your leg and the knee gets stuck in a bent position. The muscles that bent your knee are the large ones in the back of your thigh and they are all still in place and functioning. Many of the muscles that straightened your knee were severed in the amputation, so the tendency is for the knee to bend due to the unequal force of the remaining muscles. It is important to keep your knee free of contractures by forcefully straightening it. Simple stretching exercises will keep the knee mobile and this will be a great benefit to you when you start to wear a prosthesis. Be cautious as you stretch so that you don't damage the healing at the end of your stump.

Do's and Don'ts

1. DO keep your stump elevated and wrapped at all times, taking care to wrap tightly at the bottom and looser as you get closer to the knee. This helps circulation to the wound area and promotes healing.
2. DO actively work to keep the knee joint flexible and free of contractures by stretching and applying pressure to the knee to force it straight. Again, take care to avoid damage to the suture line.
3. DON'T pick at the suture line or any other abrasions or scabs. Let them heal at their pace and whoever provides wound care will debride as necessary.
4. DON'T smoke during the healing process. Tobacco is a vasal inhibitor. In other words, it will slow the flow of blood to the affected area and you will be slower to heal.
5. DON'T bungee jump or swallow swords, which is just plain good advice anytime.

Care of the Residual Limb After the Removal of Stitches

Once the stitches have been removed, you will see a puffy red wound at the end of your stump that may still be quite tender. You should still be careful not to damage the healing that has taken place, but it is time to desensitize this area as well. Extend the massaging to the end of your stump, taking care to avoid pulling the stitch line apart. There may very well be scabs and dead skin still on the site, and you should not pick at these. Wash them gently with a washcloth and soap and let them fall off. Continue the rough towel treatment and as this gets more comfortable, you can actually place your stump at the end of the towel and gently pull on the end. Let pain and discomfort be your guide as to how far to push these therapies. If it really hurts, then stop. Back off a little and continue later, but never discontinue the desensitization process. You are getting the most out of your therapy if you are on the edge of discomfort.

Your job now is to prepare your residual limb for the preparatory prosthesis and it is critical to make sure that you will not have knee contractures. If you have developed a knee contracture, it can be worked out with aggressive therapy but it is far less painful to not develop one from the beginning. It is important to continue to wrap and use your shrinker sock at all times to minimize swelling and edema. Continue to keep your leg elevated when seated or in bed. You should also be working on your general physical condition, especially some upper body exercises that will be a big assistance when you begin ambulation. Your body will have to compensate for the lack of balance and strength by relying on your upper body for stability. You should focus on mastering crutches or the walker because these devices will be the key to your transition to walking and eventually all other mobility endeavors.

Pain and Psychology

Pain

Pain is the scariest part of amputation. Sure, loss of body image, mobility, and function are not pleasant thoughts, but the fear of the pain is a terrifying proposition. For a few, amputation is an improvement in their pain situation; however, amputation for most of us is the beginning of a level of discomfort that is comparable to childbirth or an intense pain that just won't go away.

When you awake from the amputation surgery, you are still under the influence of the anesthesia and will not experience the sharp, stabbing sensations that will come later. The feeling is like you have a truck parked on your foot that you can't seem to move. You may feel your toes or foot are cramped like they are in a boot two sizes too small. As the anesthesia wears off, the pain will increase in intensity until you feel a burning at the lower extremity or if it centers on the toes, then it may feel as if they are being twisted to the point of breaking. This is not fun. Today, most hospitals utilize a self-administered morphine system that allows the patient to press a button and pain killers will be injected into the intravenous drip that is keeping your body hydrated. This is a slick system because when you administer enough morphine you just kind of fall asleep and quit pushing the button. Most good painkillers are addictive and should only be utilized when necessary and discontinued after a short period of time. My recommendation is to use the painkillers to keep yourself as comfortable as you can. The hospital healing time is not the time to be macho or brave. You might as well be as comfortable as you can while you are healing and keep in mind that healing is your only job at this stage.

The worst pain usually comes at night. The mind can deflect pain by staying busy during the day when there is something to do, such as visiting with friends and relatives, watching TV, or reading. The pain is there, but you are not paying that much attention to it so it is manageable. Then it gets late, the visitors have gone, the TV is off, and you are too groggy to be able to read. The lights go out and you are exhausted and want to sleep. That's when pain rears its ugly head and says, "Hey, you forgot about me all day but now I am here." Since there is no outside stimulus, the pain then becomes a giant white-hot glowing monster that threatens to drive you crazy. What can you do? If you can distract your mind, that works the best but often the very painkillers that cut the pain also make it difficult to focus on reading or TV. Another excellent trick is to ice your leg. Take an ice pack and place it directly behind your knee and leave it there for 20 minutes. This will numb your stump and give you a break from the pain long enough to go to sleep. I have used this successfully on numerous occasions. The ice is painful for about 5 minutes but then everything goes numb and it gives great temporary relief from pain. Twenty minutes is the maximum amount of time to leave the ice on. After that, it can cause tissue damage so be careful not to leave it on longer. Gently massaging the area behind the knee can also give minor pain relief.

Other pain strategies that I have tried or learned from other people include yoga, meditation, and TENS electrical stimulation. I have done yoga for many years. I learned it in college where I thought it was a cool way to meet girls. In all honesty, I didn't meet any girls at yoga class, but I did discover a great way to stay limber and achieve a state of relaxation. I have also practiced meditation since college because relaxing is something that I have always found difficult. Yoga and meditation can't take your pain away but they do get your mind off of it by causing you to focus and allowing the pain to pass through you. A TENS unit is an electrical device that sends a small current through the affected area, which can help block pain. It kind of feels like touching a battery, giving you a tingling feeling that is better than the pain. TENS never worked well for me; however, I was able to massage the back of my knee with my fingers and cause my stump to tingle, which was better than the pain.

Here is my personal pain philosophy that worked for me, but I don't suppose it will work for everybody. Let me preface this philosophy with the statement that, like most other human beings, I seek pleasure and avoid pain. I believe that this is the normal human response. What I discovered is that pain is like a nightmare; the more you believe in it, the greater the terror. I have learned to love my pain. I know that sounds kind of twisted but it's true. I don't like my pain, but I have learned to love it. By loving it, I am not controlled by the pain. I let it pass through me by accepting it and feeling it. This is very scary at first because it really hurts and it is not a natural reaction to pain. However, I know that this acceptance of the pain allows me to function even when the monster is alive and angry. The more I fought my pain, the bigger the monster became. Faith plays a critical role in the acceptance of pain; you must be willing to take the pain with the belief that it will lessen. A belief in God or a higher power is often the key to having the faith to accept what has happened to you, permitting you to move forward. There is nothing worse than getting stuck in a phase of grief that focuses your attention on your pain. The monster can make Bambi look like Godzilla if all you have to do is sit around and think about how badly your leg hurts.

> ### Types of Pain Sensation
>
> 1. Skin pain: Skin or surface pain is the most common preamputation pain sensation. It is the pain you feel when you cut, scrape, or burn the surface of the skin. It is sharp and irritating but generally diminishes in a short period of time.
> 2. Muscle pain: This type of sensation is more akin to the feeling of a muscle cramp. It is a soreness that is deeper than skin pain and is characterized by a dull ache as opposed to a sharp jab.
> 3. Nerve pain: Nerve pain is much more invasive to the brain than skin or muscle pain. It feels like tingling or an electric shock running through the body or limb. Sometimes nerve pain manifests itself as numbness in a localized part of the body and you may experience the sensation of your foot falling asleep. Phantom sensation is nerve pain and I will cover that in more depth in the next section.
> 4. Bone pain: If you have stepped on a stone while barefoot, then you have felt bone pain. Often times, the bruising of the bone is accompanied by a sharp sensation that diminishes quickly only to resurface several days later when you try to stand up on the foot and it is extremely sore. Bone pain is deep and disturbing and takes a long time to diminish.

Phantom Pain

This is the weirdest of all the sensations that can accompany amputation. Some people have them all of the time and others only at first. It can feel like a cramp in your toes, which of course are not there, or a tickling itch that won't go away and you can't scratch. You look down and it is obvious that the leg is not there, but you have these feelings as if it was. My experience with phantom sensation was mercifully brief and diminished rapidly after the first month following amputation, but I have had clients that still feel their toes being squished in a vice even after 20 years as an amputee.

In my professional experience, the people who had the most phantom pain were the people who spent the most preamputation time in discomfort. In other words, if you spent 6 months with a diseased foot that was constantly hurting you prior to amputation, chances are that you may experience more phantom sensation than someone who lost his or her leg rapidly or immediately. Some persons go for years with a dysfunctional foot that has sores or wounds that never completely heal and experience chronic pain throughout most of the experience. These persons have a much greater risk of continuing phantom pain than someone who loses his or her leg in an accident in which the amputation is immediate. Another major factor in the incidence of phantom pain is how the residual limb is cared for in the first month after amputation.

Massage and desensitization can go a long way in minimizing phantom sensation by helping to retrain the brain to give accurate feedback. My understanding of phantom sensation is that the nervous system is like a network of roads and the impulses are like cars traveling along those roads. When you have a lot of pain from your foot, then the impulses traveling along the nerve kind of wear a rut in the road, so to speak. The brain is so used to experiencing pain from that area that it interprets any sensation coming from the foot as pain. This is like a bad rut in the road; your wheel keeps falling into it because it is so well traveled. When you lose a body part, there are portions of your brain that have not been informed of this situation and will, therefore, still interpret signals from that area as if the foot was still there. There are some things that you can do to minimize phantom sensation and help train your brain to give you accurate feedback.

Desensitization

In order to minimize the debilitating effects of phantom nerve pain here are some simple yet effective strategies.

1. Gently massage the skin of your stump with your own hands. Begin at the knee and start to work your way down toward the suture line. If you still have stitches, then you need to stay away from this area until the wound is completely healed and the stitches are out. The massage should be gentle at first then more aggressive as you can tolerate it. It is important for you to massage yourself since the brain is getting 3 feedback mechanisms when you use your own hands. The brain can feel your hands through the skin on your stump and the hands feel the skin through your fingertips. In addition, you can see that when you touch a particular place on your stump, you understand that this no longer means back of your calf muscle; it now means front of the stump. At first this is very difficult but it gets better each time. You cannot do this enough.

2. Another great way to desensitize your skin is the rough towel treatment. Take a hand towel (the rougher the better) and gently rub it across the skin. This will be very irritating at first but it improves rapidly. Rub all over the stump, again taking care not to damage the healing suture line. Next, fold the towel and softly beat your stump with it. This will diminish the clonus reflex, which is the thing that makes your stump jumpy and twitch at the knee. Don't let the neighbors see you do this. They may think you are crazy.

The Psychology of the Amputee

When I was in prosthetics school at Northwestern, we had a lecture on the psychology of the amputee. Out of the 15 students in the class, there were 4 of us who were amputees and we were all curious as to how our psyche had been affected by the trauma of amputation. We had 2 instructors giving a lecture. The first lecturer was a very intelligent, well-read instructor who had studied all of the available literature and gave an academic presentation with the basic premise that amputees were "social deviants." Of course, this went over really big with us amputees who were muttering under our breaths that we could show this guy some social deviation. The concept was valid from an academic point of view because amputees have experiences that set them apart from other people in society and they have a visible disability that prevents integration into the rest of the community. The second lecturer was the opposite of the first person. Unlike the first lecturer, he had long hair down to his shoulders and walked up to the podium with a bounce to his step. He stood behind the podium and looked out to the class. His lecture was, "If you were a jerk before you were an amputee, you'll be a jerk afterwards." That statement sums up the psychology of the amputee succinctly. Losing part of your body gives you a different perspective on life, but it does not change who you are.

Personally, I have always considered it a blessing that at age 20 I had an experience that gave me a greater perspective on life. Most people go through life attached to the things of the world: houses, cars, toys, and status, whatever feels most important at the moment. I was slammed with the reality that what really mattered was that I was alive and could still love, breathe, and experience this time. Time was what really mattered. It was all that I actually had in life. All the other stuff was just that—stuff.

Effect of Amputation on Others

Going through amputation is a kind of hell for the person who is the object of the exercise. Something you may not realize is that it can be an even greater hell for those persons who are your family or loved ones. When it is happening to you, the whole world seems to revolve around your surgery and recovery whereby the feelings and emotions of those close to you are largely ignored. It is very tough to watch a loved one go through an amputation especially because the loved one can't do anything about it. If you are a parent whose child is undergoing amputation, there can be no greater emotional burden. At least when this happens to you, you can get better, you can heal, and you are not dependent on someone else to improve your situation; it's up to you. When the person you care about is going through such a trauma, you are helpless to improve him or her. It can be an extremely frustrating experience for the loved one.

Family support during this time is very important to the mental well-being of most people. This can be overdone, however, if the family is so traumatized by the event that they baby the amputee. The person will have a difficult time making the transition to an independent life. I have personally experienced how you can get away with actions while you are lying in bed suffering that you can't get away with normally. You can be nasty to people, short with them, and very selfish without really realizing what you are doing. Family and loved ones will generally take this type of abuse because they feel sorry for you and wish that they could do something to alleviate your pain. My recommendation to friends and family of amputees is to treat them as normally as possible and be firm, but gentle, in letting them know when they hurt your feelings. Babying the person seems like the thing to do at first but really does not help him or her in the long run.

The amputee can do a few things to help this situation and help put family and loved ones more at ease. As I mentioned before, there is one thought in common to all people who see you as an amputee, "What would it be like if that happened to me?" As you know, it is not as bad as you imagined it to be but someone who is looking at you is not thinking happy thoughts. They are terrified at what you must be going through. They may no longer see you, the human being, but instead you become this image of their fears of what they imagine it is like. Here is a strategy that works. Make a joke. It doesn't even have to be funny. The fact that you are approaching the situation with humor causes them to refocus on you and not your circumstance. If you can't think of any jokes, here are some funny things to say. When asked how you lost your leg, you can say that you didn't eat your broccoli (this works especially well with kids). When there is a somber moment, you can say that now you cannot play the clarinet. When they ask why, you can say that you never could play the clarinet. I know this sounds stupid but trust me it works. If you can get someone to smile at your circumstance, then they will realize that you are the same person you always were and that things will be OK.

CHAPTER 2

The Preparatory Prosthesis

Stories

My Experience

My first morning home I woke up and hobbled downstairs on my crutches. They were the forearm crutches, the kind that have a cuff on the arm. I was not very adept at fixing my bowl of cereal. It is nearly impossible to carry anything while crutching. I discovered what happens to a cup of coffee while trying to hop; it mostly ends up on the kitchen floor. Now, I was not known for my patience at 20 years old, so my frustration level was already at the maximum. So, like the guy I am I did something incredibly stupid, a common male reaction to intense frustration. I tried walking on my postoperative cast without my crutches. It worked. It hurt a bunch but I could do it, so the rest of the morning I cruised around the house holding onto walls and furniture, at times taking full weight bearing on my stump. I was so proud when my folks came home that evening and I showed them how I could walk on this cast with a foot on it.

I ambulated around the house for the next several days, taking care of feeding myself and other basic daily activities. I was feeling very positive, thinking that this was not so bad. My stump would hurt pretty intensely by the middle of the afternoon, but the motivation of being mobile was more than enough to compensate for the pain. I had a doctor's appointment on Wednesday and then my first visit to the prosthetic shop. The doctor was impressed with my progress so far and with very little instruction, he sent me on my way. I had gotten a beautiful girl to give me a ride to my appointments and I kept trying to get a sense of how she perceived me now as an amputee. We had never dated, but I had always had a crush on her. She seemed more reserved and cold then before but I thought that maybe she was a little nervous about the doctor's office. As we drove to the prosthetist's shop, I was looking forward to showing Grant Rice how well I was doing.

My first shock was the location of the prosthetic facility. It was in a bad section of Atlanta, where the houses in the neighborhood were run down, and next door was an auto body repair shop. I got out of the car and crutched up the steps into the waiting room. The place was filthy and smelled like the adjacent auto body repair shop. An overpowering odor of solvents and plastic pervaded the air. The receptionist was pleasant and friendly, indicating that we were to sit down in the waiting room and that Grant would be with us shortly. I looked around and was appalled at the place. There was a fish tank with a couple of dead fish floating in the greenish water, the smell was overpowering, and the magazines were ancient. After about 20 minutes of apologetic silence, I was ushered into a fitting room, a cubicle the size of a closet with '60s fake wood paneling and a naked florescent light bulb illuminating the space. I was left in the little room for about 12 days. It was probably more like another 20 minutes, but it felt like forever. There were old crutches and legs behind the door, the room was dirty, and of course the ever-pervasive odor was beginning to make me nauseous. I sat there contemplating my future. I was very disappointed and depressed. Suddenly, large crocodile tears started streaming down my face. This was only the second time that I had cried during this whole experience. I couldn't help feeling utterly devastated at the thought that I was going to have to go to a place like this for the rest of my life. I would not take my car to a garage that was this dirty and smelly, let alone have a part of my body replaced. After a few moments of misery, I heard some noise outside so I quickly wiped my face and put on my tough guy look that I'm sure Grant could see through. He came in and cut off the cast again and I could look at my stump again. It was definitely smaller now and the suture line was red but seemed to be intact and healing. I explained how I was getting around and Grant told me to take it easy and not push it too hard. This level of advice was just not adequate for a guy with my headstrong mentality. He reapplied the postop and I went home. I remember apologizing to the girl profusely about the condition of the prosthetic shop and felt ashamed of myself for exposing her to this seamy side of town and the weirdness of the facility.

The next few days passed without incident. I neglected to take Grant's advice on taking it easy and returned to walking around the house on my postop cast. It was uncomfortable, but I had gotten use to the constant pain. The only time it would stop me was when I got the zingers, those sharp shooting pains that seem to emanate from deep inside and fill my brain with electric agony. Fortunately, they did not seem to last too long and I would find myself sweating and panting in relief when they passed. Still, this didn't seem too bad. I guess I imagined that it could be much worse, and I was still so pumped up to be walking around.

On Tuesday of the following week, a couple of friends came by to visit and get me out of the house. I was a little intimidated to be in public so we decided to go out to the country. I knew of a little trail in the woods that led to a waterfall, so I suggested that we go there. When we arrived, I realized that I had forgotten my crutches so I searched the immediate vicinity for a sturdy stick to use. One of my fears was that I would never enjoy walking in the woods again, so I was curious as to whether this was possible. I found a good stick and off we trudged down the path. It was not easy. The foot was not very flexible and I kept tripping over rocks and roots but I could do it. We arrived at the waterfall after about a half an hour and I gratefully sat and rested. My stump felt like it was on fire and I had to endure a series of rapid-fire zingers that kept me gritting my teeth until they passed. Still, I was excited to be mobile and sitting in the woods, near the little grassy spot where I had once taken a girl. Memories of former lovers kind of made me sad because I just wasn't sure how women were going to react to me now. Who was going to want a guy with one leg when there were all of these guys with two legs out there? We hiked back to the car that, all told, was about a mile and a half away. I was really sore by the time we returned and was glad to get home and get my leg elevated. That night my leg really hurt. I kept being awakened by screamer pains that shot through me and caused me to sit bolt upright in bed. This did not unduly alarm me because I had accomplished so much, I was no stranger to pain, and this was still not as bad as the initial accident.

A few days later I returned to the prosthetist and this time my father took me. He was also appalled at the conditions at the facility, but the people were awfully nice, which softened the experience. When Grant came in, I eagerly related my hiking experiences to him and was puzzled by his look of concern. I was expecting him to praise me, not look like he was about to scold me. The postop cast was discolored at the bottom, kind of a ruddy brown color that of course meant nothing to me. When the cast was split, a funky odor came out and as he removed it, I could see that the entire bottom of the cast and sock were soaked in blood, most of which was dried. Grant gasped as he looked at the end of my stump. The suture line was split in 3 places and in the center you could actually look up and see my bone. Since I couldn't see this and it didn't hurt that badly, I was waiting for him to reapply the cast. He said that he couldn't do it because the wound had opened up. I was very angry with him and had him call Doc Johnson, who was away on vacation for the next 2 weeks. Grant sent me to the doctor's office and one of Doc Johnson's associates looked at my stump and pronounced that this would have to heal before I could have my cast back. I was incredibly frustrated and angry at this setback and couldn't understand what had gone wrong. I had been progressing so well.

The next 3 weeks were some of the most intensely painful moments of my life. I had to go back to physical therapy to learn how to care for my wound. My daily regimen consisted of soaking my stump in hot water and Epsom salts for half an hour, twice a day. This in itself was agony and caused zingers to radiate throughout my whole body. Then I had to use a mirror to look at the wound and debride it with a rough gauze bandage that really sent the nerves into orbit. After the debridement, I would pack the wound with antibiotic ointment and wrap it with an compression bandage, being careful to wrap tightly at the bottom and looser around the knee.

One of the things I discovered about my pain was that it got worse at night when I tried to go to sleep. It seemed that while people were around and there was something to do, I could deal with it more easily. At night, when everyone had gone to sleep and the TV was off and I could no longer read because my eyes were totally blurred, the pain that I had ignored all day would rear it's ugly head to remind me that it was still there. There were nights that I lay in bed sweating with the agony, holding onto the sheets and praying for the morning. After 3 and a half weeks of this, the wound finally healed from the inside out and my prosthetist said that he thought I was ready for my preparatory prosthesis. Once the wound was closed and while I was waiting for the preparatory limb to be constructed, Grant instructed me to massage the scar where the wound had closed. He explained that as the scar healed it might stick to the bone and that would create a lot of problems with wearing a prosthesis. I also had a major scar just above my knee where I had picked at a little scrape from the accident. It was the only place I could reach due to the hole in my postop cast where the knee poked through. Casts itch and are always uncomfortable and the tendency to want to scratch at the places that you can't get to is irresistible. I have even known people who would use coat hangers to scratch inside their casts. This is a major no-no. The damage that can be done by prematurely removing scabs or scratching is something that is avoidable.

Figure 2-1. A preparatory prosthesis with cuff strap and SACH foot. (Photo by Dale Horkey, 2004.)

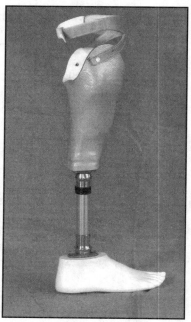

The big day came and I finally received my preparatory prosthesis. It was not pretty. It was a plastic socket with a white foam inner liner, a pipe came out of the bottom, and a rubber foot was attached to the pipe. There was a strap that went around my leg just above my knee and a waist belt with another strap that attached to the one above my knee. The strap around my knee is a cuff strap and the foot is a SACH foot (Figure 2-1). I wore wool socks next to my skin and then pulled out the foam liner (Pelite liner) and slipped it over the socks until it seemed tight. Then I slipped the liner into the socket and tightened the strap around my knee and hooked it to the waist belt. I could walk immediately and it really didn't hurt that much, just a dull ache from the compression of my stump. At first I used the parallel bars then moved immediately to the crutches, and before I even left the prosthetists shop, I was staggering around without the crutches. Grant took extra time to pound into my brain that I needed to be cautious and not overdo it, but I admit the excitement of getting to walk again was overwhelming. I think I even teared up a little when I thanked him. I was truly grateful for the ability to be mobile again.

Less than a week after I received my preparatory limb, I flew to Ohio to see my girlfriend and visit my college. The flight was very uncomfortable because I had to keep my knee bent in the airplane for the entire time, but I was glad to get there and be able to walk around. The first night in my girlfriend's apartment was nearly a disaster. Sometime in the middle of the night I had to go to the bathroom, so I hopped in the dark toward the bathroom that was in the hall. There was a slip rug in front of the sink and when I hopped on it, the rug slipped right out from under me. I did the same thing that I had done for 20 years when I was slipping: I put my right foot out in front of me to catch my fall. Unfortunately, my right foot was no longer there, so I came down directly onto the end of my freshly healed stump. The pain was monumental, as was the feeling of stupidity at not remembering that I didn't have a leg. My girlfriend rushed in and offered what help she could. Fortunately, I didn't reopen the wound but I did bruise the end of my stump rather badly. It was extremely tender for the next couple of days, but I had learned my lesson about falling; never lead with the leg that isn't there.

After a couple of days with my girlfriend I learned that even though my leg was gone, the more important parts of me worked just fine. My initial concerns about whether I would be desirable to women were at least partially diminished, but some of the things she said to me were disturbing. One thing that got to me was when she told me that her aunt had asked her if she was going to dump me now that I had only one leg. She said that her reply was of course not, but I could tell that she was thinking about it. In retrospect I guess I can't blame her. She only saw me in the beginning phases of the rehabilitation process. I still had quite a limp and was in a lot of pain all the time.

A bunch of my college buddies drove to Columbus to pick me up and take me to Oxford, Ohio where I was an undergraduate in elementary education at Miami University. We had a good old time and it felt great to be a part of my friends back at school. I stayed there for a couple of days before returning to Georgia. I had missed fall quarter of school but I was determined to return to classes by winter quarter, which were still almost 3 months away. The plane ride back was pretty depressing because of the knowledge that it would be so long before I could return to the life that I enjoyed so much.

Back in Georgia I was going a bit crazy with nothing to do. I read a lot of books and watched a lot of TV, but it was not enough. The book that gave me the most inspiration was *Alive: The Story of the Andes Survivors*, which is a story of a group of Argentinean rugby players who's plane crashes in the Andes and they are stuck there for over 3 months with no food. They end up resorting to cannibalism to survive, which seemed much worse than my situation. It was just inspiring to read of people in a far more hopeless situation than I was. Still, I was going nuts, so I began to refinish an old chair that I had found in my fraternity house when I moved in. It was in pieces and needed to be stripped as well as completely reassembled. I spent hours working on this just to have something to do. After I completed the rocking chair, some neighbors of my parents gave me some other furniture to refinish and this kept me busy until it was time to go back to school.

During this time, I couldn't wait to go back to school and it is the only time in my life that I marked days off on the calendar. It is not that I didn't appreciate being able to stay at my parent's house, but I was not a kid anymore and I needed to be out on my own. My brother and sister were great, especially my little brother who was 12 at the time. He really felt bad for me and was always there to help me with anything. My sister was 4 years younger than I and we had always fought until recently, when we had started to be friends. She put her animosity aside and helped when she could. My mother was wonderful and sympathetic as always, but my father was kind of hard core, insisting that I do things for myself. There were times when I really resented his attitude, but in the end I guess it was good for me.

At the beginning of December I went in to see my prosthetist to get my permanent prosthesis. He took my cast and when I returned 1 week later, he walked me on my first permanent leg, which used the same components as my preparatory. At first I walked on this large metal jig that was used to align the prosthesis to my specific gait pattern. Afterwards, I was instructed to come back in about a week and pick up the new leg. I couldn't wait to see it. When the day finally arrived, I was an hour early for the appointment. When I saw it, I was a little shocked. It didn't look like a leg; instead it looked like a plastic lamp base or something. I hid my shock because it felt so much better than the preparatory did and I only wore one wool sock. I was wearing up to 20 plys of socks to keep the preparatory leg snug. It felt much lighter, even though it actually weighed the same, and I could wear it without the waist belt, which was a royal pain in the you know what. This was a major improvement, and I felt that I was ready to go back to school. I had to go back to Grant on several occasions to adjust the socket. This process consisted of me getting a blister or abrasion on my stump and he would mark the place with a piece of chalk and then grind the inside of the plastic socket to give relief. This did work although after a while it seemed as if the problems just kind of moved around my stump. I had been shrinking rapidly since I had gotten my preparatory and before I left for school, I was in 8 ply of sock after only having the leg for a couple of weeks.

The time to return to school finally arrived, and my parents made a gift of the old family station wagon to me. It was a 1968 Plymouth Fury III station wagon; basically a boat on wheels, but it was a car and it ran. I know my parents must have been worried about me, but I seemed to have all the confidence in the world.

One evening my girlfriend and I walked out to a pond near her house. On the bank of the frozen pond there was a party of people who had a campfire, and they were ice-skating and roasting marshmallows. I was very curious as to whether I could still ice skate so we went back to her house where she got her skates and I borrowed her brother's skates, which were my size. I had never been a great skater but I was OK, having played a lot of pond hockey. I started out just fine holding onto her arm and shuffling along beside her. Of course with this initial success I started to become more aggressive and soon was skating off without her. On one of my turns I lost my balance and fell. As I did, the cuff strap let go and my leg came flying off. Because it was plastic, it had very little friction with the ice so it skittered across the pond until it encountered the opposite bank directly in front of the group of people roasting marshmallows. It popped up and stood on the skate for a brief second before falling in the snow. I was all right but the people on the bank were very shaken. My girlfriend had to go over and retrieve my leg for me because they wouldn't even touch it. We had a pretty good laugh about this and later I skated over to the group and apologized for any trauma it had caused; they didn't say much.

Now I was back at school and rooming with a guy whom I had met the year before. We had both been in fraternities and had tired of fraternity life. His fraternity, the Beta's, was the ultimate jock fraternity, which contrasted with the ZBT's, my house next door. If you ever saw the movie "Animal House" you have some idea of my fraternity experience. We were even kicked off of campus just like in the movie. We had a nice apartment with 2 bedrooms on the third floor. Much to my dismay, his girlfriend was living with us also. They had a very stormy relationship and the situation was tense most of the time. They showed no sympathy toward my condition, which was painful but in retrospect valuable. Miami University in the 1970s had no protocol for dealing with disabled students since, I suspect, I was the only one, so I was left to my own designs. The first challenge was the nightmare of signing up for classes. The process at that time was carried out in the huge gymnasium where each class was represented by a table with a sign up sheet that had as many lines as the number of students the class would hold. Students entered by class and rushed to the tables with the classes and times they wanted and signed up if it was not already filled. The graduate students went first then seniors, juniors, and so on. This system put me at a great disadvantage due to my slow mobility. However, as I entered I noticed my old fraternity advisor sitting at the registration desk. He was in charge of the entire process and, having heard of my dilemma, graciously offered to force add my schedule into any class I wanted.

I tried walking to class as much as I could since most of my classes were only about three blocks away. However, Ohio can be cold and icy in winter so I would have to drive the "boat" on occasion. There were no handicapped parking provisions at this time so trying to find a place to park was never easy. I would park wherever I could find space, occasionally in the president of the University's private parking space. I invariably accumulated numerous parking tickets by the end of the semester. Since I didn't know what to do, I took them to the Dean of Students. After hearing my dilemma, he graciously tore them all up. This was pretty cool getting to park anywhere I wanted, not that I ever took advantage of it.

The winter quarter went by rapidly. I managed to make most of my classes and get passing grades, even though there were times that my leg was just killing me. My stump continued to quickly shrink and by the end of the quarter, I was wearing 18 plys of sock, three 5-ply and one 3-ply. The whole sock thing was difficult. I had to judge how many socks to wear by how it felt each morning and since this was the first time I had ever been an amputee, I had a hard time getting it right. I also suffered from ingrown hair follicles and blisters that seemed to plague me continually. The other problem with the fit of the prosthesis was that my stump didn't shrink evenly; the back part kept disappearing and the bones started poking out. As I added socks to take up the space, the bones would get a lot of pressure and this is where I had most of my problems. It would be years before I figured a way to fix this myself.

Spring break was approaching and the annual decadent ritual to seek fun and adventure was upon me. A group of my friends and I decided to go on a backpacking trip to the Great Smoky Mountains at the end of March, a time of dubious weather in that part of the world. First, we went to Atlanta where I saw my family for a couple of days and picked up my vintage Boy Scout camping equipment before heading up into the mountains. Our little band was truly a sorry sight. There were 5 of us and I had by far the best equipment: a no frame pack and rain gear that was made of rubber that weighed 20 pounds. All in all, my pack and gear weighed 60 pounds, which for my weight was not bad but considering my leg was extremely foolhardy. The rest of the guys had little or no rain gear. Our tent was my father's old beach tent that took 2 people to carry: one for the 50-pound canvas tent and another for the poles. All of our food was in cans and when we arrived at our departure point, it was raining where we were and snowing at the higher elevations. About 2 miles into the soggy trip, we encountered a jeep with some park rangers that were searching for some missing hikers who had been caught in the snowstorm. They were appalled when they saw us. We told them we were only going about 7 miles in where we planned to pitch camp and stay there, taking day hikes from our base camp. They cautioned us but let us continue. After nearly 6 hours of hobbling on my walking stick through the mud, we arrived at the campsite, a dreary flat spot located at the bottom of a little draw with a rushing stream beside it. I was so exhausted from the pain that I could barely assist in setting up camp and as soon as the tent was pitched and a fire built, I went to sleep in the tent.

The next day dawned sunny and the dreary campsite turned into a beautiful tree covered spot resplendent with the promise of spring. Three of the guys decided to hike back to the car and drive to the nearest liquor store that was in another county so that we would have ample supplies of alcohol for our 5 days at the campsite. One of my buddies and I would stay, collect wood, and construct a tarp shelter beside the campfire. I was able to keep my leg off for most of the day so I actually felt pretty good by the time they returned with their burden of liquor bottles and more canned food. That night we got pretty drunk around the campfire, and I was the last one to get up the next morning. As I reached down to the bottom of my sleeping bag to get my leg, it wasn't where I had left it. I peeked out of the tent to see all the other guys sitting around the campfire glancing in my direction and I knew that they had done something with my leg. I hopped out to coax one of them into revealing where they had stashed it but no one would talk until I was actually able to grab one of my friends and persuade him with an old wrestling hold. They had buried it in some leaves nearby and thereafter I used my leg as a pillow to make sure it was still there when I awoke.

The next night we partied very hard because it was my 21st birthday and we decided to take a moonlight walk in the woods with candles and a lantern. This seems really foolish in retrospect but appeared to be a really cool idea at the time. We walked over to the stream that was about 12 feet wide and 6 feet deep and was rushing at an incredible speed because of the heavy snowmelt. The only way across the stream was a large slippery log that laid across the banks about 6 feet above the stream. What possessed us to try to walk across the log in the moonlight with only a lantern to light the way I will never know; possibly it was the whiskey that motivated us. I was behind one of the guys and doing OK, having crossed this several times during the day. Then the lantern blew out, leaving us in total blindness. The guy in front of me panicked and dropped to his knees on the log, hugging it with his arms. I just froze knowing that if I could just stand there and not fall into the stream I would regain my night vision. After what seemed like hours, I could see well enough to make my way back to the bank. I had survived that one. The other guy wouldn't move and was frozen to the log in fear until we threatened to leave him there, then he finally inched his way to the bank. For the remainder of the time we restricted our forays to daylight and I avoided drunken hikes at midnight. The hike back out was sheer agony after the first mile or so. Fortunately, the day was sunny and warm, but I lagged far behind the others. For the last mile I was barely able to hobble along on my stick and one of the guys came back and took my pack for the last couple of hundred yards. When I finally took my leg off, I discovered that there was no significant damage to my stump and after a couple of beers I began to feel better. Eventually, the endorphins overwhelmed the superficial pain and I was exuberant at my accomplishment.

Back at school I continued with my classes and life with my difficult roommates. I broke up with my girlfriend, which was to be expected, but by then I had the confidence to meet other girls and carry on. I decided to stay at Miami for the summer to catch up on the quarter that I had missed, and I signed up for the overseas teaching program that the education department offered every year. In the past it had been in Greece but because of the political climate they had made arrangements to offer a student teaching program at the American School in Monterey, Mexico. My parents thought I was crazy, but I had always wanted to travel and this would be a perfect opportunity. Besides, I was using money that I had saved over the years working summers.

I was walking back from class one brilliant spring day and I was only a block from my apartment when I heard an ominous snap. I stumbled forward, almost falling. I looked down and saw that my foot had broken off completely. I was directly in front of the campus security building so I went in and stood before a bored woman who sat at the dispatch desk. "May I use the phone?" I asked. "Students are not allowed to use the phone," she retorted with a sharp edge to her voice. "My foot is broken and I just need to call my roommate to come and pick me up," I pleaded. "Your foot is broken?" she asked in irritated disbelief. I picked up my foot that still had the shoe in it and lifted the empty pants leg onto the counter and explained my situation. In shock, she called her supervisor who personally gave me a ride back to my apartment.

Once again I was having serious leg problems and needed to go to a prosthetist to have something done. I decided to find someone local. I was up to 25 ply of sock and was in constant pain from chronic infected hairs and abrasions. There were no prosthetic facilities in Oxford, Ohio, so I looked in the phone book for places in Cincinnati, which was about 50 miles away. There were 3 places, so I took off a day and went to check them out. The first was not open and was in a worse part of town than the place in Atlanta, so I went to the second. I went in and was put into another dingy, smelly fitting room and waited until a prosthetist came in to help me. I told him my problems and showed him my leg. He said that I needed a new prosthesis but that he could adjust mine so that I would not be in so much pain. I said great and as he took the leg to the shop part of the building, I hopped behind him. He stopped and asked me where I was going. I said I was following him so I could watch him work on my leg, which was something Grant had always let me do. He said no patients were allowed in the shop area, so I grabbed my leg back and told him that I was not going to trust anyone to work on my leg who wouldn't let me watch him or her work. It was off to the third facility, which wasn't much to look at either, but they were friendly and understanding and allowed me to watch them work. The guy who worked with me was an apprentice prosthetist who was also an amputee and when I explained the kind of things that I was doing, he thought I was crazy but did a decent job.

My new leg was the same as the old one and was paid for by the State of Ohio Vocational Rehabilitation who also helped me out with my tuition and books. This was a godsend, as my father's insurance only covered the first prosthesis and then I was on my own. My lawsuit against the construction company was ongoing but could realistically last for years so I was financially strapped. I have always been indebted to this agency for their help in getting me through college and keeping me in prostheses during this time.

It was at this time I returned to competitive sports and found that I could still bicycle. I had just learned to play handball in college and had fallen in love with the fast-paced sport. One day I was walking through the gymnasium and stopped to watch some guys playing handball when I realized that the best players were not the young aggressive ones but the older, more skilled players. This fit my capabilities perfectly. I could no longer depend on my hustle to beat my opponents, but I could develop my skills and my timing to be competitive. I started playing again and discovered that even though I was not as good as before, I could play and actually win, which still really mattered to me. I had lost my leg but not my competitiveness and I desperately needed an outlet. I started playing handball twice a week. I would often be on crutches for a day afterward, but it was worth it to be able to kick ass once in a while.

That summer semester in idyllic Oxford, Ohio was a magic time. The classes were far more relaxed than during the regular school year and the professors were a lot more fun to work with. I made up the credits that I had missed the previous fall and truly enjoyed the nice weather and pretty girls that seemed to be everywhere. This was the time when I discovered that women still thought I was attractive and were not just sympathetic toward me. This was the '70s, the decade of sex and drugs, so I felt obligated to take full advantage of my circumstances by indulging in both in a moderately responsible manner.

Gary

Gary was a 63-year-old mild diabetic who lost his leg due to an infection on his left foot that wouldn't heal. The vascular surgeon did a below-knee amputation. Because he was not well versed on amputation surgery, he did not contact a prosthetist for pre-amputation counseling or a postoperative procedure. Gary awoke from the surgery with his foot gone and no clue as to what was going to happen next. His family was with him, but they were so disturbed by what had happened that they were of little comfort or practical help. His stump was wrapped in a gauze bandage with no compression stocking or compression bandage. It ached continually and he could swear that his foot was still down there. He would wake up in the middle of the night with a burning itch that he couldn't scratch or cool down and the only thing nurses could do was to give him more pain medication. The hospital's physical therapist came in twice in the 3 days he was there. He was usually so drugged and lethargic that he couldn't remember what she had told him to do from one session to the next. He was very depressed and his family shared his depression, seeing the former strength of their family so down about his life.

By the time he arrived at the rehabilitation center, he was lethargic and despondent believing that his life was over. Gary thought that he would be better off dead, a sentiment he shared with his family far too often. His unwrapped stump had started to develop a serious bent knee, or flexion contracture, and his back ached also because he was lying in bed all the time. Fortunately for Gary, he received good treatment at the rehab center. The physical therapist, Sally, immediately put him on a regimen of stretching and massage. Gary was not enthusiastic about his treatment and told the PT she could go you know where on many occasions followed by the often-familiar cry of amputees, "You don't know what it is like." Sally was a very patient person but she could only take so much so she called a prosthetist whom she knew who was also an amputee and asked him to come in and see if he could motivate this reluctant patient.

The next day in therapy the prosthetist, Mark, approached Gary as he was berating Sally for trying to get him to do his stretching. She introduced him as the man who makes prostheses and Gary made a nasty comment about what a waste of time it would be. Mark agreed with him that with his attitude a prosthesis would be a waste of time but that his life wasn't over. Gary's reply was his caustic mantra of, "Who the hell are you? You don't know what it is like." Mark calmly lifted his pant leg to reveal a below-knee prosthesis and looked Gary in the eye, saying that indeed he did know what it was like and had lived with it since he lost his leg in a lawn mower accident when he was 3 years old. Gary sat there speechless and ashamed of himself. Mark thanked him for his time and told him that it was up to him to decide whether his life was over or not, but that if he decided to get back into things, to give him a call.

Gary was silent the rest of the physical therapy session but the next day Sally noticed a change in his attitude. He tried to work on his exercises and he attempted to talk to some of the other patients in the gym. He did not berate her for her persistence in helping him and at the end of the session he did something he had never done before: he thanked her and asked her if he could talk to the "leg guy" again. Gary had always been a heavy smoker and was still smoking a pack and a half a day. His doctor and therapist had told him that it was not good for his healing but since he thought he was dead anyway what did he care. When his wife came in that morning he broke down in tears, apologizing for the way he had acted and promised that he would try hard to learn to walk and to not be so negative toward the family. His wife cried with him and both realized that this simple act of contrition was the beginning of life again.

Mark came back to see Gary the next day and talked to him about prostheses and what he could expect life to be like. After he examined the stump and in consultation with the staff physiatrist, it was agreed that a course of aggressive compression wrapping and massage would be essential for preparation to wear a prosthesis. Mark smelled Gary's stump and asked him if he smoked. When Gary told him how much he smoked, Mark said he knew it was a lot because he could smell the nicotine in the wound. Gary was shocked to find that smoking inhibited his healing process and vowed to cut back. The nicotine in tobacco is a vascular inhibitor, which means that it causes the capillaries in the body to get smaller, constricting the flow of blood to any area but especially to a traumatized area like an amputated limb. The combination of allowing the leg to hang down, lack of any compression wrap, and the smoking had created a very poor healing wound and the stitches were literally the only thing holding the stump together.

Up until this point, Gary had hardly ever looked at his stump and now he was being asked to touch it with his own hands and to massage it a billion times a day. The nurse would apply the compression bandage to the still swollen tissue, carefully using a figure 8 wrapping technique with increased pressure at the bottom and diminished pressure as she wrapped above the knee. The first couple of times the compression bandage was applied, the pain was intense but if he could stand it for about 5 minutes, the pain subsided quickly to a dull ache. After about 20 minutes, it didn't even ache and he quickly got used to the compression bandage. He was instructed to keep the compression bandage on at all times except when he was doing massage or wound care.

As the days passed, Gary noticed a dramatic improvement in how his leg felt. The wrapping had become easier and the wound actually began to heal. He had cut down on his smoking to 3 cigarettes a day instead of a pack and a half, and he actually felt better than he had in a long time. He had started to wrap his own stump, which wasn't easy at first but he got the hang of it after awhile. The key was to have the compression bandage rolled properly and to wrap tight at the bottom and loose enough to easily get your fingers inside the wrap at the knee. As his stump shrunk, the compression bandages kept sliding down off the end of his residual limb and he would typically find them in a knot at the bottom of the bed. Mark brought him a shrinker sock that fit nicely over his stump and told him that as this got loose to continue to use the compression bandage but put the shrinker over the top of the compression to hold it in place. This worked well and the doctor took out his stitches after 4 weeks.

Gary was discharged home having mastered the walker for ambulation but still using the wheelchair often. He had lost a lot of his strength while in the hospital, and he found that just getting on and off the toilet was difficult. Sally had come to his home on the first day back to do a home visit, which was designed to help Gary and his family adapt their home to his current state of mobility. Gary's son was there and volunteered to make the minor renovations to the house that would make it more easily accessible. He constructed a temporary ramp on the 2 steps leading into his garage and put grab bars that he bought at a hardware store on the door entry and next to the toilet in the bathroom. Their bathroom had a tub with a high sidewall so they purchased a rail that clamped onto the side of the tub and put a stool in the shower. All of this cost around $150 and took only 2 hours to install and it made the house accessible. Sally's parting words were not to Gary but to his wife, "The most important thing you can do for Gary is not to do everything for him but to make him do things for himself." This is never an easy thing for loved ones to do because natural human emotions are to care for someone who is injured or disabled, but she promised she would do her best.

During the week that he had returned home, he went for the first time to the prosthetist's shop. It was in a decent part of town and the facility was clean and medical. Mark, who had seen him in the hospital, came in and examined his stump. It looked a lot different than it had 4 weeks ago. The suture line was well healed and it actually had a little taper to it instead of looking like a bowling ball hanging off the end of his leg. Gary had been wrapping and massaging diligently, and Mark told him that he was ready for his preparatory prosthesis. They went into another room that had an examination table and Gary was helped up onto it. Mark told him that he was going to take a cast of his stump with which he would use to make his leg. Gary didn't completely understand what was going on but he trusted Mark. First, Mark slathered Vaseline (Cheesbrough-Ponds, Greenwich, CT) all over Gary's skin from just above the knee all the way to the bottom. Then, Mark took a thin gauze sock out of a bucket of warm water and stretched it over Gary's stump, attaching it to a stretchy fabric belt that was around Gary's waist. Next, Mark took a blue pencil and drew all over the sock. When Gary asked him what that was for, Mark said that he was marking the bony prominences and that the indelible blue markings would then transfer onto the cast when he poured it full of plaster. Next, Mark took a roll of plaster bandage and dipped it into the water, then gently wrung out the excess water. He started at the bottom of the residual limb and wrapped the plaster bandage all around Gary's stump, taking care to cover the entire surface with the plaster. The plaster felt warm and comfy to Gary and was very similar to wrapping his stump with the compression bandage except this felt better. Mark wrapped another roll of what he called rigid plaster on the first wrap and then used his hands to mold in the cast. He made dents beneath Gary's knee and in between the two bones in the front as well as a gentle pressure behind the knee. The plaster set after only a few minutes and Mark went off to wash his hands. When he returned, he unfastened the belt and slipped the cast off of Gary's stump. It didn't hurt at all and the warm plaster actually felt good. Mark took a warm towel and washed the plaster and Vaseline off of the stump, but the blue indelible pencil marks were still there. Mark said not to worry; they'd wear off in a couple of years, which made Gary laugh. Gary was told to come back in 3 days to be fitted with his preparatory prosthesis and to make sure that he brought a pair of shoes with him. Mark emphasized that the shoes should be lightweight yet sturdy in construction, recommending a good pair of tennis shoes. Gary said that he had some almost new ones and would remember to bring them.

Waiting for his leg to be made was not easy. Gary was excited but also nervous. He feared that it would be painful, and he had a very difficult time imagining walking on something that wasn't part of his body. He faithfully stuck to his therapy regimen and finally the day came. His wife and son accompanied him to the appointment, and he used his walker to get into the fitting room, which was different from the casting room. Instead of an exam table and sink, there was a long corridor with parallel bars extending almost to the end of the room and large full-length mirrors on both ends. He was ushered into a chair that sat at the end of the parallel bars, setting his walker to the side. Mark entered carrying Gary's leg. It was a flesh-colored plastic socket with a pipe attached to the end and a foot on the bottom. He carried a multitude of socks in a bag and something in a large rectangular box. Mark handed the leg to Gary and told him to examine it. It was not as heavy as Gary imagined it to be and Mark said not to be put off by the appearance of the pipe. When they finished the fitting, Mark said that he would put a temporary cover on it so that it would at least have the shape of a leg. Mark took Gary's shrinker sock off and took what looked to be a giant rubber sock out of the shoebox and turned it inside out with the shiny rubbery side out. He explained that the material was a gel and asked Gary to touch it. It was soft and a little slimy feeling, but Gary could immediately see that this would be comfortable on his stump. Mark next took the inverted liner, as he called it, and rolled it onto Gary's stump. It rolled on with a little difficulty but actually felt good and secure, but it was so long that it came halfway up Gary's thigh. Mark made a mark with his pencil and rolled the liner off then cut the sleeve cleanly with a very large pair of scissors. When he rolled it back onto Gary's stump, it went on easier this time and came to just above his knee.

Mark took a white foam pad that he called an insert out of the plastic socket of the leg and slipped it over top of the gel sleeve that was on Gary's stump. It was a little loose and so Mark took a sock out of a plastic bag and had Gary slip it on first. When the insert was put back on Gary, it felt snug so Mark next slipped it into the socket of the leg. He instructed Gary to put pressure down onto the leg and as he did, Mark rolled another gel-like sleeve up over the socket and onto Gary's thigh, extending halfway up his leg. When Gary lifted his thigh, the leg lifted with it. It felt heavy but not as much as he had imagined. Now Mark asked Gary to stand with all his weight on his arms on the parallel bars. Gary was standing for the first time in almost 6 weeks and as he glanced over at his wife, he could see tears in her eyes and he had a hard time maintaining his emotions. Mark asked him to put some weight on the leg. Much to Gary's surprise, it didn't hurt. He felt pressure and a bit of discomfort but no pain. Almost without realizing it, he started to take some steps before Mark told him to slow down. First, Mark had to adjust the height of the leg, which he checked by having Gary stand with his feet together and equal weight on both legs. Then, Mark put his hands onto the sides of Gary's pelvis and pushed hard on the two bones that poke out of the side of his hips. Mark looked at both sides then placed a thin board under the prosthesis and said that that was better, although to Gary it felt like the leg was too long. Mark said that the leg would feel a little long until Gary's pelvis was used to being supported again, explaining that Gary's hip on his amputated side had been hanging for almost 6 weeks and was now used to that position. Mark said it was normal for it to feel like the leg was too long but that it was important for the prosthesis to be long enough to make the pelvis level. He further explained that if the pelvis wasn't level, the spine would be bent and this would cause damage to the spine as well as back discomfort if it were not correct. Mark also explained that if Gary didn't feel normal in a week, Mark could shorten it a bit but not too much.

As Gary took his first steps, Mark emphasized that he should take short even steps and that the tendency of amputees was to take a long step with the prosthesis and a short step with the good leg. He explained that contrary to the way that sounded, it actually caused the amputee to spend less time on the prosthesis with each step. Each time Gary would walk to the end of the parallel bars and back, Mark would have him sit back down in the chair and he would take an Allen wrench and make tiny adjustments to the screws at either end of the pipe on the leg. After each adjustment, Gary's gait would get smoother and smoother until by the end he was only just barely holding onto the bars. Mark then had Gary sit back down and remove all the stuff off of his leg. He examined the stump and pronounced that everything looked fine and then walked Gary through the reapplication of the liner, then the sock, then the insert, then into the socket, and finally pulling up the suspension sleeve that held the leg on. Mark explained that the suspension sleeve held the leg on by not allowing any air into the socket, which held the leg on by a kind of suction. He then explained how to care for all of the materials that he had given to Gary, emphasizing that he had to wash the liner every day with warm water and an antibacterial soap. The suspension sleeve should be washed at least 3 times a week and the socks at least weekly. He went over how to add socks based upon how the leg slipped into the insert. He showed him the array of socks that were provided with the leg, 1 plys, 3 plys, and 5 plys that were to be used to take up the space in the socket as his stump shrank. Gary asked how much he could still be expected to shrink, and Mark explained that depended on his activity level and how good his circulation was.

As Gary was preparing to leave, Mark handed him a brochure that explained many of the things that he had mentioned in the fitting. Gary was grateful because it had been a lot of information. They set up a return appointment in a week so that Mark could check on Gary's progress and make sure things were going right. Mark said that he would want to see Gary every week to 10 days for the first month until he was confident that Gary had the hang of how to adjust his own fit. He also recommended that he return to outpatient physical therapy to work on gait training and so that there was someone else keeping an eye on the fit of the prosthesis. Finally, Mark took the leg back into the lab and returned 15 minutes later with a foam cover over the pipe and a couple of socks over the foam so that it had the shape of a leg.

On the way home, Gary and his wife talked about how their lives had changed since he had accepted the prosthesis and how much easier it had been than they expected. They both felt very lucky to have met Mark and were determined to do the best they could. This change in attitude is the key to turning a tragedy into a blessing and both Gary and his wife grew stronger and more intimate for the experience.

Gary returned to outpatient physical therapy and although he no longer worked with Sally, his new therapist Dave was just as positive and helpful. The sessions were full of exercises on balance and negotiating steps and ramps. Gary did well with his walker and within 2 weeks had progressed to a cane. At times, when he was around the house, he even went without his cane just to see if he could do it. Between the visits to the physical therapy and his checkups with Mark, he maintained a good fit in the socket and at the end of the first month he was wearing almost 10 ply of socks, two thick wool 5 plys, which were hot in the warmth of spring. Gary realized that this constant socket adjustment with socks was important. Mark had told him that he might have to adjust socks for years until his stump had stabilized so he was prepared. During his second month with the preparatory, he was discharged from outpatient physical therapy and only saw Mark every 2 or 3 weeks. On one of these visits he was up to wearing 14 ply of socks and Mark said that he needed to line the insert of the socket to take up some of the space. He took the leg into the lab and glued a piece of soft leather around the inside of the insert. When Gary put the leg back on, he discovered that he only needed to wear 5 ply of sock again. The leg felt so good that he started to walk without his cane more and more. During another visit, Mark commented on how the liner was no longer fitting properly anymore. Gary had noticed how the liner was gapping at the top and from time to time air would "fart" out of it. This was a little embarrassing, but he did have fun with it around his grandchildren who thought that the idea of a farting leg was pretty funny.

After 6 months of wearing the preparatory, Gary went in for one of his routine checkups and Mark said that it was time for Gary's permanent leg. Gary first asked if this would be the last leg that he would ever need, and Mark said that it was likely that Gar would need a new leg every 3 to 5 years for the rest of his life. This surprised Gary who had no idea that they would need to be replaced so frequently, but then Mark added that he might not need to replace the entire leg but just maybe the socket. They spent almost an hour talking about the various options that were available to Gary for his permanent prosthesis. In the end they decided that the liner and insert with the sleeve suspension was a tried and true combination and Gary was confident in the way it worked as well as its operations. They did, however, decide that a new more dynamic foot would serve Gary well in the activities in which he wished to engage. Gary had expressed a desire to go for walks with his wife and grandchildren, to work in his garden, and to begin fishing again, a passion that he had felt that he would ever enjoy again. The new foot would be an energy storing foot that also had multiaxial ankle motion that simulated the motion of the real ankle. This would make it easier to walk on uneven ground that he would definitely encounter when hunting for that perfect fishing hole. Mark told Gary to go to his doctor and get a prescription for the new leg, as that was the only way that his insurance would pay for the leg.

Gary returned the following week with the written prescription from his doctor and Mark took a new cast. This time, Mark casted slightly differently than before. He made a plaster splint of just the front of Gary's stump, which was much more defined now that it had shrunk, exposing the front bone. A week later Gary returned for a test socket fitting, which was a clear plastic socket that he stood in and Mark evaluated the fit from what he saw in the clear test socket. Mark wasn't completely happy with the first fit so he did a second test socket, which was more comfortable when standing and put no pressure on Gary's side bone (the fibula), which had become increasingly sore in the preparatory. Gary returned in a week for the fitting of the new leg and after the initial alignment, he was walking almost as well as he had with 2 legs. Gary and his wife couldn't believe it. He took the new leg home with his old cover on it for a few weeks of trial wear. When Gary returned, Mark made a few adjustments to the alignment and then took the leg for finishing, which he said would take a few days. Gary would have to wear his old preparatory leg in the meantime, which now felt like it weighed a hundred pounds and really made his fibula sore. After he received the new leg—completely finished with a latex cover on it—he had to go show off. The first place he went was the rehab center to show Sally, the person who had turned his life around.

Gary walked into Sally's office without his cane and with a barely perceptible limp. She recognized him immediately and broke into a broad grin at the realization of how far he had come in such a short time. She told him how wonderful it was to see the results of what she had initiated because generally she only saw the patients when they were at their worst and rarely after they had recovered. Gary told her about the process and thanked her over and over again, offering to help her any way he could. She said that as a matter of fact there was a way that he could help her. She had a client who had recently lost his leg and was very depressed about it and would Gary come and talk to him. Gary followed her into the physical therapy gym and there, in a wheelchair looking despondent, was Harold who had just been transferred from the hospital. Gary asked Sally if that is what he looked like and she said that he looked even worse. He spent a half an hour talking to Harold about life as an amputee and at the end he could tell that Harold felt better and was more enthusiastic about his rehabilitation. Gary returned to the rehabilitation center more often to talk to Harold and other amputees. Each time he felt more positive about himself as he saw how his words changed the way people viewed themselves.

The story of Gary's rehabilitation is not unusual. Most amputees go through a time where they get depressed about their situation. The trick is not to spend much time in the depressed phase but to pull out into the active, rehabilitation phase. Gary had given up on life because he was afraid of the unknown: life as an amputee and the fear of how people would see him without his leg. What he discovered was that life was just as rich as before the amputation and in some respects, he no longer took for granted his relationships with his wife and family. Volunteering to help others helped Gary see where he was and how far he had come, which did a lot for his self-esteem.

Preparatory Prostheses and Rehabilitation

Why Preparatory Prostheses?

There are many prosthetists today who skip the preparatory limb (Figure 2-2) and go straight into the permanent prosthesis. The justifications are that they want to create as little transition to the permanent as possible and the use of the same components means that there are no adaptations for the client. The other reason that preparatory prostheses are sometimes not used is due to the funding of the client. If the client's insurance will only cover one prosthesis, then the prosthetist will not have other options. What a prosthetist can do is to replace the socket frequently to accommodate atrophy in the stump, which accomplishes the goal of keeping a well-fitting socket on the patient.

In my experience, the preparatory prosthesis is very important, not just for the transition to the permanent but also as a future backup leg when the permanent is being repaired. In my practice, we generally utilized a soft, lightweight, multiaxial foot for a preparatory limb. This made it easy for the amputee to learn to walk while he or she was still gaining strength and stability. I discovered that if I was too aggressive on the foot by using a spring-loaded component, then the client might have difficulty getting the most from the foot. Young, highly motivated clients can make the adaptation, but older, less dynamic clients tend to develop bad gait patterns because they do not pos-

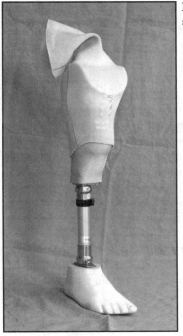

Figure 2-2. A preparatory prosthesis with a suspension sleeve. (Photo by Dale Horkey 2004.)

sess the strength and balance to operate the foot. I found that patients who had learned to walk on a more forgiving foot and developed good gait patterns were more easily able to make the transition to an energy storing foot because they had the muscles and timing to get the most from the dynamics.

I have always believed that every amputee should have a backup leg. How many people drive around without a spare tire in their car? Prostheses are mechanical devices that cannot fix themselves so they need periodic maintenance. You can't rent one for the day and you can't borrow a friend's prosthesis if something goes wrong with yours. In my private practice, I always tried to make sure that my clients had a decent backup prosthesis, usually an old leg that had been adjusted to be comfortable enough to wear for days if their other prosthesis was "in the shop," so to speak. This can occur for several reasons. If the foot or suspension lock mechanism breaks, then it may take days for the replacement parts to come in and the prosthetist to be able to repair it. If the cosmetic cover needs repair or replacement, then it may take 3 to 5 days to fabricate a new one and the leg would not be available. If you do not have your leg, then you are disabled and someone else has to do things for you. If you have children or a job, how will you perform? I believe a backup prosthesis is essential for all amputees and the preparatory prosthesis makes a good initial backup.

These are just 2 examples of preparatory prostheses. Each prosthetist is most comfortable with feet and suspension techniques that he or she has had the most success with in the past. My opinions are based on my personal experience and preferences and are not the only things that will work or provide optimal outcomes.

The Team Approach to Rehabilitation

When I was in prosthetics school, the rehabilitation process of the future was the team approach. This system of managing amputees utilizes the doctor, prosthetist, and physical therapist to provide the optimal rehabilitation program with all of the relevant caregivers having input. "What a concept!" I thought, "This is the way that amputees should be cared for." In the '80s I worked at facilities that had contracts with rehabilitation centers or clinics and there were always doctors and physical therapists around to give prescription input that was often invaluable to the prosthetist. The veterans' hospitals utilized the team approach to care for their amputees by holding a clinic with an orthopedic surgeon and physical therapist in attendance as well as multiple prosthetists who received patients on a rotating basis. This environment was excellent for the amputee who received the benefit of the experiences of the entire team. The only down side was when competition between prosthetic facilities got in the way of caring for the amputee, but if there was a strong clinic leader, this rarely occurred.

As managed care took over health care in the '90s, the team approach began to disappear. Competition between providers caused more and more facilities to issue exclusive contracts to prosthetists, which eliminated the healthy interchange between professionals that, I believe, truly benefited the amputee. Unfortunately, the managed care companies chose their providers based upon the amount of discount that they would give with little regard for quality and service. Rehabilitation centers neglected to develop protocols to insure that amputees received proper care, and the prosthetists who were being squeezed by the managed care companies to cut costs could hardly afford to provide the kind of services necessary to fill the void. Many amputees do not receive the proper follow-up or consistent care that leads to optimal rehabilitation.

There are still rehabilitation centers and hospitals that use the team approach. If you are the recipient of this benefit, then you are indeed fortunate. If your care does not include the doctor, physical therapist, and prosthetist, then take it upon yourself to make sure that these people are communicating with one another. In today's health care climate, you must be more aggressive to insure that you are receiving optimal care because most insurance providers have a very short-term perspective on your health.

Choosing A Prosthetist

Most urban areas of the United States have a variety of prosthetic providers from which to choose. Some are really good and care for their clients and others are leg mills that just crank out a product designed to last for as short a time as possible. How can you tell the difference? It is hard, if not impossible, to distinguish between a good prosthetist and a poor one because the bottom line is that you have never done this before. How would you even know what to look for? Many of you will not even have a choice of prosthetists due to your managed care company who has contracted with a facility to provide exclusive service to their clients. This choice of providers is done almost solely on the basis of cost; whoever puts in the lowest bid gets the contract, which is not always a wise way to choose a body part provider. Nevertheless, this is the system and you will have to work with it in order to get the best care that you can.

The standard of professionalism in the United States is certification in prosthetics. It is offered by 2 entities, The American Board of Certification (ABC) and the Board of Certification (BOC). A certified prosthetist is one who has either studied prosthetics at a university or one who has apprenticed under a certified prosthetist and has passed the national exams. The exam consists of 3 parts: written, oral, and practical in which the candidates are expected to have mastered the skills and knowledge to prescribe and fabricate devices that are comfortable as well as functional. I went through the apprentice program in the early '80s and attended the prosthetic school at Northwestern University in Chicago for a 6-month certificate program. I learned a great deal and actually thought I knew something when I got out of school. Unfortunately, it took me almost 2 years before I realized that I really didn't know anything and that the only person who did know something was my client and I better start listening to him or her. Education is a good start but experience is what leads to continual problem solving and an open mind, allowing the practitioner to keep learning throughout their career.

If at all possible, you should meet the prosthetist as soon as you know that amputation is looming or in the case of the emergency amputation, as soon as your doctor permits. I met my prosthetist at my first cast change. The doctor chose him for reasons that I don't know but he turned out to be great. This is not always the case, however. Prosthetists are just people and some have great talent and are personable while others may possess talent but no personality, and still others don't have either. Generally, you can tell if someone is personable by his or her demeanor and how he or she relates to you. Do you feel comfortable with him or her? Do you feel like you can trust him or her? The relationship with your prosthetist will be very critical to your continued progress because he or she will be the primary source of information about prostheses and your options. You should make the decision very carefully because most people stay with their first prosthetist for the rest of their life. Make sure you are comfortable with the person you choose!

What can you do if you don't like your prosthetist? You always have the option of going somewhere else even if it is not convenient or on your managed care list. If the facility is not a preferred provider, they still may be able to make your leg but it may cost you more out of pocket. You must be honest if there are problems because once the prosthetist has started your leg, he or she will initiate the billing process and it may be difficult if not impossible to change once the leg is in process. When the prosthetist takes your cast, he or she has begun the process and once you accept the prosthesis and leave the facility with it, he or she has provided what the law says is his or her service. If you're not sure about the prosthetist, don't let them take a cast and especially do not take delivery of the leg because once you do, you bought it.

Legs are expensive. Costs for a preparatory prosthesis can range from $3500 to $6500 (in 2004 dollars), depending upon the type of componentry and suspension that is used. Your insurance provider will not pay for a secondary device just because you didn't like the prosthetist after you accepted the prosthesis. You will be stuck with it. This can be a very devastating experience if you receive a leg that doesn't fit and is not suited for your activity level. Some people just give up at this stage and are confined to the walker and wheelchair for the rest of their lives.

Probably the best source of information regarding prosthetists in your area are other amputees. If you are in the hospital and you don't know another amputee, ask the prosthetist, nurse, physical therapist, or surgeon to have an amputee come and visit you. One of those sources will know someone who can talk with you about the prosthetists in the area and network you to other amputees. If you are fortunate enough to have an Amputee Support Group in your community, then this is an excellent source for information about your area. The Amputee Coalition of America has chapters all over the United States that disseminate information about amputees and various products that can help you out (see Chapter 12 for more information). If you have the opportunity to attend an Amputee Support Group meeting, then you should make the effort. They are generally filled with well-meaning people who have suffered a similar experience as yourself and can share what they have learned. Beware that these are not professional counselors and their advice is from their experience. Some of these groups can degenerate into gripe sessions in which everyone sits around and complains about their prostheses and their lives, but this is not the normal scenario.

There can be a large difference in the quality of follow-up care from facility to facility. In my private practice we unconditionally guaranteed our work for 6 months to a year, depending upon the type of prosthesis. We provided routine maintenance and adjustments free of charge for the first year as well as provided a large quantity of supplies designed to last for a year of use. If a client was not happy with the result, we would give him or her the money back and I actually did this 3 times in my career. There was another local facility whose owner had great personality and charm; however, he provided the opposite type of service. He would come to your home to measure and cast your prosthesis and then mail the finished product to you weeks or months from the time of initial casting. He provided no follow-up care and although there were many complaints and even an investigation by Medicare, he had broken no laws and delivered the products for which he had been paid. As a matter of fact, he got paid the same amount of money for his products as we did and we provided consistent follow-up service. This may sound sick, but that is the reality of the system in the United States as it is today.

Choosing a Prosthetist

1.   Do you feel comfortable with the person? Can you trust him or her?
2.   Can he or she answer your questions in a manner in which you can understand?
3.   Will he or she refer you to other amputees that he or she has worked with in the past?
4.   Is he or she certified by the American Board for Certification (ABC) or the Board of Certification (BOC)?

Warning Signs

1.   Does he or she insist on taking your cast right away without explaining everything to you?
2.   Does he or she use terms and language that you cannot understand and then cannot explain it in simple terms?
3.   Does he or she seem uncomfortable and unsure of him- or herself?
4.   Does he or she offer to come to your home and tell you not to worry about the billing?

Rehabilitation and Gait Training

One of the most important things you can do if you're awaiting your preparatory prosthesis is to keep the rest of your body active and limber. The key to compensating for the loss of your leg is to have a strong body so that it can take the added stress of learning how to walk again. If you were able to walk before you lost your leg, then chances are you will still be able to walk again. The body remembers how to do this. The greatest barrier is fear of what it will be like. When I first stood a new amputee up in the parallel bars or on his or her walker, I would tell him or her just to bear a little weight on the prosthesis and to tell me how it feels. If there was no pain, then I instructed him or her to shift weight onto the prosthesis then onto the good leg, kind of like a two-step if you are a country western dancer. Some patients want to just take off and I have to hold them back to keep them from overdoing it, while others are so afraid of pain that they won't put any weight on the leg. The more reluctant patients will eventually weight bear if they are not in pain. If the leg hurts, take it off and try to find out what is causing the pain.

Pain is the body's way of telling you when something is wrong. **Listen to it!** A prosthesis shouldn't hurt. It may feel uncomfortable, tight, or really weird, but it shouldn't be excruciating. If it is excruciating, something is wrong. Take off the prosthesis and examine the stump. Are there red marks on the skin? Some socket designs leave red marks beneath the patella (kneecap) and this is OK unless it is causing an abrasion. Red marks on the bone on the side (fibula) or the tip of the stump are not supposed to be there and need to be adjusted. Most of the time, simply adding a sock will relieve the pressure at the end of the stump. Other times, an adjustment to the socket by grinding the plastic or heating it and remolding it is necessary. The bottom line is that when the amputee stands up, the prosthesis should be relatively comfortable and free of sharp pain. It can feel tight, tender, sore, or weird and these sensations are normal. If the amputee has not done desensitization exercises, then there could be intense phantom pains or the feeling of electric shock and these sensations can be very distracting. It is never too late to do desensitization exercises such as vigorous massage and the rough towel treatment.

Once the amputee is relatively comfortable and able to stand and transfer weight back and forth between legs, then he or she is ready to take his or her first steps. I usually had the patient take a step with his or her prosthesis first then step back, alternating between legs and stepping out with each but not going anywhere, just like the hokey-pokey. This gives the sensation of alternately weight shifting onto each leg. If he or she mastered this quickly, I usually told him or her just to walk to me at the end of the parallel bars or on his or her walker. I reminded him or her that he or she knew how to walk, just let the body do what it remembers to do. Fear is the greatest barrier. After he or she had walked up and down one time, I asked him or her to sit back down and let me look at the stump and double check his or her height. If there were alignment adjustments, then I would make those adjustments at that time. I checked the stump for any marks that should not be there and then had the amputee re-don the prosthesis by him- or herself, assisting him or her if necessary. It is important that the prosthetist is confident that the amputee can put his or her leg on independently.

The typical routine in my private practice was to set up a follow-up appointment for a week to 10 days, depending on whether the amputee had other follow-up care, such as out-patient physical therapy or in-home physical therapy. We would see the client every week to 10 days for brief follow-up appointments to check to see whether he or she needed to adjust socks or to have alignment changes. We checked the height of the prosthesis about a billion times on each client (slight exaggeration) because the height could change with the addition or subtraction of socks or the settling of the stump into the socket. The most common problem that I saw in prostheses that came in our door was that they were too tall or too short. This can be a major problem if the height discrepancy is more than a centimeter (quarter of an inch). In order to check height, we measure the level of the pelvis by sticking our fingers onto the pelvic crests and standing back as far as our arms allow and eyeballing whether the pelvis is level. If something is off, we place wooden boards beneath the short side until the pelvis is level and then adjust the prosthesis accordingly.

The height of the prosthesis is critical to the performance of the rest of the body. Nearly every amputee experiences the sensation of his or her first leg being too long when he or she puts it on. This is due to the fact that the amputated side of the pelvis has not been supported for a while and the body gets used to the way that feels. This is the body's homeostasis, or feeling of normalcy. When the prosthesis supports the pelvis and elevates it to level, then the body sends a message to the brain saying, "Hey this leg is too long." It generally takes several hours to a day for the body to develop a new homeostasis and for the feeling to subside. I have seen people function for years with a prosthesis that was as much as 6 centimeters (2.5 inches) too long. The person had terrible back problems but had adapted to the height. If a person has worn a leg that is too long or too short for a long period of time, then he or she may not be able to adapt to a radical correction. We oftentimes had to shorten them by 1 centimeter (0.25 inch) increments over a period of several weeks to achieve the proper height correction.

Determining the Correct Height of a Prosthesis

1. There are three anatomical bony landmarks that will help you to determine the level of the pelvis. The first is the pelvic crests, which are usually easily felt by poking your hands onto the top of your hips until you feel bones. If you are overweight and have love handles, then you may have a difficult time finding these or it may tickle or actually hurt some.

2. The second anatomical feature is the anterior superior iliac spine (ASIS), which are the bones that poke out the front of your pelvis just inside and down from the crests. These are a bit harder to find but can also be used to determine pelvic level.

3. The third is the posterior superior iliac spine (PSIS) that can be easily found on most people from behind by looking at the base of the spine. There are two dimples on most people on either side of the spine and are another good bony landmark to judge pelvic level.

4. Finding these bony prominences will only help if you can see level. What is seeing level? Can you tell when something is flat by looking at it? This is a skill I developed when I built my own house, and most good carpenters have the ability to see level. I have worked with prosthetists who could not see level if their lives depended on it. They generally didn't stay in the field that long. There are devices that assist the prosthetist and don't be surprised if someone holds a device with a carpenter's level (bubble) onto your hips.

5.   If you are experiencing any soreness in the lower back, that is a pretty good indi-
      cator that you may have a leg length problem. You can experiment on yourself by
      standing in front of a full-length mirror and place a magazine underneath the
      short side to see how that feels. If it helps, glue the magazine to your shoe. No, just
      kidding. What you can do is to place a thin pad into your shoe. If you are wearing
      tennis shoes and the prosthetic side is too long, take the thin insole out of the
      shoe for a while and see how that feels. If it is too short, take an insole from an old
      pair of shoes and put it beneath the prosthetic foot. If this is better, tell your pros-
      thetist so that he or she can make a permanent adjustment.

6.   If your pants leg is consistently different from one side to the other, this may be
      an indication that the leg is off. Go through step 5 to determine if there is a prob-
      lem.

7.   A leg length discrepancy of more than a centimeter (quarter of an inch) can cause
      a permanent curve of the spine if left untreated for an extended period of time. I
      cannot emphasize the importance of this simple correctable problem.

8.   The height of a prosthesis can change with the addition or subtraction of socks or
      even a socket adjustment. Check the height regularly to assure that you have a
      level pelvis.

Hygiene and Care of the Stump

Caring for your residual limb needs to become a daily ritual for any amputee. You
need to realize that this part of your body, the skin of the lower leg, was never
designed to be encased in silicone, wool, or plastic. It was originally made to hang out
with lots of air circulating around it and other than the occasional leg massage it was
not intended to withstand pressure or friction. In the prosthetic socket, that same skin
is surrounded by nonorganic materials; under extreme pressure; and in a warm, dark,
moist environment with sheer forces that would tax skin that was designed for pressure. This environment is very similar to a petri dish, which biologists use to grow bacteria and viral cultures. It is easy to see that the skin of your stump is being stressed
to the maximum, and care of it is essential to the continued success of wearing a prosthesis.

Keeping the skin clean and free of harmful bacteria is a major factor in caring for
your stump. You need to wash the skin with some type of antibacterial soap at least
once a day. Whatever soap you use on the rest of your body should be OK unless it is
a heavily perfumed or dyed soap. These dyes and perfumes can irritate the skin under
the pressure and perspiration of the socket. There are several soaps that kill many of
the bacteria on the skin surface that can be bought over the counter such as Hibiclens
(GC America Inc., Alsip, IL), Betadine (Purdue Frederick Co., Norwalk, CT), and
Phisoderm (Chattem Inc., Chattanooga, TN). These soaps kill bacteria on contact but
unfortunately, once you put your prosthesis back on the bacteria can regrow and
repopulate your stump within hours. Rubbing alcohol is not recommended because
although it does kill lots of bacteria, it also dries out the skin and can cause as much
harm as good.

Washing the residual limb thoroughly is important. Use a rough wash cloth and
scrub vigorously all over the skin, especially behind the knee and the bottom, which

are places that are difficult to see. If the amputation is still fresh and the stitches were only recently removed, then you need to scrub the suture line gently to remove dead skin and scabs. I emphasize that you should not pick the scabs from the suture line. Soak the skin in warm water for a while and let the skin fall off naturally. Within a week of vigorous washing, the dead skin should be gone and the suture line should be pink with new healthy skin. Just as important as thorough washing is drying the skin completely to prevent trapping moisture in your socket when you re-don your leg. If there are patches that don't look healthy, then you should go see your doctor to make sure that the skin at the end of your stump is viable and healthy.

When I first lost my leg back in the Cretaceous Period, there were not too many products that one could use to keep the skin clean. I also just wore wool socks next to my skin, which once they had been worn and washed a couple of times tended to get very hard, to the point where they would stand up by themselves. I also must admit that my washing skills as a 21-year-old college student were not the best. Infected hair follicles or pimples that would come up plagued me in areas where there was a lot of pressure on the skin. This may not sound like a big deal to the nonamputee, but if you have ever tried to walk on a big old zit, then you may have a little empathy for what amputees go through. It is extremely painful and it is a sharp, invasive pain that you experience strongly each time you weight bear on the prosthesis. The worst thing you can do for pimples on your stump is to pick or pop them. Your fingers are probably the dirtiest parts of your body and when you squeeze the pimple and you open the skin with your dirty fingers, there is a high probability of infection. A pimple is bad and painful but nothing compared to the pain of a full-blown stump infection. I confess that I am guilty of popping pimples on my stump. Sometimes it just seemed like the right thing to do at the time (the same can be said for bungee jumping). The pimple is the body's attempt to isolate a local infection of the skin. The white pussy stuff that shoots out when you pop it are white blood cells that have been attacking the infection. When you pop these things, then you have opened the body up to infection. The worst-case scenario, which unfortunately I have stupidly done, is to try and pop a pimple and to have it pop on the inside, which disperses the infection underneath the skin, spreading it to the underlying tissues. My stump was swollen for almost a week afterward and I could not wear my leg for the duration. **Don't pop pimples on your stump!**

When you get chronic pimples in one area, this is an indication of a concentration of pressure and the prosthetist needs to adjust the socket. What can also develop in areas of chronic skin pressure are tiny grains of what look and feel like sand but are really just a hard mass of dead skin and white blood cells that are left whenever a pimple occurs. The body can dispose of them with vigorous washing but the temptation to try and dig them out is great. The other problem with these little hard granules is that they form a source of irritation for another pimple to form. When this happens time after time in the same place, then it is an indication that there is something wrong with the fit of the prosthesis and needs adjusting. Some of the worst places that I saw in my career were behind the knee in sockets that were either too high and bound behind the knee or cut too low so that there was no counterpressure to the patellar tendon area (the space just below your knee cap). Large cysts would form in these areas where the body was trying to contain infected hair follicles or old pimples. Sometimes they would get so bad that they would have to be surgically removed; however, this was often not a great solution because the resulting scar tissue was inelastic and prone to continued breakdown. I will cover these phenomena in more detail when I discuss socket design in the next chapter.

The best antibacterial soap for the stump is Phisohex (Sanofi-Synthelabo, Inc., New York, NY). Unfortunately, it is a prescription item because it contains hexachlorophene, which is a controlled substance. An amputee veterinarian told me about it after it cured his infection problems that had plagued him for many years. Phisohex does not kill as many bacteria as Betadine or Hibiclens; however, the hexachlorophene sets up an environment in which bacteria do not like to grow, which means that the stump has a much lower bacteria count than with other more potent agents hours later. After I started using Phisohex, my pimple problem pretty much cleared up and I didn't have to resist the temptation to dig little hard things out of my skin. Another product that has come along in the last several years that could have been made for the amputee is waterless hand cleanser. This is a clear, alcohol-free liquid that dries rapidly when rubbed onto the skin and comes in small, easy to carry containers. It is perfect for cleaning your stump during exercise or just when it gets all hot and sweaty, and it does a great job at reducing the bacteria count on the skin. I now utilize it to clean my stump just before I go to bed. I keep it on the nightstand and use it every night. It can also come in handy when you need to clean a sheath or liner quickly and do not have access to a sink and soap.

Just as important as caring for your skin is the caring and cleaning of whatever your prosthesis uses next to your skin. Whether this is a sock, sheath, gel sheath, silicone liner, or gel liner, whatever goes next to your skin should be cleaned as often as you clean your skin. The manufacturers of the various liner products all have recommendations on the care of their products, so read the instructions carefully and follow them. I know no one actually follows the directions on the box, but I do highly recommend reading the suggestions and developing a routine that includes daily cleaning of your liner. If you don't wash your liner (defined as whatever you put next to your skin), then you will begin to concentrate the salts and acids from the perspiration in your body. There will be a residue of perspiration on the surface each time you take the liner off. As the perspiration evaporates, particles of salt and acid are left as a residue on the liner. The next day when you put your liner back on the new perspiration dissolves the salts and acids and when you take it off again they are left behind again as a residue, except this time they are concentrated with the leftover stuff from the day before. Each day you do not wash your liner you are concentrating salts and acids next to your skin, and after a week of this you can imagine what the skin is having to try to process.

When I first lost my leg, I was told by the doctor that my stump would have to get tough before I would be able to wear a leg. I took this to mean that I would need to have calluses and thick skin to be able to weight bear on the skin so I was pleased to see thick tough skin develop on the end of my stump. Nothing could be further from the truth. The best skin for weight bearing is soft supple skin that has its full elasticity. Calluses are the body's reaction to pressure and friction, which are things that need to be adjusted in the socket, not toughened up by the skin. If you get calluses on your stump, they are telling you that this is an area of too much pressure or that there is movement in the socket and the skin has to get thick to accommodate. You can use a hand lotion on the skin at night to soften the tissue and use a pumice stone when you wash to gently remove the callous. I have tried many different skin lotions on my stump, but the best products that I have used are Eucerin (Beirsdorf, Inc., Wilton, CT) and Lubriderm (Warner-Lambert Consumer Healthcare, Morris Plains, NJ). Whatever you use as a lotion on the rest of your body you can use on your stump. There are only two specific body parts that have the specialized skin necessary for weight bearing, the bottoms of your feet and the palms of your hands. All the other skin was designed as a covering and not to walk on. Take good care of the skin on your stump. Keep it clean and soft and it will provide a good basis for wearing a prosthesis.

Ambulatory Aids

There are 3 basic ambulatory aids that amputees use: walkers, crutches, and canes. Each has a place in rehabilitation with the ultimate goal of not having to use an ambulatory aid for getting around. Most people learn to walk using parallel bars, which are great for training but I don't know of anyone who has parallel bars in his or her home. In my practice, we rarely trained people on the bars because we wanted them to learn to walk using the same device that they used at home. Still, they are useful as a training tool but prosthetists should be careful to make sure that the amputee can use another ambulatory aid before sending him or her home with a prosthesis.

Walkers are a great aid to the amputee who has strength or balance problems and needs a firm base of support to learn to ambulate. The walker should be adjusted so that the amputee can stand as erect as possible and still keep it in front of him or her. If the walker is held too close to the body, it becomes unstable and can cause the amputee to lose his or her balance. My personal experience with walkers of any type is that they promote a hunched over gait pattern, which causes some very bad walking habits to develop if used for a long period of time. Some geriatric amputees will never progress beyond the walker due to balance and strength issues and this is acceptable, but if it is possible to progress to crutches then their gait and the posture of the rest of the body is vastly improved.

Crutches are the next step in ambulatory progression and provide the amputee with greater mobility than a walker, as well as a better physical posture. There are two basic types of crutches: the underarm crutch (the most common) and the forearm or forearm crutch. The underarm crutch gives the amputee maximum stability and does not require the arm strength of the forearm crutch. They should be adjusted in height so that the top pad rides about 10 centimeters (4 inches) below the armpit. If the crutches are too high and actually come into the armpit, they can inhibit circulation and will be less stable. One of the advantages of the underarm crutch is that it is possible to carry something very carefully with your hand while you clamp on the crutch with your armpit. It isn't easy but it can be done and it is definitely preferable to spilling the coffee while you hop or scooting the cup across the floor while you crawl. Just like the walker, it is important to keep the crutches in front of you for balance and like the walker the underarm crutches will promote a hunched forward gait in which the back is not straight but leaned toward the front.

The forearm crutch requires a great deal more strength and balance than the underarm crutch or the walker. The forearm cuff should be adjusted so that the cuff is a bit more than midway up the forearm on the largest part of the forearm muscles. They should be lengthened until the amputee is standing fully erect and the crutches are just touching the floor. This is one of the ambulatory aids that does not promote a hunched forward gait pattern and allows the amputee to walk as close to normal with maximum stability. Again, it is important to keep the crutches in front of the amputee at all times, as this provides the greatest base of support. Forearm crutches are worthless for carrying anything because both hands have to be on the arm grips for them to work. I have personally spilled many types of liquids and solids while trying to move them with forearm crutches. This ambulatory aid is the optimal gait-training device because it allows for an upright posture and promotes the most natural walking pattern.

   The final ambulatory aid is the cane. It does provide some stability for the amputee as well as an ability to slightly take weight off of the prosthesis for a brief period of time during gait. Canes have been around a long time and some can be as fashionable as they are functional. The cane should be long enough for the amputee to be able to bear some weight on it without bending forward. There are many varieties of canes that have specific handgrips as well as tips that can have a 4-pronged bottom to provide a more stable base. There are varying philosophies on which hand to hold the cane in, with the physical therapy world saying that it should be the hand that is opposite the amputation. This certainly makes sense from a gait pattern point of view. I always carried my walking stick in my right hand, the same side as my amputation, mostly because this provided the greatest unweighting of my prosthesis. I used a walking stick instead of a cane, which was nearly as tall as my shoulder, and I held it at almost shoulder height mostly to take some pressure off of my leg and for stability on uneven ground.

The Mirror Trick for Gait Training

   Since I really had no formal gait training from a physical therapist, I had to learn to walk on my own. The method that I used was to watch myself walk while looking into a mirror. I bought an inexpensive full-length mirror and placed it at the end of the hallway of my apartment where I could get the longest stretch of open space. Each time I walked in front of it, I would try to walk with no limp or gait deviation. I was very critical of my stride, making sure that I was taking even stride lengths, which I later discovered were the most common gait deviations of below-knee amputees. When I didn't have a full-length mirror, I would watch myself walk in storefront windows or classroom windows, trying to walk with no visual difference in the 2 legs. I would also watch my feet as I walked in corridors with evenly spaced tiles, using the lines in the tiles as a guide to make sure I was taking an even length step on both sides. This system worked very well because I have no visible limp now, unless I am wearing my pirate costume peg leg.

Bilateral Amputee Gait Training

   If you have lost both legs, then you are faced with a completely different set of balance circumstances. The best analogy for being a bilateral is if you ever tried walking on stilts as a kid, you will have some idea of what it is like to walk on 2 prostheses. It is tricky but not impossible. As in single leg amputees, the bilateral will rely heavily on the upper body strength to compensate for the lack of stability in the legs. It is even more important for the bilateral to maintain good arm strength and flexibility. The energy expenditure for bilateral leg amputees is far greater than that of a single leg amputee, so the general physical fitness of the amputee is more important. He or she will work more than twice as hard as someone with 1 leg.

We were taught in prosthetics school that when working with a bilateral amputee we should always shorten the legs to lower the center of gravity of the amputee. This makes a lot of sense to anyone who works with the amputee—the shorter the person, the more stability he or she will have. Most prosthetic systems have easy adjustment of the height of the prostheses so this becomes a simple matter to change the height of the limbs as necessary. The prosthetist should take particular care to check the pelvic level of the bilateral because with the added strain of the balance and stress on the spine, a leg length discrepancy can have a disastrous effect on their performance. My personal opinion is that bilaterals should utilize the same type of prosthetic feet and suspension on both sides when possible. This increases the feel of consistency in the way the person walks and how the prosthesis feels to the amputee.

Most bilateral amputees will generally develop a gait pattern that has very little limp. This is due to the fact that a limp is perceived as some difference in motion of the two halves of the body. The human eye is looking for equal motion on both sides and when it sees that one shoulder dips slightly or one arm doesn't swing quite the same as the other, it causes the observer to scrutinize the individual more closely. This is not necessarily a conscious act on the part of the observer; it is just a natural reaction to something that the human eye is expecting. Because bilaterals limp equally on both sides the human eye doesn't perceive it as a limp, it may just appear to be an unusual gait pattern. Gait training is basically the same procedure as the unilateral amputee with more attention to the fit and comfort. Ambulatory aids are generally used for a longer period of time until the amputee has mastered the balance and trust issues of not being able to feel the ground beneath them.

Although it is recommended and it makes common sense to shorten the bilateral amputee to give him or her more stability, this has not been my experience as a prosthetist. Nearly every bilateral that I know wanted to be taller. At first I fought with them over this because of what I had been taught at school, but I learned that motivation is often the most powerful rehabilitation tool that exists. Here is a story that changed my view.

I had been a prosthetist for 5 years when I began working with Aaron, a very wealthy man who had lost one leg to diabetes. He had many other medical issues such as a bad heart and liver so within 2 years his other leg had to be removed. He had been very successful as a unilateral amputee and when I first saw him after the second amputation, I was surprised at his negative attitude. Aaron was at the bottom of a hole in his life. Despite his wealth, he felt that his time was over. His wife had left him, he had just had triple bypass surgery, and he saw no future as a legless man. I explained to him that we would be shortening him by a few centimeters, and the look on his face betrayed his disgust for his life. Trying to be funny, I told him that I could make him taller if he wanted and then made some crack about the Boston Celtics needing a new power forward. All of a sudden, his demeanor changed completely. He asked if I could make him almost 2 meters (6 foot 1 inches) tall, which was a good 7 centimeters (3 inches) taller than he had been with 2 legs. I told him that I could but it was not recommended. He said he didn't care, that he could make it work if I would only make him taller than his 2 sons. This went against everything I was ever taught, but I gradually increased his height over the next 6 months until he was slightly taller than his sons. The change in Aaron was dramatic. He was a handsome man in his sixties and now with his new height, his confidence had returned. I was convinced that the power of motivation was one of the real keys to successful rehabilitation and that biomechanical advantages were outweighed by attitude.

Gait Considerations of Child Amputees

Children who lose limbs almost always perform at an outstanding level with a prosthesis. Their motivation is high and they can adapt to learning to walk with far greater ease than adults who have experienced life with 2 legs and regret the life they have lost. In my experience the biggest problem is when prosthetists or health care professionals limit them by telling them all of the things that they can't do. Child amputees participate in nearly all types of sports and recreation and although they put their prostheses to the test, they seem to find a way to do anything. Encouragement and creativity are the 2 factors that help children to live normal lives.

Since motivation is rarely a problem with children, the problems come from developing bad habits with their prostheses because they are too busy doing stuff to worry about how they walk. At the expense of being a nag, it is important to keep their gait pattern in the front of their minds by reminding them of how they are walking. Height is a big problem because they are growing all the time and not evenly. They may grow 1 cm (0.5 in) one year and 7 cm (3 in) the next. Parents have to take some responsibility for keeping the leg within the 0.5 to 2 cm (0.25 to 0.5 in) range that often times is not easy at all. Routine pelvic level checks are important to make sure that the child does not go too long with an uneven leg length. Children generally will need prosthetic replacements on an average of once a year and some years even more, so parents should be prepared both financially and logistically.

Another factor that is unique to children is that since they are still growing, the bones in their stump are also still growing. This can cause a situation called osseous overgrowth where the bone continues to grow at the bottom of the stump, stretching the skin to the point where it can no longer cover the bone. Most child amputees will have to have revisions to their stumps at some point. If this is left undone, it will render the child unable to wear the prosthesis due to intense soreness at the tip of the stump because the bone is trying to grow out the end. Once the skin gets thin and red, it is time to consider revision.

There are many great components available for children today. As with adult prostheses, the fit of the socket is still the most important factor in the success of the amputee. In my private practice, there were 2 special considerations that we built into all children's prostheses. These were height adjustment and dual inserts in the socket. We would use a pylon system anytime we could fit it into the shank of the leg so that we could more easily lengthen the prosthesis when necessary. If the leg were too short to use a pylon system, we would have to add pieces of wood or foam to lengthen when necessary. When we made the socket, we would always use some type of soft liner, usually pelite (a soft white foam material) and made 2 inserts, one inside the other. When the child no longer fit the liner due to growth, then it was a simple matter of pulling the inner liner out and just using the outer liner that would often give the leg another few months of function.

It has been my experience that children function well with a prosthesis if they are given encouragement and assistance. Today the world is much friendlier for a child amputee than in the past. Children will tease them some in school, but the public's perspective on the amputee is much more accepting than ever before. Still, there will be times when they ask why did this happen to them. I don't have any answer to this question. It is a matter of your personal faith and needs to be answered with as much honesty as they can understand. Sheltering your child from the world due to an amputation will not serve him or her well as an adult. Be as real and honest as you can.

The Art of Distraction or How Not to Limp

1. A limp, as perceived by the observer, is some difference in the way the 2 halves of the body move. If you don't want to limp, then walk the same way with both sides of the body.
2. Use a mirror to watch yourself walk. If you can't see a limp in your gait, I promise you that no one else can. You will always be the most critical observer.
3. The best way to keep someone from looking at your leg is to look him or her in the eye. If you look people in the eye as you approach them, they will always do one of two things. They will either look you back in the eye or they will look away. Either way they are not looking at your leg.
4. Another way to keep people from looking at your leg is to use the art of distraction. A Carmen Miranda fruit hat will generally do the trick or a talking parrot on the shoulder (a favorite pirate distraction) will cause people to focus away from your leg.
5. Much of people's perception of you will be created by your perception of yourself. If you are ashamed of your leg and you are looking down at it all the time, people will look down to see what you are looking at.
6. I have worked around people all day long in shorts with my leg hanging out in the open and it would be hours before they realized that it was a prosthesis. I just didn't give them a reason to notice.

CHAPTER 3

The Permanent Prosthesis

Stories

My Experience

My first permanent prosthesis was just like my preparatory, except that it did not use a permanent waist belt. The socket was made from plastic with a foam liner made from a material called pelite. Pelite is white or sometimes pink and is soft and squishy to the touch. Prosthetists like to use it because it is heat moldable and easy to work with. The foot was still a SACH foot that bent at the toe and had a cushion heel. The suspension was the old cuff-strap that when pulled tight above the knee held the leg on with some degree of confidence. I could attach a waist belt to it if I wanted so when I engaged in more strenuous activities I could use the belt to make sure the leg would not fall off. One of the disadvantages of this type of suspension was that my stump moved up and down in the socket with each step, causing what is known as pistoning. The shank of the leg was shaped to roughly look like a leg and laminated in a hard shiny pink plastic, giving the appearance of a countertop as opposed to a piece of living body. I was able to get around with this leg much better for my spring quarter of college and the first half of the summer.

Unfortunately for me, the type of amputation surgery performed on me was having its effect on the stability of my fit. My stump, which had none of the muscles attached below the knee, was shrinking rapidly. My activity level was also contributing to the rapid atrophy of the remaining muscles; the more pressure on the tissue, the more it would tend to shrink away. Because the muscles had nothing to pull against, they could perform no work, so under the pressures of the socket they would deteriorate until eventually they atrophied to the muscle fibers with no bulk. This rapid change in volume was not evenly distributed on my residual limb either. The big muscles of my calf lost their bulk rapidly, which caused the bones to begin to protrude, especially the fibula, which pokes out of the side of the leg. This rapid change meant that any time I got a new prosthesis, the fit was only good for a couple of weeks and then because of the new pressure on my stump, more atrophy occurred and the fit deteriorated.

What this all meant was that I needed new prostheses every 6 months or so to keep up with the changes in my residual limb. My second permanent prosthesis was made in the summer after I had returned to Georgia at the end of the class sessions. It was totally different than the previous prostheses and got rid of the straps and belts for which I was glad. I had returned to my original prosthetic facility because I had more faith in their abilities than the place in Cincinnati. This type of leg utilized a wedge above the knee to hold it on and is called a supercondylar suspension. The technical name for this type of suspension is SCSP, which translated into the common tongue means supercondylar superpatellar. This type of leg came all the way over my kneecap and encapsulated my entire knee. There was a wedge built into the insert that dug into the still intact muscle above the inside of my knee. This soft wedge, made out of pelite that was glued together, hung on the condyle and prevented the leg from coming off. I was able to don the prosthesis by first slipping the insert over my socks then putting the insert into the plastic socket. The plastic socket was just tight enough to prevent the insert from slipping out but loose enough to allow me to get my leg into the socket. The big advantage of this system was that there were no belts and straps needed to hold the leg on. It was easy to get on and take off, and it provided a lot of protection for my knee because the entire knee was surrounded by hard plastic. The disadvantages of this system were that it hurt like hell for about a week because of that pressure on the inside of my knee, but after the second week, the pain subsided as the muscle shrank. Since the leg was so easy to get off, this also meant that it fell off easily, especially when I bent my knee just right. It was nice to be able to easily slip the leg off whenever I sat down and since it was not particularly comfortable to sit with this was almost a necessity. The new leg also had a different foot for me, a Griesinger foot (Otto Bock, USA), which is a multiaxial device utilizing rubber bumpers to cushion the heel and allow the foot to move in all directions. This simulated ankle motion and took a lot of torque off of my stump by allowing the forces to be absorbed by the ankle instead of the socket. The foot screwed onto the bottom of the shank of the leg and my prosthetist, Grant, showed me how it worked and how to take it apart to perform minor repairs. This was a major step for me in my mobility because the foot gave me ankle motion that made walking on uneven surfaces much easier and improved my handball game immeasurably. The shank was still the hard plastic with the color of doll skin, but Grant had laminated a loop attachment into the top of the socket in front of my knee that allowed me to use a waist belt if I needed to.

Mexico

I embarked on my first overseas adventure armed with my new leg. I left Oxford, Ohio to perform my student teaching in the American school in Monterey, Mexico, a large industrial city about 100 miles south of Brownsville, Texas. I was with a group of student teachers from Miami that included 2 other men (this represented half of all of the men majoring in Elementary Education) and 8 women. This was my kind of odds, plus one of the men was a good buddy of mine and we decided to drive down to Monterey after stopping in Atlanta to see my family. Dave was a former Miami football player and a really great guy with which to travel. First I drove up to Akron, Ohio to pick him up and I also decided to visit my former girlfriend who also lived up there.

I had this need to show her that I wasn't the crippled man that she had seen when I first lost my leg. In retrospect, this has been one of the powerful forces in my mania to excel in sports and activities. I had to show people that I was just as good as anyone else. As a matter of fact, I unconsciously developed a philosophy of having to be better at something than anyone else just to be equal. I reasoned that having only 1 leg put me at a disadvantage in competition for everything: girls, jobs, sports, and girls. Needless to say, girls were very important and I was still struggling to come to grips with how I appeared to women. I strove to walk with no limp and rarely showed my pain in public, reserving it for when I was in the relative safety of my home.

Dave and I drove south in the mammoth Fury III station wagon; after stopping to see my family, we headed for Mexico. We arrived in Mexico and moved in with our family, the Morales, who gave us 2 of their bedrooms to live in. Dave and I occupied 1 bedroom and Mike roomed with the supervising teacher, who was a milquetoast kind of guy. Mike was another real man's man and he and I had some adventures together. Before we started classes, we had a couple of weeks to do some sightseeing, so we took a bus to Mazatlan, a beach resort on the Pacific that at that time was mostly Mexican tourists. We had some adventures, and I met some girls and had some romances.

Back in Monterey, we began our student teaching experience. I was assigned to a fourth grade class of mostly Mexican kids who spoke English. I developed my strategy for dealing with children and prostheses at this time. Invariably within the first week of class one of the kids would discover that my leg was hard and ask me why. I would sit down with the entire class and take my leg off and answer any questions that they had. I would let them touch my stump and pass the leg around the class to satisfy their curiosity. Most kids thought it was pretty cool, but a few were a little shocked by the whole idea of a missing limb. This honesty and openness worked well because from then on the kids treated me normally without regard for my disability. This contributed immensely to my healing process and gave me effective tools to use with adults as well.

While in Mexico, I accomplished a few "firsts." I did some climbing in the local mountains, not technical stuff but very challenging for me considering the newness of the prosthesis and of my amputation. As in many of the endeavors at this time of my life, they were motivated by trying to impress a girl. I also got the opportunity to visit Mexico City, a sprawling metropolis of 12 million people even in 1975. As part of my visit there, I went on a tour of the ruins at Teconuxian where I climbed my first pyramid, taking one step at a time but eventually getting to the top. I was fascinated by the ancient city dominated by the great pyramid that towered over the entire plain and tried to imagine what it must have been like 600 years before. I also had to deal with going to the beach, something that had not occurred to me as to how I was going to get into the water without a leg. The first incident occurred in Mazatlan where we stayed in a hotel right on the sand and since I could not get my leg wet, I decided to just hop out to the surf until I was in water deep enough to swim. This was no easy chore; hopping on sand is difficult as you lose a little on each hop. I perfected a clever strategy to not only help me get to the beach but also meet girls. I would walk onto the beach and scope out the best looking girl who seemed to be by herself and then ask her to assist me in hopping into the surf. It was not foolproof, because once the girl was not alone and when her very large boyfriend showed up he was not so sympathetic to my situation. However, I did get a few dinner dates due to my boldness.

My 5 months in Mexico were a huge confidence builder for me. I learned that it was my attitude about myself that determined other people's attitudes toward me. I believed that I could do anything that I set my mind to, which all by itself was an enormous change in my life perspective. There was a lot of pain involved in being active and having responsibilities, especially with a prosthesis that never fit properly due to my continued stump atrophy. I met teachers who had traveled all over the world, teaching in exotic places and living fascinating lives and I determined that this was what I wanted to do.

I returned to my parent's home in Georgia just before Christmas and decided to take a backpacking trip in the Smoky Mountains with my 13-year-old brother, Bill. The weather was terrible, snowing and windy the entire 3 days of our trip. One night after we arrived at the shelter where we planned to spend the night, there were already some other people in the shelter getting out of the weather. There was a teenager standing by the fire, boasting about all of the equipment that he had, dropping the names of his pack, his canteen, and just about every piece of stuff he had. I just stood there not saying anything, wishing he would shut up. I reached over to the pile of wood and picked up a nice size stick and proceeded to break it over the shin of my prosthesis. The teenager's jaw dropped and I looked up at him, pulled up my pants leg, and said, "Atlanta prosthetics leg." He never said another word. We had to hike uphill most of the day, and my stump socks were soaking wet as I laid them out to dry in the cold damp air. My brother and I had poor sleeping bags, so we joined ours together and wrapped plastic around us for more warmth. The next morning I awoke to find that my stump socks were frozen stiff. It was not a happy thing to have to put them down into the sleeping bag to thaw them out.

Bill and I took off for the hike to the car that was mostly downhill. This was more difficult than I expected since the trail was steep and very deeply rutted. It was more like an icy toboggan run than a trail. I slipped and fell of course and my leg came flying off. It skittered down the trail and disappeared around a corner of the descending path. We had not seen another soul the entire morning, but as luck would have it, there were 2 hikers coming up the trail just around the bend. You can imagine their horror to see a leg come screeching down the path. Bill and I heard terrified screams and I yelled down to them to stop the leg. They brought it up to me but were visibly shaken. My brother and I got a good laugh at this, but when I put the leg back on I knew that I was in trouble. When the leg slipped off, it had taken a big chunk of skin off of the front of my stump and we still had 4 miles to go before we reached the car. I was leaning heavily on my walking stick and didn't know how I was going to make it but also realized that no one was going to be able to give me a ride so I was going to have to stick it out. Bill was as helpful as he could be, and I could see the pain on his face as he tried to empathize with my dilemma.

I made it back to school brimming with confidence and full of adventure stories for my friends. I also knew what I wanted to do with my teaching career; I wanted to teach overseas in someplace like Kuala Lumpur, Malaysia, or Katmandu, Nepal. I was not going to be satisfied with a position in Middletown, Ohio or Conyers, Georgia, so I paid a visit to the placement office at Miami to enlist their help in finding a teaching position overseas. The placement person had my file open on his desk and listened patiently as I explained my desires. When I finished, he patronizingly got up from his desk and patted me on the shoulder, telling me that the basic requirement for overseas placement was 2 years teaching experience and that I should forget the idea since I didn't have this. He suggested that I go back to Georgia and maybe I'd meet some nice girl and forget the crazy idea of teaching overseas. This was all I needed; someone to tell me it was impossible. I was now determined to make this happen for me.

I discovered that every year there is a convention of overseas directors of American schools and that this particular year the convention was held in early February in

Atlantic City, New Jersey. I cut off my long curly hair, donned the only suit I owned, made up a resume, and then hitchhiked to Atlantic City. There I found a room a couple of blocks from the hotel where the convention was being held. Atlantic City in 1976 was a deserted, slum-ridden town, but I was fortunate enough to have a great landlady who straightened my tie each morning and fed me a bagel. I showed up at the convention with nothing to lose. I stole a nametag from a table of tags for people who hadn't shown up yet then flipped it over and put my name on it. I hung out in the hospitality room and just started going up to directors and promoting myself as a teacher with experience in Mexico. I ended up getting 11 interviews and 3 job offers. 1976 was a year when there was a serious teacher glut in the United States and Miami, which normally places 90% of their teachers, had only placed 10%. I accepted a position as an elementary school teacher at the American School in Cairo, Egypt. It was the only overseas teaching position offered to a graduating senior in the United States. My confidence was very high.

Back in school I was having the time of my life. Classes were easy, good friends surrounded me, and the girls were friendly. One night a good buddy and I decided to go sled riding at a small hill on campus. We had no sleds, so we went to the dining hall and stole a couple of the large trays to use as sleds. We arrived at the hill and it already had a large group of underclassmen having a blast "traying" down the hill. After a couple of runs, the group formed a train by sitting one behind the other and locking their legs around the person in front. I immediately sought out the best looking girl and got behind her, hoping to make her acquaintance. We all locked legs, my buddy behind me, and we took off down the hill in a big train of trayers. The train started to break up at the back toward the bottom of the hill. To my dismay, my buddy fell off, dragging me with him. My leg came off under the arm of the pretty blond in front of me. She made it to the bottom of the hill about 15 feet in front of me, so I yelled down to her, "Hey you pulled my leg right off!" Laughingly, she turned around to look at me, expecting me to be right behind her since my foot was still under her arm. The look of incongruity on her face was priceless as she tried to figure out how I could be 15 feet away and yet she still had my foot. She screamed and dropped my prosthesis in the snow and all of the other people on the hill froze in their tracks. My buddy and I almost split our guts laughing at the dilemma as I scooted down the hill to retrieve my leg. Later, I went up to her to apologize for any embarrassment that I caused her and she forgave me for coming apart in her hands. This was not the traditional way to meet girls, but I figured that I needed to take advantage of any opportunity that presented itself.

Real Tragedy

One thing losing my leg did for me was to teach me that one can never be too sure of what life will throw at you. It was a Saturday morning, and I was awakened early by the phone ringing. It was my mother telling me that my 13-year-old brother Bill had been shot while visiting our grandmother's house in Virginia. Apparently, he was spending the night at a friend's house and they went downstairs to play in the basement. As the friend passed the rack where the family firearms were stored, he picked up a new pistol and pointed it at my brother. He pulled the trigger as my brother was turning and the bullet went through Bill's windpipe and esophagus, lodging in his spine and causing paralysis. He was taken to the local hospital but was in intensive care and only my parents could visit him. I immediately wanted to come to him but my parents asked me to wait since his condition was stable and he was going to need a lot of care once he returned to Georgia. A week of pure hell went by as I tried to understand how something so stupidly tragic could happen to Bill, the kindest, most empathetic kid I had ever known. The following Friday, my mother called to say that Bill's condition had gotten worse and that I should come as soon as I could. I drove all night to arrive in Bluefield, Virginia by morning. Spinal meningitis had set in and Bill was dying a terrible death. I cannot even write this without tearing up; it was so tragic and senseless. I was with my father when the doctor came in to announce that he was gone. My father collapsed into my arms like a child and I felt that I had to take over as the strength of the family for a while.

The funeral was a few days later and to my utter surprise, 8 of my college buddies drove the 10 hours to Virginia to be with me during this time. I will always be indebted to them for their kindness and understanding during a time when my brain was trying to make sense of the incomprehensible. I discovered that losing my leg was definitely not the worst thing that could happen to me. Losing a loved one is far worse. When something happens to you, you can do something about it, you can overcome adversity. Yet when someone dies, you can't make it better, you can't say you are sorry for the things you did, you can't tell them you love them. I got hard. I couldn't cry. I couldn't laugh. Nothing was funny anymore. I went back to Georgia for a week to help my parents. I did one of the hardest things I have ever done in my life. I cleaned out my brother's room, each item tearing a new hole in my heart as I packed it up. I was trying to be strong and I held my emotions in check, not knowing that this would ball up inside of me for years until I finally chose to grieve for Bill. My family is one of deep faith and we leaned on one another during this time, but a deep chasm had been opened in our hearts that only time would heal. I can only now imagine my parents' grief at losing a child after having another lose a leg—all in the space of 18 months. I have the deepest respect for their faith and determination to carry on in the face of abject tragedy. Maybe it's the mountain heritage that gave them the strength to endure the unendurable. I pray that my kids will have similar strength and understanding.

Back at school, I was a shell of the man I had been. My infectious good humor was gone and replaced with a grim determination to succeed in my quest to accomplish my goals. In retrospect, it was probably a necessary defense reaction to shield me from my grief. I graduated in the spring and said farewell to my friends, determined to keep in touch with them no matter where I was in the world. I returned to Georgia and spent the summer working as a house painter, climbing ladders and trimming windows. I got a new leg made before my trip to Egypt and it was just like my previous prosthesis except it was a better fit. I also stocked up on parts for my foot that needed constant maintenance to keep it from squeaking loudly. Grant introduced me to one new component that definitely improved the comfort of wearing my prosthesis. It was a sock system by a French manufacturer named Daw that included a nylon sheath that went next to the skin and provided a friction barrier from the sock. In addition to reducing friction to the skin, the sock and sheath combination also minimized the moisture build up next to the skin by wicking the sweat away from the skin and into the sock, kind of like a diaper does. This new sock system did a lot to give me a more comfortable fit in my prosthesis.

House painting was probably not the best choice of summer jobs for a guy who was not quite 2 years postamputation. I really didn't have stability problems on ladders since I discovered that I could lean the shin of my prosthesis against the rungs of the ladder and it didn't hurt like it does when you have 2 legs. I mostly did trim and cut in so that my partners could roll the flat spaces. I had to be very cautious and conscious of where my prosthetic foot was at all times. It was very easy to trip over a curled drop cloth or bucket of paint since I could not feel subtle changes in the ground beneath me.

As the summer progressed, I slowly began to regain my sense of humor and outlook on life. I had not really grieved the death of my brother. Instead, I had walled it off in my psyche and tried not to think about it. I thrived on activity and pain, which feed on one another very well as well as being an extremely effective block to feeling. I focused on the upcoming move to Egypt and avoided mention of my brother. My sister was very devastated and closed up except to the family who she embraced as her strength. My mom cried a lot, especially when something reminded her of Bill. My father regained his usual outer strength but I think he went for 2 years without sleeping. The demons were always waiting for him in his subconscious where he could not control them. After I left for Cairo, my parents sold the house in Conyers and moved 20 miles away to Covington, the town where they filmed the TV show, "In the Heat of the Night." They had a little farm there with a barn and a creek, a very pretty place.

In late August 1976, I sent my steamer trunk of possessions off to Cairo. The school paid for 2000 pounds of personal effects to be shipped over. I did not own 2000 pounds of stuff so I went out and bought a new stereo and anything else I could think of to make Cairo like home. I had no idea what I was getting into. I accumulated as many prosthetic supplies as I could: extra socks and sheaths, spare parts for the foot, and an extra waist belt. Lastly, I carried a half-dozen jars of Ampubalm (Southern Prosthetics Supply, Atlanta, GA), a salve for the stump that was the only prosthetic specific medication that was available at the time. Ampubalm is a lumpy, lanolin-based salve that also lists mutton tallow as one of its major ingredients. Yes, it is made from the hooves of sheep. It smelled terrible and that smell actually got me into trouble once. When I was in my senior year, I was dating several women who were not particularly aware of each other. I had spent the night at one girl's house and the next night a friend of hers (whom I was also dating) came by her apartment to pick up a book. Upon entering the bedroom, she remarked at the strange odor. The other girl replied that the odor was from her boyfriend Rick Riley. They discovered my duplicity and it was the fault of the Ampubalm. Still, it was all that I had to soothe the sores, infected hairs, and abrasions that continually plagued my stump.

In early September I left my still grieving family to embark on my biggest adventure, life in Cairo, Egypt. I was almost exactly 2 years postamputation, I had my teaching degree, and I was embroiled in a lawsuit against the construction company that had been in charge of my accident scene. I was seeking adventure and, in some respects, running from my own demons. I will discuss my adventures overseas in following chapters.

Dave

Dave lost his leg at the age of 62, the result of a blood clot in his right calf that cut off the circulation to his foot. The deterioration of the leg occurred rapidly and although the vascular surgeon that he had been seeing did everything he could, so much tissue had died that he had to amputate only about 23 cm (3 in) below the knee. The vascular surgeon viewed the amputation as a failure of his efforts and when it came to the actual amputation surgery he allowed an intern to perform most of the work. No myodesis or myoplasty was performed and Dave's stump began to shrink rapidly.

Dave went to the prosthetist that his doctor referred him to and they did an adequate job in providing his preparatory limb. Dave did well at first, ambulating in his walker or in the parallel bars but his 15-degree flexion contracture did not contribute to his stability or comfort. As his stump shrank, he became more and more uncomfortable in his socket due to the fact that his bones were now becoming exposed beneath the skin and since his stump was so short he had very little leverage with which to move the leg. His first permanent prosthesis was very lightweight with a cuff strap suspension and a Seattle foot, an energy-storing foot designed to give spring off of the toe. At first this leg worked well and he seemed to make some progress but he experienced continual pain as the more integral fit caused more shrinkage.

Dave was no stranger to pain. He was raised in central Texas, in a small town northeast of Dallas. His father was an honest to God Texas Ranger. He and his brothers grew up on a cattle ranch and learned how to ride and rope as a matter of daily life. Dave was never a big man (1.7 meters [5 ft 7 in]) and when he was young only 150 pounds. However, when he joined the Army in 1942, he enlisted as a combat engineer. The invasion of Normandy found Dave on a landing craft at Omaha beach with 120 of his comrades. The shelling was intense and when the door of the landing craft opened, he experienced the greatest horror of his life; a German machine gun nest was directly in front of their landing craft shooting straight into their midst. Dave was in the very back of the landing craft and all around him blood was flying and people were dying. The big sergeant next to him grabbed him by the backpack and threw him over the side of the craft. Weighed down by his gear, Dave found himself over his head in the water, unable to get his head above the surface. Bullets were streaking through the bloodstained water and although he felt the bile taste of panic start to rise in his mouth, he kept his cool. He unfastened his pack and dropped it as he kicked himself up to the surface to gulp a breath of air. The carnage of the battle was overwhelming above the water and he knew that he was dead unless he could get to the beach. He began the tortuous slow motion crawl through the surf that was thick with the bodies of his fallen comrades. Upon reaching the beach, he ran for the nearest hole and jumped into it, not realizing that it was a 3.5-meter (12-ft) deep antitank ditch. As he landed, he realized that he had injured both knees in the fall but what the hell, he figured he was dead anyway. There was another live man from his company in the hole and he asked him where the rally point for the unit was. As far as the other man knew, he and Dave were all that was left of their entire 120-man company. After what seemed like days in the trench under constant fire from the pillbox and well-sighted artillery, they decided to do something. There were no officers to give them orders and although they heard the cries of the wounded, they didn't see any other Americans. For all they knew, they were alone. Dave said that he wasn't particularly brave, he just figured that he was dead anyway, and in the typical way of thinking of a Texan, he was going to take a few of those bastards with him when he went. On the back of one of the dead soldiers in the ditch was a satchel charge, basically a backpack full of explosives that can be detonated with a timer. He and the other soldier crawled from their hole and made their way through another shallow depression in the sand to the corner of the pillbox. They could see the barrel of the machine gun still spitting death to anyone who raised their heads. They set the timer for immediate explosion and tossed the satchel charge through the gun slit as they dove for cover. A large muffled whump threw them to the ground, temporarily rendering them deaf but the pillbox was no more than a tumble of concrete. It took a few minutes for the impact of the removal of the pillbox to take effect. Dave and his buddy just sat there in the sand in shock, as the beach seemed to come alive with soldiers. They came out of their holes like ghosts and began to advance up the beach.

Like I said, Dave was no wimp but the constant pain of the prosthesis caused him to give up and stick to his wheelchair only wearing the leg when he went out. In the 2 years since his amputation, his residual limb had atrophied to basically skin and bone with the sharp edges of the bones protruding underneath the skin, making it painful to weight bear on the prosthesis. He went back to his prosthetist on numerous occasions, trying to get some relief from the constant ache whenever he wore the limb. His prosthetist was nice but he was also just out of prosthetics school and was becoming visibly frustrated at his inability to solve Dave's problems. The prosthetist started to insinuate that Dave was not trying hard enough. Both Dave and his wife began to notice that "not you again" look on the prosthetist's face when he came in for adjustments. At one point he suggested that possibly Dave was not a candidate for a prosthesis and would be better off in a wheelchair. Dave's wife, Bobby, was very sensitive to Dave's pain and suffering and felt that there should be some way to make a comfortable prosthesis so that her husband of 45 years could get out of the wheelchair. Bobby is a fiery redhead and became quite indignant with the attitude of the prosthetist. She started to make inquiries as to other prosthetists in the local area and who was good.

That is when Dave showed up in our facility. He was a little old man in a wheelchair, not much to look at except the twinkle in his eye. We listened to his explanation of how he had lost his leg and what had been done to try to give him a comfortable fit. The prosthesis that he was wearing utilized a cuff strap suspension and had a Seattle foot (the original energy-storing foot, very lightweight but not very flexible). He wore a 9 mm (0.3 in) thick gel liner next to his skin but went into a hard socket with no padding or insert. The leg was an endoskeletal design with a soft foam cover and the prosthetist had shortened the leg by over 1.25 cm (0.5 in) because the cuff strap suspension allowed the leg to piston so much. Dave used a walker to ambulate in our lab, but you could tell from the look on his face that he was in extreme discomfort with each step. When Bobby indignantly told us that the prosthetist had begun to insinuate that Dave was not trying hard enough and was being oversensitive to the pain, I perceived that the problem was probably in the prosthesis and not in Dave's attitude. We explained that we thought that we could do a better job (a claim all prosthetists make) but would need to take time to make a proper prosthesis and that they should take their time to make a decision.

Bobby called the next day and set up an appointment for a casting. We took a cast using an old-fashioned 3-part casting technique directly onto the skin. When we explained the test socket procedures to Dave, he was surprised at our technique, saying that the previous leg was casted over the 9 mm (0.3 in) liner and the test socket was also fitted over the liner. I explained to him that my philosophy of socket design was to fit the stump first and then add the cushion of the liner and/or insert and that this was particularly important in his case since his stump was so bony. Three days later we fitted his first test socket, which was a clear plastic socket made from Surlyn (basically thick plastic wrap from the kitchen). He stood on the hard plastic socket with most of his weight on the walker and as he tried to bear more weight on the test socket, I could see him wince in pain. As I looked at the changing color of his skin, I immediately saw the source of his discomfort. The fibula (the side bone) was cut slightly longer than the tibia (the shin bone) and whenever he bore weight on the prosthesis he was putting pressure on the cut end of the fibula. I had personally experienced fibula pressure, and it is a very difficult problem to diagnose because the pain has no precedence in your experience. You can't describe it but it is a sharp ache that radiates from the bottom of your stump and really plays havoc with your ability to function since it hurts for hours even after you take the leg off. In order to test my theory, I took the test socket and spot heated the place where his fibula had been hitting and I gently pushed out the plastic in that spot. I put it back on him after the plastic had cooled, and this time he could put almost full weight on the leg.

Solving the problem of the fibula only brought up other discomfort issues, which I marked on the test socket so I could make those corrections on the second test socket. I felt that we had discovered what had been causing him the pain: that he just could not tolerate pressure on the end of the fibula. I arranged to have him return in 2 days for a second test socket fitting. One of the lessons I learned as a prosthetist is that people generally only feel the pain that is the most intense. This was illustrated to me personally after my accident when I was lying in the hospital on the fifth day. The doctor came in and said that he was going to take my stitches out. I looked at him through my morphine haze and was puzzled because he had previously told me that it would be 2 weeks before he would take out the stitches in my stump. When I asked him about it, he replied that he was going to take the stitches out of my arm. I was totally unaware that I had 12 stitches near my right elbow where I had landed on my arm. As a prosthetist, I knew that often times solving one source of pain might indeed bring up others of which the patient was unaware. Dave had lost his faith in the prosthetic process, and I knew that he was going to have a tough road ahead of him to be able to get out of that wheelchair. In addition to the fitting problems, he now had a nasty flexion contracture on his right amputated leg. His previous prosthetist was not a bad practitioner or a mean person; he just did not have a lot of experience. In his frustration at Dave's case not following what he had learned in school, he became defensive. This has happened to every practitioner out there; the good ones recognize it and strive to listen and learn from their experiences instead of blaming others for failure.

The second test socket was more comfortable and Dave was actually able to weight bear evenly on both legs. He was still quite sensitive and dubious about the entire process, but I could tell that he was beginning to regain some faith. Convincing Dave that he could wear a prosthesis after he had been told that he couldn't was not going to be easy, but I believed that he had what it takes to make it happen. The third test socket was actually comfortable and I could see from the look of surprise on his face that it really didn't hurt. We placed a suspension sleeve onto the plastic test socket and actually had Dave walk a little on it. After several trips up and down the parallel bars, he was getting sore and tired but the look of hope on his face said it all. From now on we just had to keep the positive experience going and this guy was going to ditch his wheelchair. We made a fourth test socket to fit with his locking liner since it was my experience that the liner would compress soft tissue and changed the fit enough that it was best to make sure that the fit was intact.

Dave's new leg was a significant change in design from his last leg. Due to his short residual limb, I brought the leg up over his knee on the sides that would give him a lot more stability. This was not a complete supercondylar design because there was no suspension from the high sidewalls; however, it increased his surface area of contact with the prosthesis. The locking liner was the primary suspension, but I also utilized an auxiliary suspension sleeve to minimize the distal or downward pull on the skin of his stump. I discovered that the underlying layer of fascia, the tissue that separates skin from bone, gets used to being stretched in one direction and it can cause an intense burning sensation when it is stretched in the opposite direction. The skin of Dave's stump had been stretched upward toward the knee for 2 years but the new locking liner suspension would stretch the skin downward, pulling it toward the floor. This opposite stretch can create unbearable pain and cause a person to reject the prosthesis, even though it will subside in a few weeks if the patient can tolerate it. The auxiliary suspension sleeve minimizes the downward pull by taking some of the downward forces away, allowing the wearer to ease into the system.

The fourth test socket was good. I only had to tighten up the posterior or back part of the socket to compensate for the compression of the liner. Dave was able to walk up and down the parallel bars on the test socket without any discomfort. I knew that if he was comfortable in the test socket with no insert, he would be comfortable in the final socket. We rescheduled him for his fitting in a week and set about making his leg. He arrived on the day of the fitting, full of the optimism that I knew was the key to experiencing success. The fitting went smoothly with almost no discomfort. He was ambulating around the office with his walker by the end of the session. He even wanted to wear it home, which I discouraged since his drive home was about 45 minutes and a new leg that is bent in a car seat could get uncomfortable and there is no way to take it off if it hurts. He agreed to take it easy and wear the leg for no more than 2 hours at a time before taking it off and checking for red marks. He was excited about the new leg and sometimes this is a very dangerous time for an amputee because he or she will overdue it, especially when there is someone to show the leg off to, like friends and family. We scheduled him to come in for adjustments in a week to check on his fit and alignment. The leg was not finished but wrapped in a fiberglass reinforcing material that held everything together well enough for him to test it out but allowed us to remove the wrap if we had to change the alignment more than the adjustments permitted.

One of the biggest mistakes that I had seen made in our profession is the premature finishing of prostheses. Prosthetists seem to be in a hurry to put the final lamination or cover onto a prosthesis. The problem is that whenever an amputee is given new or different components or socket design, he or she needs some time to adjust to the new system. If the prosthetist has finished the leg in his or her own mind, he or she is very reluctant to tear off the cover or strip off the lamination to realign the leg to the adjusted gait pattern. I saw quite a few of these types of mistakes in my private practice and our solution was to put off final finishing of the prosthesis until the client said that it was perfect. Sometimes the process took weeks or even months, but the end result was a prosthesis that really did fit and was aligned as optimally as possible. Another trap that this process avoided was after a month of wear, the amputee would reject the new system and want to go back to his or her old type of suspension. Since we had not finished the leg, there was no real barrier to making a new socket and, therefore, keeping our clients happy. There is no worse feeling for an amputee than to feel that he or she is with a prosthesis that does not work for him or her and it is very unlikely that he or she will return to that prosthetist for future work.

When Dave returned for his check up a week later, he had been wearing the prosthesis for most of the time and entered the shop on his walker instead of the wheelchair. This in itself was a good sign. He had a couple of minor red marks on the stump that I was able to relieve to his satisfaction but nothing that would prevent him from wearing the leg. Since he was up on his walker more and stretching the leg out, his hamstrings had loosened up some and he had a little less flexion contracture. I told him to wear the leg now as much as he could and only take it off when it hurt. I also suggested that he get a little physical therapy to help him work out the flexion contracture in his knee, which would be a key factor in his ability to ambulate well. I aligned his foot so that when he stood with full weight on the leg, his heel was just slightly off of the ground and it was a slight strain to stand flatfooted. I told him that this was on purpose to help work out his flexion contracture but that a little bit of therapy at this point would speed up the process immeasurably. He agreed to see a physical therapist and we set up another follow-up appointment in a couple of weeks to make sure that no problems were preventing his progress. After we had finished with most of the work on his leg it was lunchtime and since I was sending out for sandwiches, I offered to buy them a sandwich and have them join us for lunch. He and Bobby agreed and that is when Dave started to tell us his stories. At 65 years of age, Dave did not look like a particularly impressive man, but that did not tell the true story of his life.

We saw Dave every other week over the next 3 months and I started to budget an extra half hour to listen to Dave's stories. Like most people, he had a fascinating life that was dying to be told if only someone would listen. His previous prosthetist missed out on some great entertainment because he never took the time to get to know Dave. He only saw a stump that didn't behave like the book had told him it would. We finished his prosthesis after 3 months of wearing it and adjusting it to accommodate his diminishing flexion contracture and in that time we heard some really great stories.

Dave told us many other stories that kept us entertained with his slice of history that he had experienced and I learned a valuable life lesson. Everyone has a story to tell and a life they have lived if we can only take the time to listen. I started to make a real effort to learn and listen to my clients, which had the effect of making me closer to my clients and personalizing our experience. I found that people responded positively to being listened to and would tend to share their prosthetic problems in a more understandable fashion, allowing me to solve their problems more effectively.

Margaret

Margaret was a 65-year-old single woman who lived in Florida with her 3 cats and a parrot. She lived in a retirement community where she enjoyed a number of good friends with whom she played canasta and bridge on a weekly basis. She had lost her right leg to diabetes at 60 years old and had adapted to wearing a prosthesis with the same gusto she had lived her life. None of her girlfriends would have ever guessed that Maggie had traveled the world in her youth.

Margaret was born in Italy in 1919 to a family of circus performers and due to her incredible flexibility she was a contortionist. She performed with her family until she was 18 years old and then went off on her own, touring Asia and dazzling Chinese warlords and Indian princes. One such prince was so taken with her performance that he convinced her to stay in his palace in the north of India where she had a romantic liaison with him for several years. As the prince fell from favor, she perceived that it was time to move on and began to travel around India. After several months of traveling, she came upon the entourage of Mahatma Gandhi and was taken by the gentle strength of the leader of the Indian independence movement. She traveled with him for weeks. She eventually left India. Margaret went to the United States because WWII was beginning in Europe and she felt she could stay out of the conflict in the United States. Margaret had a gift for languages and spoke Italian, German, French, Hindi, and English with only a trace of an accent.

She married a businessman from Atlanta and settled down to live a more normal life, keeping her wild youth a secret from her husband and her 2 children. After her husband died, she moved to Florida to be near her daughter and settled into the little retirement community where she made some good friends and was quite happy. She took the loss of her right leg in stride and was still able to take walks with a cane and tinker in her garden growing tomatoes and peppers. She had been very fortunate to be sent to a local prosthetist named Tony who was strikingly handsome and was only one generation removed from his Italian heritage. She found that she could confide in him the story of her life. She told Tony things about herself that she had not even told her husband and certainly not the bridge ladies who would be appalled at the exploits of her youth.

Margaret's diabetes, even though closely controlled and monitored, caused her to begin to have real difficulty seeing. She wasn't blind but even with her reading glasses she began to have difficulty reading anything. When her doctor changed her diabetic medication she was too proud to let on that she could not read the directions and started to take too small of a dosage. The result was that her left leg began to get very bad; sores started appearing on her toes, and she could not cut her toenails properly since her eyesight was so poor. The resulting abrasions would not heal and when she returned to the doctor, he was alarmed at the deterioration in her remaining leg. Even though she embarked on a crash course to try and regain the lost circulation in the leg, it had to come off 2 months later. Tony was with her in the hospital just before she went in for surgery and explained to her that he was going to apply a postoperative cast on her stump and that she would be back up and walking in couple of months. Margaret trusted Tony and even though her daughter and son were with her, she took the most comfort in the knowledge that Tony would be taking care of her.

Margaret progressed nicely under the care of Tony and with the help of the physical therapy staff at the rehabilitation hospital. She had a preparatory prosthesis that allowed her to begin the task of using a walker. At first she had a very difficult time just getting up because the time in the hospital had weakened her but day by day she regained her strength. She was discharged home after 3 weeks with the aid of a home health nurse. Tony came to her house from time to time to make adjustments to her prosthesis but mostly just to talk awhile and listen to her stories. Six months after the second amputation, Tony told her she was ready for a permanent prosthesis on the left side and that he would need to also replace the right prosthesis as well. He explained that the alignment and components for a bilateral were different than that of a unilateral amputee and it would be best if he made two new prostheses for her that were designed with her situation in mind.

Tony had his own method of casting and test socket procedure that had worked well in his practice in coastal Florida where the vast majority of his clients were geriatric. His laboratory was able to make a prosthesis from start to finish in less that 5 days. Margaret came into his office and he explained what the procedure would be for getting her new legs. He would be casting one leg at a time so that she could have her prosthesis on for stability. Since he was going to use locking liners for her prostheses, he already had those prepared and fitted them first, making sure that there were no gapping or loose places on the liners. Next, he had Margaret take them off to make sure that she would have no problems with donning and doffing.

She was accustomed to the locking liners from her other prosthesis and had no difficulty inverting the liner and rolling it onto her residual limb. She remembered when she first tried to roll one of those things onto her stump she felt as if she were handling a slimy fish or something; it just took a bit of getting used to. Next, Tony took a piece of plastic wrap, placed it all around the liner that was covering her stump, and then pulled a tube sock over the plastic wrap that was about twice as long as her stump. He then placed a roll of fiberglass wrap material in some cold water and then wrapped it all around her leg, making sure that there were no gaps or holes in the wrap. After completing the wrap, he molded the fiberglass as it set to delineate the bony areas and contours of her residual limb. The fiberglass set in 5 minutes and he gently slipped the cast off of her stump. He took out a pair of bandage scissors and began to trim the fiberglass socket to use as a test socket, cutting down the back to allow her knee to bend. After he completed the trimming, he slipped the socket back onto her limb and checked the fit by sticking his fingers into the edges and looking up into the hole that was left at the bottom where the tube sock poked through. He made some marks on the fiberglass cast and then repeated the process on the other leg. He set up an appointment for her to return in 2 days for the fitting and told her that her new legs would be totally finished in a week if the fitting went well.

When Margaret returned in 2 days, the new legs were waiting for her in the fitting room, a long narrow room with parallel bars and 2 mirrors at each end of the bars. Tony first had her don the locking liners that were thicker in the front and thinner in the back, which he told her was necessary to allow her to bend her knee easier. The legs had pipes coming out of the sockets with lightweight energy storing feet on the bottom that had nice toes, something that Margaret thought was important. The pipes had adjustments at the top and bottom to allow Tony to change the alignment to suit her gait pattern as well as adjust the height. He showed her how the locking mechanism worked and she felt very comfortable with operating the lock since it was like her old one. She put the legs on and was very surprised at how light they felt. Tony explained that they would only weigh about 2 pounds when finished and that they would feel lighter since they fit her well.

Next, he checked the height and made an adjustment so that her pelvis was level. She then started walking in the parallel bars, holding on tight to make sure she didn't fall. Each time she returned from a trip down the bars, Tony would make a little adjustment to the legs and each time it would be easier to walk. After a half an hour of this, she was walking in the bars with only a slight touch on the rails. On the last pass, she walked without touching the bars at all. Tony pronounced that he was happy with the alignment and told her to return in 2 more days to pick up the finished limbs. Before she left, he took her outside and they used some plastic color swatches to determine the skin color that the legs would have.

Margaret returned 2 days later and was ushered back into the fitting room where in the corner stood her new legs. They were beautiful, long and slender with none of the varicose veins that had streaked her real legs. She put her new shoes onto the legs with the help of the metal shoehorn that Tony had given her and stood up on them for the first time. She felt as if she could take off and run, but Tony told her just to walk slowly in the parallel bars for a bit to get used to the new legs. They were so light she couldn't believe it, and her gait showed only the barest trace of a limp. Best of all was that in her knee length skirt you could not tell that she had both of her legs missing. After Tony made sure that she had all of her supplies and set up a follow-up appointment, she threw her arms around him and planted a big kiss on his cheek, whispering to him, "If only I were 40 years younger!" and winked at him. As she went out the door, Tony's tanned face had turned a deep red but he was grinning from ear to ear.

How Prostheses are Made

The Socket

The most important part of any prosthesis is the fit of the socket. Let me repeat that in another way, "It's the fit that counts." I don't care if your leg can play the star spangled banner and cost $50,000; if the socket doesn't fit, than the leg will not be functional. When the fit is not good, the amputee will be in pain and living with chronic pain makes people fussy at best or downright impossible at worst. What is the key to getting a good fit in your prosthesis? It comes down to the skill of the person making the limb and their diligence to teach you how to maintain the fit as your body changes. The first part, getting a good fit, is the easiest since it is a matter of persistence and utilization of the tools with which the prosthetist is most comfortable. The second part, maintaining a good fit, is more difficult because it requires an intimate knowledge of the likely changes that will occur in a residual limb and the ability to explain to the amputee how to make adjustments.

There are many ways to make a good fitting socket and I will attempt to describe as many as I am familiar with. Most prosthetists find the socket fabrication method that they work best with and refine that technique over time to achieve the optimal result. There are 2 basic ways to get the raw model of the residual limb. One is to make a cast of what is left, and the other is to digitalize the surface of the residual limb using a computer aided design (CAD) system. The casting technique is still the most common and will probably be the way that most legs are made; however, the CAD systems are gaining in popularity as well as coming down in price, so they may be the wave of the future. CAD systems utilize an infrared light source to map out the surface of the residual limb and digitalize the data, inputting it into a computer. This produces a 3-dimensional replica of the remaining leg on the computer screen. The prosthetist then uses a light pencil or mouse to modify the replica, which is then sent to an automated milling machine that carves the shape out of wax. A test socket is then generally made from this model and fitted to the client where it is marked and modified until a suitable fit is achieved.

The old fashioned casting technique is the method with which I am most familiar and is still the standard way of getting a positive model of the residual limb (Figure 3-1). Casting involves using either plaster bandages or fiberglass wrap to encase the residual limb and then removing the wrap to obtain the impression of the stump. There is a great variety in the way that prosthetists take casts, from a simple circumferential wrap to a 3-part cast focusing on the contours of the bones. Some prosthetists

Figure 3-1. Modifying a plaster cast. (Photo by Steven Spinetto, 2002.)

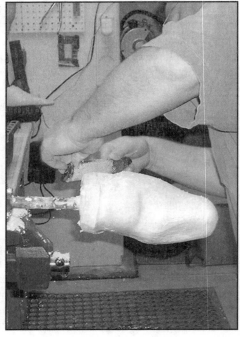

cast the patient while he or she is wearing the gel or silicone liner and others cast directly over the skin. When the amputation is new and the tissue is so swollen that no bones are visible or can be felt through the edema, then a circumferential plaster or fiberglass wrap is sufficient.

I have a gift for communication and was generally able to draw out information from my clients as to where they could tolerate pressure or where they were sensitive. However, I learned the hard way that feedback from amputees could be misleading if not verified by physical examination. Many years ago, when I was a thin cross-country ski racer, I began to get a very sharp and severe pain in the front of my stump. It occurred on top of the flare of the tibia (shinbone) just below my kneecap. I would examine the area for a pimple or abrasion but could not discover any cause for the pain. This pain went on for months; it would come and go with no warning or sign of abrasion. I adjusted the socket by relieving the area but this had no effect on the instance of the pain. I was very baffled since I was a prosthetist and should have been be able to figure it out. One day I was picking at my stump (something you are not supposed to do) and had it twisted around so that I could examine the back of it behind my knee. I have a large scar where I had two neuromas removed and have almost no skin sensation near the scar. As I twisted my knee to examine closer, I discovered a small but inflamed pimple near the scar. When I touched it, I received a very sharp pain in the front of my stump where the chronic problem had been. I couldn't believe it. I kept pushing on the pimple and my stump would hurt about 7.5 cm (3 in) away on the front of my stump. I could only surmise that my body searched for the nearest intact nerve to transmit the pain and my brain interpreted the pain to come from a totally different source. Right then I learned that the residual limb can give inaccurate information if the prosthetist isn't careful to verify the source and type of pain sensation.

Test Sockets

After I have modified the cast to my liking, I smooth it out with sand screen and water and then prepare it for fabrication of the test socket. There are many materials with which to make a test socket; we preferred to use Surlyn , which is thick plastic wrap, because it comes out very clear and has enough flexibility to allow for difficult donning. We also used a more rigid plastic on occasion that was like glass and was also very clear. It was difficult to remove from the cast without damaging the surface. The prepared cast is taken to the lab where a vacuum pump is attached to the pipe that is in the cast. The plastic, which comes in sheets of varying thickness, is cut to size and placed in an oven where it is heated until it becomes very soft and pliable. At just the right moment, the plastic is draped over the cast and sealed. The vacuum is then turned on and the plastic is sucked down to the surface of the cast. When this cools, the plastic is trimmed and the cast is either broken out of the socket or if the shape is very tapered, it can be knocked off with a hammer. The edges are smoothed and the test socket is attached to some type of adjustable alignment device that allows the prosthetist to change the alignment of the test socket to fit the person.

Test sockets, regardless of how they are created or used by the prosthetist, are one of the most important advances in the fit of the socket and thus the comfort of the amputee. It is a significant improvement over the old method of fitting the prosthesis and seeing where you get blood to make an adjustment. The other problem of the old method of socket fit was that every time the prosthetist makes an adjustment to the prosthesis in one area of the socket it can and often does create a problem somewhere else. The socket is a dynamic mechanism and to carve a hole in the front can cause movement and problems in the back. The test socket procedure allows the prosthetist to experiment with pressures and reliefs to achieve an optimal fit without damaging the overall fit of the socket design (Figure 3-2).

Test sockets will go a long way to ensure that the final socket fit is intimate and comfortable. If you are experiencing a high degree of discomfort in the test socket, there is a good chance that the actual finished prosthesis will not be a good fit. Make sure that you are comfortable with the test socket before you let the prosthetist make the definitive socket. If you have tried several test sockets and they are not comfortable, it may be wise to just start the process all over again by taking a new cast. In my private practice, we had to do this from time to time if the socket just got off of where we were trying to go with it. It is much better to get the bugs out of the fit at the test socket juncture than to wait until the leg is made then decide that it is not a good fit. Prosthetists are just people and they do not like to make things over again once it is finished, so use the prefabrication process to make changes. Some prosthetists allow their clients to leave the lab and walk around with the test socket to make sure that it fits over time. It is necessary to reinforce the socket with fiberglass wrap or some other material in order to use a test socket for ambulation. If your prosthetist sends you home with a test socket, take it easy and have an ambulatory aid handy in case something breaks.

The Below-Knee Socket

Once the prosthetist has achieved a good fit in the test socket, it is time to fabricate the actual socket that the leg will use. There are 2 basic types of sockets that are in

Figure 3-2. Test sockets with fitting markings. (Photo by Dale Horkey, 2004.)

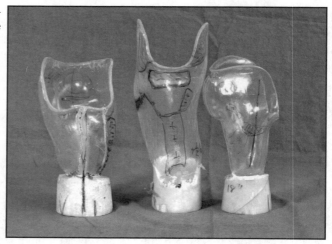

primary use today, the laminated socket and the thermoplastic socket. The laminated socket is made from cloth fibers of different types that are impregnated under vacuum with a resin that is catalyzed and promoted to harden over time. The thermoplastic socket is fabricated in much the same manner as the test socket by heating a piece of plastic in an oven and vacuuming it onto the cast.

Regardless of how the socket is made, the next step is to pour the test socket full of plaster with a pipe in it so that there is a positive model of the definitive cast with which to work. The test socket is removed, and the plaster model is adjusted according to any new information from the last test socket and smoothed up. Laminated and thermoplastic sockets require an extensive preparation of the cast before actually pouring the liquid plastic into the prepared mold.

Soft Inserts

Many below-knee prostheses utilize a soft insert that is an independent part of the prosthesis and is custom fabricated to fit inside the socket. In order to make an insert, it has to be fabricated onto the cast before the socket can be either laminated or thermoformed. Most inserts are made from pelite, a soft foam material that is easy to work with and can be molded when heated by a heat gun or in an oven. The material comes in a variety of colors but is usually white or beige and has a soft feel to it that provides extra cushion for the residual limb in the relatively hard socket.

There are many other types of inserts that are part of the prosthesis. Other materials that can be used for inserts are Kemblo (Griswald Rubber, City of Industry, CA), silicone sheets, and an injection-molded type, usually made from silicone. All custom inserts have lost popularity due to the advances in gel and silicone technology, which have produced a variety of roll on liners independent of the prosthesis.

Soft Inserts

1. A soft insert is a cushion device that is fabricated into the prosthesis and provides a layer of padding to the skin and bone of the residual limb. It reduces torque (twisting motion) to the skin and absorbs impact to the bones.
2. Custom fabricated inserts can be made from foams such as pelite, PPT foam (Langer Biomedical, New York, NY), and Kemblo. Utilizing other fabrication techniques, the inserts can be made from silicone gel, sewn sheets, or injection molding, which creates a custom insert in the shape of the socket.
3. Amputees that have bony stumps or lots of scar tissue or even sensitive nerves may find that an insert can give added comfort to the daily use of a prosthesis.
4. Inserts when used in conjunction with pin suspension systems can be useful as a means of assisting in guiding the pin to the lock mechanism.
5. Inserts in most cases allow a greater ease in adjusting the prosthetic fit since they make it easier to pad or remove material in the socket.
6. New amputees find that inserts allow them to attain a good fit prior to donning the leg since they have to put the insert on first. It is easier to tell if the right numbers of socks are being used.
7. Inserts are less often used today due to the advances in gel and silicone technology, which provide roll on liners with varying degrees of thickness.

Double Wall Sockets

Another very popular socket design is the double wall socket. This involves fabricating an inner socket of a softer material than the outer rigid socket that allows for more cushioned edges as well as the ability to relieve the outer rigid socket without changing the shape of the inner socket. The double wall design needs to be made from 2 different materials to truly achieve the intended effect of creating a contained but adjustable socket. These are very common in our industry due to the fact that there is a reimbursable code for them and if done properly, they can allow for long-term changes to the fit of the socket without altering the original container.

One of the major advantages of the double wall socket is that the prosthetist can make reliefs to the outer socket without changing the inner shape. The inner socket maintains its original volume and since it is flexible, it will have some give in it to allow for slight movement when the rigid outer socket is adjusted. This has a particular advantage when the amputee has a very bony stump and has a protruding tibia or fibula that needs relief. The prosthetist can actually grind a hole in the outer rigid framework, allowing the more flexible inner socket to protrude through the hole but maintain the initial socket fit. Another big advantage is that the edges of the socket are more flexible due to the lower trim line of the rigid framework and can reduce wear and tear to liners and sleeves.

A true double wall socket that uses 2 different materials can also alter over time due to the pressures on the inner more flexible material. If the inner material is too soft, then it will slowly creep through the reliefs in the framework and create pressure ridges at the edges of the reliefs. It is difficult to cut a hole in the framework that does not create pressure ridges over time. The edges of the relief need to be tapered and smooth to minimize this effect. Otherwise the edges of the holes in the framework

Figure 3-3. The parts of a below-knee limb socket, insert, and locking liner. (Photo by Dale Horkey, 2004.)

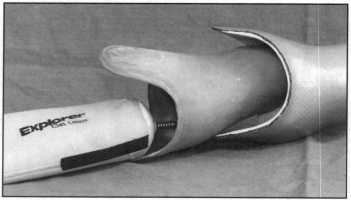

become pressure problems where the softer inner socket bulges through. Another big advantage of the flexible inner socket is the back wall of the prosthesis. This can be cut lower in the framework, allowing for greater knee range of motion without compromising the important containment function of the back wall.

Assembly of the Parts

Now that the parts are fabricated, it is time to put them all together (Figure 3-3). The laminated or thermoformed socket is completed and trimmed out with all of the edges smoothed and if there is a custom insert, it is cut off of the cast. Generally, if there is a soft inner liner, there won't be a double wall socket. The edges of the socket must be smooth and free of burrs or rough spots since most wear and tear on suspension sleeves or locking liners occurs at the edge of the socket. Some materials smooth easier than others. Thermoplastics can generally be buffed to a clean edge while laminates with carbon fiber almost never get totally smooth. If there is an insert, it will typically be trimmed a bit longer than the socket so that the insert pokes up above the edge, creating a softer buffer for the locking liner or the residual limb.

Many prostheses that are built today utilize locking liners. This is a roll on, prefabricated liner made from silicone or gel that has a serrated locking pin fabricated into the end of it. When the amputee rolls it on, the pin should be at the very bottom of the stump, looking a little like a unicorn with a funny horn. As the amputee inserts the residual limb into the socket, the pin at the end of the liner engages into a locking mechanism that is fabricated into the bottom of the socket. The locking mechanism is known as a shuttle lock and has become a very popular method of suspension in the last 10 years. I will discuss the various means of suspension in a later chapter. The actual locking mechanism is manufactured by over a dozen companies and comes in many different varieties, utilizing varying materials and engineering. Some shuttle locks are fabricated into the socket during either the lamination or vacuum forming process, while others are inserted after the socket is made.

Once the locking mechanism is in place, the next step is to attach the pylon or shank to which the foot will be attached. This process varies considerably from facility to facility, depending upon the type of foot to be used and the type of fabrication process. Many thermoformed sockets will actually place a coupler at the bottom of the cast and vacuum form the coupler directly into the socket. Some couplers are built right into the shuttle lock mechanism. This works if the amputee's alignment happens to be directly below the end of the residual limb, a circumstance that is very rare in my experience. Others will form the end of the socket with a rigid foam and after that has hardened, they will sand it flat and glue the coupler onto the bottom of the socket. If the prosthetist is confident in the alignment position, the coupler is laminated to the socket or it can be temporarily attached using a fiberglass wrap material. If the attachment coupler is permanently attached to the socket, then there is no room for changes to the alignment except for the changes that can be made in the pylon system.

Socket Design

There are many different socket designs that utilize unique strategies for creating a comfortable and stable container for what's left of someone's leg. After WWII, the most common type of socket was what is known as the plug fit; the name says it all. It was a container made from wood with an open end so that the amputee stuck his or her stump down into a tapered wooden socket that was typically lined with leather. A large thigh corset was held in place by means of metal joints that were screwed into the sides of the socket and extended up onto the thigh of the amputee. A large leather corset was attached to the joints and laced up the front, allowing most of the weight to be born on the thigh and not on the residual limb. This system had some serious drawbacks but was the best that could be done considering the state of the art in materials at the time. Because there was no contact with the end of the stump, the blood and fluid would tend to pool at the tip and often times a condition known as varicose hyperplasia would occur. This is a painful condition in which the continued pooling of fluid causes the skin to react by callusing and hardening to the point where it actually cracks and bleeds as well as creating a warty discolored area where there is no skin contact with the socket.

Like most professions, prosthetics has devised its own language to describe the types of socket designs that are being used. Some of the names of the designs are patellar tendon bearing, patellar tendon bearing supercondylar superpatellar, total surface bearing, and the original plug fit with thigh lacer. All of these designs have applications today, and most prosthetists utilize a combination of them to achieve the best fit for the individual amputee. Remember, the fit of the prosthesis is the most important part of any limb and since no 2 residual limbs are the same, there is no perfect socket design—only a perfect fit.

Socket Designs

1.   Patellar tendon bearing (PTB) is a socket design that uses the joint space below the kneecap to bear the majority of the load of the prosthesis. Crucial to the success of this design is the posterior or back wall of the prosthesis that must be high enough to provide counterpressure to the patella tendon bar.

2.   Patellar tendon bearing supercondylar superpatellar (PTBSCSP) is a design that comes above the knee, providing enhanced stability as well as suspension. It utilizes the same basic socket design as the PTB but is distinct in that it encases the knee completely in the socket. In addition to the side-to-side stability, it can provide a stop to hyperextension at the knee by preventing the knee from bending backward.

3.   Total surface bearing (TSB) is the most recent design for the below-knee socket. As its name implies, it attempts to distribute the pressure over as much of the surface of the residual limb as possible.

4.   Plug fit with thigh lacer and knee joints is a socket design that was popular for many centuries prior to the widespread use of plastics and foams. It is an open-ended socket, often times made of wood with a leather lining. Metal hinges are attached to the socket and extend upward to the thigh where a leather corset is laced around the upper leg. This design seeks to unweight the stump and take the majority of the load on the thigh. The knee hinges provide lateral as well as hyperextension stability to the knee and are particularly useful for short stumps or heavy-duty activities.

There are 2 tendons that run behind the knee and they are the major flexors of the knee joint. Bend your knee and feel behind the joint and they are easy to find. If these tendons are restricted, then the ability of the amputee to bend the knee will be inhibited. I always created channels for the tendons to run in and this allowed for maximum knee flexion without having to compromise the counterpressure to the patellar indent. It never ceases to amaze me how different human anatomy is from individual to individual, and this is evidenced by the position of the tendons. Some amputees have tendons that are on the outside of the knee, but once in a while there would be a stump that had the large inside tendon almost in the middle of the knee. This made socket design very challenging and sometimes compromises have to be made in order to attain the optimum for the amputee.

I embrace the concept of the TSB socket but it has one serious drawback: the residual limb rarely cooperates with the design of the socket. What I mean is that the stump is a living, changing thing and the socket is a dead lifeless thing. As prosthetists, we design sockets for the shape of the residual limb that we have in front of us but as all prosthetists have seen, these stumps change over time. A total surface contact socket that is perfect when the amputee walks out of the door may not fit well at all 3 months later and if the socket design is such that there is little ability to adjust it, then the amputee can be stuck with an ill-fitting limb.

Socket Suspension

Suspension of the prosthesis is one of the most critical aspects of the design of the socket. It effects how the socket is designed, directly as in the case of the PTRSCSP as well as indirectly by the trim line of the top of the socket. I have worn most of the suspension systems that are used in prostheses over my 28 years as an amputee and know that if the leg doesn't stay on, even the best socket design is worthless.

Story Time

It was the summer of 1979 and I was on one of my 2-month bicycle tours that I was able to take since I was an elementary school teacher. I had just decided to get out of teaching and apprentice in prosthetics but took the summer off to bicycle around Oregon and Washington with a college buddy. We had stopped in Eugene, Oregon to visit some friends of his and they had taken us to a rodeo and square dance outside of town. I wore a prosthesis that was the PTRSCSP type, clamping above my knee to hold it on. We were taking a break from watching the bull-riding and were sampling lots of the local beer in the gymnasium where a square dance was going on. While standing in line for another beer, I met a very attractive woman and I asked her to dance. I had not square danced since high school but it didn't matter, since this was Oregon in the '70s and the style of dancing was less than formal.

The woman was full-bodied and strong for her size. As we swung each other around, I ceased to exercise much caution. As a matter of fact, I was just a little drunk and on one of the swings, I picked her off of her feet and swung her around. She laughed and thought that was good fun, so on the next swing she picked me up and swung me around. As I was flying through the air, I felt my leg slip off under my long white painter pants and as she released me, I flew across the floor and knocked over an entire table, 3 people, and a pitcher of beer. The leg, with a life of its own, skittered across the gym floor to come to rest in front of the band. The band stopped. The dancing stopped. Everyone just stood there frozen as they stared at this leg lying in the middle of the dance floor. I picked myself off of the floor and looked at the woman standing in front of me with her mouth wide open and said, "Darlin, you danced my leg right off," which caused everyone to laugh. Fortunately, the people whom I knocked over forgave me as I offered to buy them a new pitcher of beer and as I sat at their table, a young man walked over to me holding my leg. "Is this yours?" he asked with a look of sheer terror on his face. I looked around as if I wondered whether he was talking to me and replied, "By God, I think it is." This made him smile and put everyone at ease. Now this story nearly had the ultimate happy ending. A few minutes later the good looking woman was sitting on my lap and I thought she was going to invite me home. Just then a rather large and burley logger walked up and asked his wife what she was doing sitting on my lap. This was a minor detail that she had neglected to tell me before we started dancing. The logger gave me a break and didn't kill me for having his wife on my knee and my friend and I skipped out of there as quick as we could.

Another Suspension Story

Bobby T. is a rough and ready biker who just could never stay out of trouble. He is the only other human I know who knows where Cucumber, West Virginia is located and actually lived in the same town where my father was born.

Bobby was on his Harley, long before they became the toys of lawyers and doctors, and was on his way to a billiard tournament where he hoped to win some beer money. A cuff strap held on his prosthesis, a leather strap that wraps above the knee and provides adequate suspension. As he motored across the Nevada desert along an empty country road, he subconsciously sang an old rock tune in his head, the thump-thump of the motor keeping time. He started to tap his feet to the rhythm in his head and before he realized it he had hooked his prosthetic toe beneath the shift bar. As he tried to unhook the toe, he jerked upward on the leg. To his horror, the cuff strap slipped off and his leg tumbled onto the pavement. He immediately slowed the bike and turned around where he saw the leg lying in the middle of the road. In a panic that another car would come along and run over the only leg he had in the world, he decided to try and kick it off to the side of the road before any traffic came along. The old Harley was so heavy he knew that once he stopped he was going to have to lay down the bike so he wanted the leg in a safe place.

After 3 passes on the bike trying to kick at the leg with his good foot, he decided to go really slow in order to be sure to get it this time. As he slowed to a crawl, he actually kicked at the leg but all it did was spin instead of move and since he was focused on the leg instead of the bike, the monster Harley tumbled over on him in the middle of the road. He hopped to his good foot and although a little bruised he was OK. He hopped over and picked up his leg. Just at that moment, he heard a car coming and hopped over to his overturned bike with his leg in his arms as a car crested the small hill in front of him. The car came to a halt about 30 meters (100 ft) from him and an Asian man got out of the drivers side and stood there in disbelief. Here was Bobby standing in the middle of the road with his leg in his arms, waving at the man to stop. The man let out a shriek, got back into the car, and drove back the way he had come. Bobby managed to get his leg back on and his bike back up and made it to the pool competition where he won his beer money and entertained the crowd with his story of the Asian man and the leg. I made legs for Bobby for many years and this was his favorite story.

Types of Suspension

There are five 5 types of suspension for the below-knee amputee. They are belts, straps, wedges, locking, and suction. A sixth type is not very common and requires a particular type of residual limb that, in my experience, is rare and that is muscular contraction. These suspension types fall into 2 categories: mechanical, which uses belts, straps, wedges, and lock; or suction, which uses negative air pressure to hold the leg on. The mechanical methods provide adequate suspension but the leg hangs off of the body, whereas the suction suspension gives the most positive sensation that the leg is part of the body. All suspension methods have their pros and cons and if the amputee is aware of the limitations of each, he or she can make an intelligent decision as to which method will work the best for him or her. Another option is to combine suspension methods to insure that if one fails, then the leg will not fall off.

Belts

Belts have held prostheses on for many centuries and provide one of the most positive sensations of suspension that an amputee can experience. The belt goes around the waist just on or above the pelvic bones and an elastic strap extends down on the amputated side to attach to an inverted Y strap that is attached to the leg. The upside-down Y strap is usually attached to the elastic belt by Velcro or a buckle and the elastic allows the knee to bend with minimal restriction. Belts have one big drawback: the constriction around the waist is not comfortable and most amputees will try any other means of suspension to get away from the belt. I personally wore a belt for the first year of being an amputee, but preferred the wedge even though the leg fell off all of the time. Belts show through clothing and tear up pants and skirts as the buckles or loops wear on the inside of the fabric.

Still, I have a waist belt that I use for heavy-duty activities such as downhill skiing or pushing a wheelbarrow where I don't have the option of my leg coming off. My belt is removable and attaches to the leg by means of a Velcro strap that wraps around the bottom of the socket. If an amputee has to wear a belt, it should be padded and lined with leather so that it minimizes the discomfort of the edges of the belt digging into the skin of the waist. No matter how comfortable a belt can be made, it still has a pull on the pelvis and will cause the back of the wearer to get sore over time.

Belt suspension is the primary method of holding on prostheses for wooden legs that use the thigh lacer for unweighting of the residual limb. The belt runs over the leather corset and buckles on the front so that the amputee can tighten the belt if necessary or remove if he or she doesn't need to wear it. Thigh lacers can also provide limited suspension, especially after they have been worn for many years due to the atrophy of the thigh muscles. The metal knee hinges can be bent to follow the contours of the sides of the knee and the corset can come down to the top of the knee to provide suspension without the use of the belt. Most thigh lacer legs use a belt, especially under more strenuous circumstances.

Straps

One of the most common methods for suspending a prosthesis is the cuff strap. This is a leather or nylon strap that attaches to the socket in 2 places on the side of the knee joint and then circles above the knee and is fastened by either Velcro or a buckle. This style also provides adequate suspension but does allow for a degree of pistoning in the socket. There are many versions of the cuff strap that all have varying advantages for individual amputees, such as the figure 8 style or a wide strap around the knee.

There are problems with the cuff strap. The major one is the amount of pistoning that this means of suspension permits. The problem stems from the fact that a cuff strap is attached to the prosthesis at 2 points and the flexible leather or nylon allows the knee to bend as well as rotate around the pivot point. The knee unfortunately does not bend in a single axis of rotation; it bends in an arch of rotation, which cannot be duplicated by any single point of attachment. In order to get the cuff strap to suspend well when the amputee is standing as well as allow for the bending of the knee, there will be looseness somewhere. Usually this means that the strap is loose when standing or walking so the stump moves up and down inside the socket, causing friction to the skin or bony prominences. Another problem is when the strap binds behind the knee while sitting, causing friction or bunching of the skin that can result in cysts or pimples. Cuff straps are notorious for this condition, which often results in surgery to remove chronic impacted cysts.

Belts and straps have another negative effect on the anatomy of the residual limb. They constrict the growth and development of the muscles above the knee. The cuff strap actually keeps the quadriceps muscles from expanding because the strap is tight around the lower fibers of the muscles. The belt with the elastic strap actually helps to extend the knee that causes the body's natural musculature to atrophy for lack of use. I have always been of the philosophy that the amputee should use the remaining muscles to their full capacity and avoid methods that restrict their use.

Wedges

The wedge or supercondylar suspension uses a soft wedge of material that fits snugly over the top of the inside of the knee. Take a moment and feel the inside of your knee. You can easily find the spot where the wedge fits; it is a slight indentation just above the condyle or bulge of the knee. When the leg is straight or nearly so, the wedge holds the prosthesis on by clamping above the knee. Important to this design is the outside wall of the socket. It is critical that it provides a counterpressure to the inside wedge. This design is often combined with a superpatellar knee encasement that brings the socket up over the kneecap and as long as the leg is straight will suspend above the kneecap. This total covering of the knee is called the supercondylar superpatellar (SCSP) socket and was a design that I wore for over 5 years.

Constructing this particular type of prosthesis requires great skill by the prosthetist since the motion of the knee inside of the socket must be provided for in addition to holding on the prosthesis. The margin of error in the fabrication of this type of socket is very small and will permit adequate suspension yet still allow for sitting without the leg being held straight. A minimum of 1.25 cm (0.5 in) of difference between the measurement of the width of the knee and the width above the knee is necessary for this type of suspension to work. Even then it is an iffy thing and the greater the difference, the better chance of success. In my particular case, I had exactly 1.25 cm (0.5 in) difference between my condyle measurement and the space just above it that predisposed my leg to come off at the wrong time.

This design does eliminate the need for the strap or belt and personally that was a huge improvement over my previous means of suspension. Still the leg hangs off of you and has a tendency to fall off at the wrong time. It was always very uncomfortable for the first 2 to 3 weeks until the muscles on the inside of the knee shrank enough to permit the wedge to suspend adequately. Generally, most amputees who wear the PTS slip their leg off whenever seated as this socket is not that comfortable while sitting for an extended period of time. Movies, airplanes, and classrooms were always a problem for me but since the leg slipped off easily, I would normally take it off in those circumstances. The socket design also has the effect of restricting the use of muscles by compressing the muscle fibers of the medial or inside quadriceps. In addition, if the socket design incorporates the superpatellar portion, it will also cause the quadriceps as a whole to atrophy since they will not have to act as a hyperextension stop to the bending of the knee.

In my experience, the SCSP socket design works well for persons who are not going to be very active or who have short stumps. It definitely increases the surface area of the limb with which to distribute weight bearing and if there is instability at the knee, it can provide a much more secure structure to contain a loose knee joint. However, as a means of suspension of the prosthesis there have been some dramatic improvements in the way legs can be held on that have less constriction of the natural anatomy or restriction of the motion of the knee.

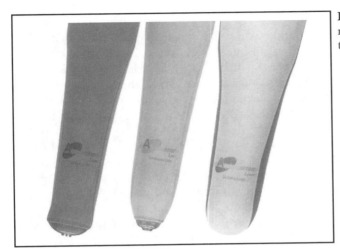

Figure 3-4. Locking liners and nonlocking liners. (Photo courtesy of Ohio Willow Wood.)

Locking Systems

The locking liner system (Figure 3-4) has been one of the most innovative suspension designs in recent times. I first became acquainted with this method in the early '80s when a manufacturer asked me to try it out. Surprisingly, it actually held my prosthesis on even though I have a severely tapered stump. The technique uses a liner made of silicone, urethane, or gel that has a pin attached to the end of the liner. When the liner is rolled onto the residual limb, it has the look of a unicorn with the pin sticking out of the end of the stump. Embedded into the bottom of the socket is a locking device that engages the pin and locks it into the socket. When the amputee lifts up the leg, the pin holds the prosthesis on by means of the suction or skin traction of the liner.

Locking liners have become very popular in the United States and provide a good level of suspension for many amputees. Each manufacturer has a line of prefabricated liners that come in varying sizes that are accompanied by a unique locking mechanism. The locking system suspends without belts, straps, or suspension sleeves and is quite adequate provided that the amputee is not engaged in heavy-duty activities. The suspension is based upon the tightness of the liner that holds the pin and can fluctuate depending upon the amount of tissue that is on the individual residual limb. Large fleshy stumps that are not very firm will experience more movement in the socket or pistoning than firmer residual limbs. This is due to the amount of movement of the skin on the stump since the liner is holding on by grabbing the skin. Like a suction suspension, there is no airflow beneath the liner, so in warm, damp climates this system tends to produce moisture and can slip when enough perspiration accumulates beneath the liner.

When I first used the locking liner suspension, there were no locking mechanisms, only a loop at the end of the liner and a pin that inserted across the shank of the prosthesis that engaged the pin therefore securing the liner. This system was quite frustrating at times because everything had to be perfectly aligned for the pin to go through the loop. Sometimes it took me 20 minutes to get it in the exact right place. The liners were all custom made and were not particularly comfortable and the improvements in mechanisms and liners have made this a very viable system.

Another Suspension Story

I used to mountain bike with a buddy who was in good shape even though a little older than me. He was a sniper in Vietnam but was quite short for a Marine, and he and I were very competitive whenever we biked or skied. He couldn't stand the thought of a one-legged guy beating him and I couldn't stand the thought of a curly haired guy beating me so we always beat each other up. He and I were mountain biking in the hills behind his home one afternoon and I was up front, pushing myself and trying to not let him pass me. I was wearing the locking liner with the old pin system in it and a latex suspension sleeve to provide dual suspension since I knew that I would be sweating a lot. I tried to hop over a ditch and crashed into some sagebrush on the side of the trail. My prosthetic foot was strapped onto the pedal of the bike so when I crashed it pulled my leg off. I got up bruised but unhurt and disengaged my leg from the bike and to my horror the pin that holds my leg on was missing. I searched the ground for some time trying to find it but a horny toad or something must have eaten the pin because it had disappeared. I was OK because I knew the suspension sleeve would hold my leg on but in order to hold suction I had to seal up the hole in the side of the leg where the pin inserted. I searched my kit but there was no duct tape (the standard repair kit of all amputees). The only thing I could find was a Power Bar (Power Bar Harvest Corp., Berkeley, CA), one of those energy bars that are supposed to taste like chocolate but remind you of eating shoe leather. I chewed up a small piece of the bar and shoved it into the hole and it sealed up nicely. The next day I was back in my lab and tried to remove the Power Bar plug but it wouldn't budge, no matter how much I heated it or picked at it. I eventually had to drill it out since it had hardened to the density of the plastic around it. That marked the last time I ever ate a Power Bar again.

The locking liner system works great if you have the right type of residual limb and your activity level is moderate. If you utilize this system and want to engage in more strenuous activities, I recommend a secondary means of suspension such as a suspension sleeve that can be worn over top of the locking liner. This can also be helpful to persons who have worn other types of suspension and are switching to the locking liner system. All other systems pull on the skin of the stump in an upward direction. The underlying layer of tissue that separates the skin from the bone is called the fascia and it gets used to being pulled in a constant direction. The locking liner pulls the fascia in a downward direction and can result in a burning sensation that is very uncomfortable. If the amputee is not expecting this, he or she may reject the system due to the pain. However, if the fascia is gradually introduced to the downward pull, the pain will be minimized and will generally go away after a couple of weeks. The use of an external suspension sleeve for the break-in period will allow the amputee to make a smoother transition.

Not all liners are of the locking variety. Most manufacturers have nonlocking liners (see Figure 3-4) available in the same sizes as their locking styles. Nonlocking liners can be used with any other suspension system and are especially well suited to suction, which I will talk about in the next section. I wear nonlocking liners in both my everyday walking prosthesis as well as my shower/swim leg.

Suction

Suction suspension is used to describe any system that utilizes negative air pressure to hold the prosthesis onto the body. This is most commonly achieved through the use of suspension sleeves that have the effect of preventing air from entering the socket, therefore not allowing the leg to come off. If the socket does not have any air entering it, then the leg cannot come off. It's like holding a glass of water upside-down with a piece of glass covering the opening; the water cannot come out since no air can enter the glass and take up the space of the water. The suspension sleeve acts like the piece of glass covering the open end of the glass of water; as long as it is intact and has no holes, then it will suspend by negative air pressure. Unlike the glass of water, however, once a suspension sleeve gets a hole in it, the leg does not necessarily come off. It will generally hold onto the body by the mechanical structure of the sleeve.

Suspension sleeves have come a long way since I first used a latex one back in the early '80s. Latex is basically rubber and is very abrasive on the skin as well as subject to tearing when stretched too much or punctured. Those types of sleeves would tear my thigh up and leave welts or blisters on my skin where heat and friction would cause dermatitis. Today there are numerous suspension sleeves made from such varying materials as urethane, silicone, and gels. Urethane feels sticky on the skin and generally persons with good skin are most comfortable using them. Silicone is a bit harsher on the skin but has the added benefit of extreme durability. Gels are more comfortable than any of the other materials but do not have the durability of the silicone materials.

The great advantage of using a suspension sleeve is that it really does hold the leg onto your body with no belt, strap, or wedge and the prosthesis feels more like a part of the body than with any of the other methods of suspension. It also requires no effort on the part of the amputee to hold the leg on and most people who switch from some other system claim that the prosthesis feels lighter with the suction type of suspension. Another advantage, especially over the wedge or strap style, is the increased range of motion that the suction allows. Generally, prostheses that use suction have lower socket trim-lines and also look more cosmetic since there are no buckles or bulges in the upper brim of the socket. Another important benefit of the suction socket is that it holds the residual limb more firmly in the socket and, therefore, reduces pistoning and friction between the skin and the socket. Most amputees who wear suction sockets do not remove their prosthesis during the course of the day and are able to sit relatively comfortably in a chair with their knee bent at a near normal angle.

The disadvantages of wearing a suction suspension prosthesis are primarily the build up of heat and perspiration inside of the socket. Since no air enters the socket, there is no cooling effect of perspiration on the skin and no place for the sweat to go. If enough perspiration builds up, the socket can begin to slip off of the stump and the suspension sleeve will need to be removed for drying. This is a particular disadvantage in warm humid climates and needs to be a major consideration when deciding whether to use this type of suspension. Another disadvantage is the durability of sleeves, which will start to lose their suction advantage if punctured. This makes getting down on hands and knees a tricky maneuver, since even a small hole in the sleeve will allow air to enter the socket, therefore destroying the suction. Some suspension sleeves also restrict the range of motion at the knee because of rigidity or thickness and it is always a trade off when choosing which type of suspension sleeve is best for you.

There are 2 types of devices that assist the suction in a prosthetic socket. One is the expulsion valve, which is a one-way valve that allows air to leave the socket but does not allow it to enter. This valve increases the actual suction inside the socket, creating a true negative air environment, therefore, eliminating pistoning. There are many different types of expulsion valves, but I prefer the more simple ones that require minimal maintenance. The other system that aids suction actually uses a miniature pump to expel the air from the socket, maintaining a constant negative air pressure at all times. This system requires some elaborate mechanisms that add weight and complexity to the prosthesis but some amputees swear by the system.

The Future of Prosthetics

The field of prosthetics has come a long way since I lost my leg over 30 years ago. Advances in materials and components have changed the expected functional capabilities of the amputee in ways that I couldn't even imagine when I first became an amputee. It has truly been an exciting time to be in a profession where the sky has been the limit on innovation and accessibility to new and exotic resources.

What does tomorrow bring for the below-knee amputee? I believe that there will be a continued development of foot components that will more closely mimic the actions of the real foot. They will probably be mated with microelectronics that will monitor the dynamic needs of the prosthesis and utilize the foot capabilities to their fullest. There are already great strides being made in microprocessor usage in knees and has been functional in arms for decades. It is only a matter of time before this technology will find an application for the below-knee amputee.

The real potential for dramatic change in the comfort of the amputee will be in the socket. I envision a socket of the future that actually changes shape depending on the needs of the residual limb inside. The technology already exists to monitor the shape of the stump and change the socket to accommodate the movement. Imagine a socket that lowered the back wall when you sat and gave you a little more room at the tip of your stump. When you stood back up, the socket changes to give your stump the maximum contact and control for walking. Socket changes can be programmed into a microprocessor and adjustments could be performed by remote control anywhere in the world. If you could plug your leg into a laptop connected to the Internet, then you could have your prosthetist make socket adjustments based upon pressure readings that he or she could download as well as your feedback. This is a potential future for our industry.

Another area in which I foresee big changes happening is the cosmesis of the leg. Skin coverings will continue to improve in both durability and realism. CAD will enable prosthetists to digitalize the good leg and have a milling machine reverse and duplicate the shape onto the prosthesis. There will be advances in materials that will actually darken when exposed to the sun, mimicking the color changes of the human body.

There will be continued improvements in the types of materials that can be used as an interface with the human body. Silicones, gels, and urethanes will continue to be improved and mixed to give the ultimate in comfort as well as durability. The future looks bright for the potential of prosthetic improvements provided that the market is willing to pay for the innovation.

Conclusion

Socket design and suspension are the cornerstones of a good prosthesis. If these things are not right, then all of the other stuff that can be added to a prosthesis will not make it successful. There is no magic machine that produces a good socket. It is a function of the skill of the prosthetist, his or her experience, and openness to hybridizing designs to fit the amputee's individual needs. Even when all of these factors are in place, the amputee will still experience problems. After all, the prosthetist is fitting a living, changing body part into a lifeless piece of plastic and composite materials. Amputees who have a realistic understanding of this situation will get the most out of their prosthesis and live full lives with little restriction. Science cannot put legs back on yet, but life as an amputee is far better then even a short 25 years ago and there is no reason that it won't improve further. In the next chapter I will deal solely with components, feet, and other mechanisms that are used to provide smooth and efficient gait.

CHAPTER 4

The Prosthetic Prescription

My Travels

At the ripe age of 22, having no idea of what I was getting into, I packed up my few possessions and traveled to Cairo, Egypt. The year was 1976 and I arrived late in the afternoon at the beginning of Ramadan. I did not know what Ramadan was, but it is the major religious holiday for Muslims in which they fast during the day, abstaining from food, drink, and sex for the daylight hours over a period of 50 days. The scene was very surreal as we left the airport for my apartment in Maadi, a suburb just south of the city where the American School is located. The ride from the airport was unforgettable and exotic. It was night by the time we left and the streets were crowded with people and the mood was definitely that of a huge party. Everything smelled a bit like a barn, but all of the people were genuinely friendly and I decided that I could make this place my home for the next 2 years.

Teaching was easy since my fourth grade class contained only 15 kids and I had wonderful experienced teachers to help me through all of the things that I didn't know. I lived in a nice 2-bedroom apartment on a street shaded by flame trees that turned deep lavender in the spring. I had a small garden in the back with mango and lime trees as well as a gardener to maintain it. In addition, I had a maid who also cooked for me as well as a laundry boy and grocery delivery person. Compared to my old college life, this was grand. I made some good friends with some of the teachers there at the school but discovered that I was closer in age to the high school students than to most of the other teachers. I started playing handball with one of the other teachers at a rather snooty club in Maadi where I also swam several times a week.

I was playing handball 3 times a week. Unfortunately, it was on a squash court, which is not the same, but it was something. About 2 weeks before Christmas vacation I was getting my butt kicked by Warren, one of the other teachers who was 45 years old but in great shape, when I heard a nasty "crack" as I bent down to take a shot. I looked at my prosthesis and discovered a large break in the inside wall of the socket. This crack in the plastic lamination allowed the side wings of the socket to spread, which loosened the supercondylar suspension to the point where my leg would not stay on unless I also used a waist-belt. I was in a bit of a panic. The pain that I lived with was very invasive. Somehow the pull upward that was exerted by the waist belt caused a sharp pain in the back of my stump where my major nerves ran up my leg. After a week of living with this, I determined that I would need to go back to the United States to get a new leg made.

I flew back to Atlanta and got to spend Christmas with my folks while Grant made me a new leg. I had him duplicate it so that I would have a backup leg in case I had another break. I returned to Cairo with a bunch of stuff that was unobtainable in Egypt. I had a waterbed in my pack and a new bicycle that someone had generously given me when I told them I wanted to bicycle the Alps that next summer. I think that I had the only waterbed in Egypt and I thought I was pretty cool.

Upon my return to Cairo, I started a high school wrestling program. Unfortunately, the nearest American high school was in Tehran, Iran so we contented ourselves by wrestling against local clubs who wrestled Greco-Roman style. This was really weird since I was only familiar with American wrestling, but it was great training for my high school wrestlers who often had to wrestle men who were in their 20s and 30s.

In addition to coaching wrestling, I also ran the chess club and science club. Between my teaching duties and all of the extracurricular activities, I was a very busy guy. I got to do a lot of sightseeing while living in Cairo. On one such excursion to Alexandria and Marsha Matruh, on the Mediterranean Sea, I was out walking on the sand dunes. I decided to go for a walk on the beach and so I took my shoes off to keep them dry. My foot was set up for a 2.5-cm (1-in) heel height so I had never walked barefoot before. Since the sand was soft, I could walk on the beach without my shoes on. I exulted in the feeling of being barefoot and couldn't believe how light my leg felt without the shoe on it. I got so excited that I started running down the sand dunes and found that I could still run if I had something to absorb some of the impact. Unfortunately, soon thereafter, I developed an extremely sore lump behind my stump, just below the head of my fibula, the side bone. The lump got bigger over the next several months and became excruciatingly painful. I went to a local surgeon to get an evaluation and he informed me that I had a neuroma. He explained that this is a condition that is not uncommon in amputees. It occurs when a large nerve, in my case it was the peroneal nerve, becomes irritated beneath the skin and lays down scar tissue. This was why the lump was growing and was so painful. Nerve tissue can lay down scar but cannot remove it once it is formed. The only way to treat the problem was to remove the nerve bundle. I agreed to have him do the surgery and met him at the Maadi Hospital accompanied by my girlfriend, Heidi, one of my nefarious affairs. The surgery went smoothly and I was back home that evening, although I should have been more wary of the lack of sanitation in the hospital when I noticed that the operating room window was wide open and there were flies everywhere.

Five days later, my stump ballooned up to the size of a cantaloupe. I returned to the doctor and he drained several cups of bloody fluid from my stump. I panicked and was afraid that I was going to lose my leg above the knee. At the advice of the director of the school, I flew to Thessalonica, Greece to recover from the surgery in a hospital that was clean and staffed by more Western-style doctors. While I was there for almost 2 weeks, my buddy Warren also arrived to have a hernia repaired so at least there was one other person who spoke English.

Nonetheless, I made it through the first year intact and decided to join 2 other teachers on a bicycle tour of the Alps for the 3 months of summer vacation. Warren, the 45-year-old handball player, had bicycled around Tuscany and had some experience and Sue, who was a second grade teacher and had never really done anything athletic in her life, were to be my partners in this adventure. I had been training around

Egypt by taking some long rides along the Nile and into the desert, but there were no hills to practice on and certainly nothing to prepare me for the Alps. I wrote to all of my old college buddies, encouraging them to join me for this trip but they all had lame excuses like they were working for their fathers for the summer or something. None of them were actually working in the field that they had studied in college. The day before we left for Athens, Greece, I received a letter from a buddy named Aaron who expressed interest in bicycling. I couldn't call from Egypt so I called him from Athens and invited him to join me on the adventure. He didn't have a passport or a bicycle but said he would meet me in Treviso, Italy less than 2 weeks later.

One of my experiences of Greece came as we were boarding the ferryboat for the 2-day cruise to Venice. As I was carrying my bicycle through the crowded terminal, the back tire of the bike accidentally bumped against a Greek man who took offense at the gesture. The next thing I knew, I was grabbed by my shirt and slammed up against the wall where this mean looking guy was yelling at me in Greek and had his fist back preparing to slug me in the face. I was holding my bike on my shoulder and had my saddlebags on the other arm so I couldn't even get my arms up to protect myself. I readied my face for the blow when all of a sudden some woman yelled something to the man and he stopped and looked down at my leg. I was in shorts so my prosthesis was pretty obvious. He immediately started apologizing to me and then took my bike and carried it for me the rest of the way. Saved by the leg. Unbeknownst to us, we were embarking on an Israeli registered ship and as we tried to board, the security forces singled us out of the line and took us to a separate building for interrogation. This was not long after a major plane hijacking and the abduction of the Achille Lauro cruise ship. Since our passports had all of these Egyptian visa stamps on them, they really put us through the third degree.

We finally got onto the ship and found our berths, which were not really berths but chairs. I discovered that when you sail deck class you get a chair on the deck of the ship. I determined that I was going to find a bed to sleep in no matter what. It just so happened that I met a young American woman, Frederica, who was traveling back to the United States after traveling around Europe in her MG for a year. When we arrived in Venice, she stayed with us while we traveled north to Treviso where Warren and Sue bought new bicycles from Pinarello, one of the premier bicycle makers in Italy. Frederica was driving north from Venice and followed us on our shakedown ride into the mountains north of Venice. It was the kind of romantic liaison that poems are written about and it sure was a nice way to start off the adventure.

Two days later we met Aaron, who had managed to obtain a passport and a bicycle in the 10 days time since I had spoken with him. We took off bicycling across northern Italy, stopping at guesthouses and pensions along the way. We were attempting to bicycle around all of the lakes of northern Italy and the scenery was spectacular, the food and wine were unbelievable, and there were girls, lots of girls, who were friendly and weren't wearing veils. I would have been in heaven if not for my leg. After the first week, I started getting nasty pimples and blisters. We were biking nearly 100 km (60 miles) a day and this was the Alps, so the terrain was mountainous. I got used to the dull ache of an infected pimple and after a while could even muscle through the blisters. By the second week I was in trouble. I would take off my stump socks and they would be soaked in blood and I knew I couldn't keep this up. We arrived in Bergamo, a beautiful town where we stayed just off of the main square and decided to take a couple of days off to rest and recover.

Even though my leg was giving me fits, the ability to accomplish this had done a great deal to boost my ego. One afternoon I was sitting in the square having a coffee when I spied a beautiful blond woman sitting on the steps of the church. I boldly walked over to her and invited her to my table for a cup of coffee. She accepted and that began my romance with Giovanna, the best woman chess player I ever met. My stump was still a mess when the rest of the gang decided to continue the trip. Giovanna offered to take me to Milan where I could get some work done on my prosthesis. I accepted her generous offer because it also meant that I could spend a little more time with her, so we took the train to Milan. No one at the prosthetic facility spoke English so I was dependent upon Giovanna to translate my needs. After a frustrating several hours at the facility, I could tell that these guys didn't know what to do with me so I took my leg in disgust and Giovanna and I took the train to try and catch up with my buddies.

Having rejoined Warren, Sue, and Aaron and saying goodbye to a tearful Giovanna, we returned to our grueling bicycle routine. I could keep up but after 2 more days of bloody stump, I got really depressed. One night I was sitting on my bed looking at my leg and the 25 plys of socks that I had to wear to keep it snug on my stump. As I stared at the leg and wondered if I could keep this up I lamented the fact that if I only had a grinder, I could grind out the plastic in this one area that was giving me fits. All of a sudden it occurred to me that instead of grinding the plastic, I could cut a hole in one of my 5-ply socks and that would give me the pressure relief that I needed without permanently grinding a hole in my socket. I pulled on the initial 5-ply wool sock and found the sore spot. I then drew a circle around the affected area and cut a hole in the sock slightly smaller than the hole I had drawn. When I put the leg on, the pressure was much less so I cut another hole in the second sock and when I put on the leg there was no pressure on my sore spot. Over the subsequent weeks of bicycling I cut holes in most of my socks and just moved them around whenever I got an infected hair or blister. In this way I was able to continue to bicycle with my friends and the pain became manageable.

We bicycled across northern Italy until we got to the Grand St. Bernard Pass. This was one of the most brutal mountain passes in the Alps but we all made it and crossed over into Switzerland. At this point the party broke in 2, with Warren and Sue heading to the Matterhorn while Aaron and I detoured to Montreaux where the annual jazz festival was about to begin. We arrived at the casino where the festival was to take place and decided to do a little scouting to see what we needed in order to attend the festival starting the next week. Aaron was on a tight budget and could not afford the ticket price for the concerts so we hatched a plan to get us in. We called a friend of ours from Denver and asked him to send a telegram to the festival announcing that a writer and photographer would be arriving from a fictitious radio station and would require press credentials. We took off for a week of bicycling that took us to Interlaken and Grindlewald and upon our return we had been paged for 2 days. The telegram had arrived and we picked up our press kits and badges to pretend to be journalists for a couple of weeks. This time was major fun as we got to hang out in the musician's bar as well as enjoy our seats in the press box. I had to fake my way through interviews of Ella Fitzgerald and Count Basie but we pulled it off while basically having the time of our lives.

After 2 weeks of scamming the jazz festival, we decided that it was time to go. We headed for Germany to bicycle the Black Forest Region and to try some of the German beer. Over the next month, we wove our way through the incredible serenity of the

Black Forest and down through Western Austria to the border of Italy again. There we decided to attempt to bicycle over Stelvio Pass, the highest mountain road in the Alps. The day we bicycled the pass it was rainy and foggy but since we would not be going very fast on the way up that was no problem. There were 42 individual switch-backs on the way up and it took us over 5 hours to reach the summit where even in August there was snow and people skiing. The ride down was harrowing due to the slippery road surface and the bad visibility, but back in the little town of Gloria Glorenza we put away a beer or two in celebration. It wasn't until the next morning that I noticed a familiar agony when I put my leg on. The neuroma had returned. Behind my knee just above the scar from the first removal was a new lump the size of a large marble that caused me to grind my teeth when I applied pressure to it.

After a lengthy discussion with Aaron, I knew that I could no longer continue to bicycle with this lump of nerve tissue screaming at me all of the time. We decided to part company. I was heading back to Greece to go to the clinic where I had been before to see if they could remove the neuroma and have me back on my feet again before classes started again in 3 weeks. Aaron would head to Israel to visit his sister who was living there. As we parted, we knew that communications would be difficult since Egypt and Israel were still technically in a state of war so that any mail correspondence would have to go first to his parents in New Jersey, then between us.

I took the train that crept along for 2 days to Thessalonica where I checked back into the hospital. The surgery took place the next day and after 2 weeks my incision healed so I could head back to Cairo. While I was stuck in my lovely hospital room where I had a balcony overlooking the bay, I decided that after my second year in Cairo I was going back to Georgia to build a house. Drawing up the plans gave me a nice alternative to the 3 books that I had to read and the time passed quickly.

My second year teaching went a bit smoother since I had more of my systems in place. At Christmas break I decided to go on safari to Kenya with a tour group of 15 other teachers from the school. We flew on a really funky airline, Air Ethiopia, and had quite the adventure landing in Addis Ababa where we were stuck for 8 hours. Upon our arrival in Nairobi, we checked into the Pan Afric Hotel and were informed that the next day we would head to Mombassa.

While in Mombassa I had the first fight of my adult life. I am not a fighter, never really enjoyed it, figuring that even when you win a fight your knuckles are beat up and somebody's brother is trying to kill you. I had met a German girl, Ushi, and had asked her to take a walk with me on the beach in the moonlight. We stopped to sit on a low stone wall next to our hotel compound and while sitting there we were approached by 2 native looking fellows. One man who was dressed in a trench coat told us in impeccable English that we were trespassing on the property of Mzee Jomo Kenyata, the ruler of Kenya. I explained that we were just staying in the hotel next door and that we would leave. He said he was a police officer and when I asked him for some identification he pulled a 45-caliber pistol from his trench coat pocket and leveled it at my abdomen. Ushi started to panic but somehow I remained calm, staring at the cold barrel of the gun. At that time of my life, I always carried a walking-stick, which I used for balance. As I stood before this man, I clutched it in my right hand. I spoke softly to Ushi to try and calm her down, but I never took my eyes off of the gun. The supposed police officer was telling us that he needed to take us to the police station and as I was agreeing with him he inexplicably lowered the pistol and slipped it back into his pocket and glanced off to his right. Without thinking, I used my walking stick much like a quarter-staff and brought it crashing into his left temple as he turned back to face me. He dropped like a sack of potatoes and I turned to the other man and growled while thrusting my stick at him. He took off running as fast as he could. I reached over to the collapsed man in front of me and pulled the gun out of his pocket, checking the chamber for bullets. The gun wasn't loaded and didn't even have a clip in it. Just then two uniformed guards with carbines ran up to us yelling in Swahili. I handed them the gun and grabbed the still-screaming Ushi and walked back to our hotel. Whew! That was a close one. There were lots of mosquitoes out that evening and I distinctly remember being bitten on numerous areas of my body.

There were more adventures in Kenya but nothing to compare with the adventure that I got to experience upon my return to Cairo. After about a week, I came down with flu-like symptoms that seemed to abate after a day so I didn't think much about it. I took a day off and the librarian came by to pick up my lesson plans, but I told her there was no need since I would probably be back at school the next day. That night I went to bed early since I felt a little weird and about 11:00 that evening I woke up with a fever and was feeling a bit disoriented. I took my temperature and the thermometer said 106°F. I knew that this was not good, but it didn't completely register and I felt powerless to affect any change. I didn't know it but I was beginning one of many delirium fevers that I would experience fighting malaria. Fortunately for me, the librarian came by to pick up my lesson plans and found me babbling and drooling in my bed with the same horrendous fever. The first doctor who came to see me had done his residency in a tropical disease clinic in London and after taking one look at me said that I had malaria. I was transferred to the librarian's house where they had 2 beds and a washing machine that ended up being necessary since I would drench a set of sheets in about an hour. I suffered through 5 more severe fevers that came on every 22 hours and I had lost 50 pounds at the end of a week while turning a pale yellow.

I took another week off to recover and then I was back at school, teaching and coaching again but weakness plagued me for another month. Since I was young, healthy, and stupid, I had no idea what I had just survived. I had contracted falciparum malaria one evening on the beach in Mombassa when one of those evil mosquitoes had bitten me. I would not really understand the long-term ramifications of my bout with malaria until I was in my 40s and discovered that the high fever had melted some of my kidneys.

A month later I had a funny experience with my class of fourth graders. At around 10:00 each morning I would go to the teachers lounge for 5 minutes to get a cup of coffee. I couldn't help noticing that whenever I returned from those coffee breaks, all of the kids in my class were in their seats reading their books like little angels. This made me suspicious since I had basically been a bad boy in school and every time the teacher left the room created an opportunity for mischief. Totally unrelated to this, I had been to the beach the weekend before and my foot was filled with sand and grit. The Griesinger multi-axial foot (a mechanical foot that simulates ankle motion by using rubber bumpers and gaskets) that I wore had a lip around the ankle part of the prosthesis and dirt tended to get into the rubber bumpers. It was squeaking pretty bad so one evening I took the foot apart, lubricated the bumpers, and cleaned all of the sand out. It was now quiet as a mouse. The next morning I took off for the lounge to get my cup of coffee. As I returned and opened the door to my classroom, one of my students tumbled out of the room. Apparently, my class had been posting a scout by the door to listen for my squeaky foot coming down the hallway and issuing a warning so that when

I returned from my coffee break they would all be in their seats. The lesson here is to keep the foot clean and squeak free if you need to be able to sneak up on people!

The wrestling season ended with the big tournament in Tehran, Iran, the home of the largest American school in the world in 1978. I flew with my team to the tournament and since there was only one flight a week between Cairo and Tehran, we were stuck for a couple of days with not much to do. One of my wrestlers who had previously lived in Tehran invited me to go skiing with him and his buddies. I had never skied in my life, having basically grown up in the Southern United States or in Northern Ohio where skiing is not a big sport. I decided to be manly and stupid, so I went with him on the excursion. He helped me to get my equipment together and then took off to ski with his buddies. I tumbled down the slope having no instruction other than having watched this sport on television. I was wearing my supercondylar suspension leg with an auxiliary waist belt and my multi-axial foot, which is not what you need to ski with. My real challenge was the poma lift, which looks as if you should sit on the little disk attached to the moving rope. Wrong. It took me at least six tries before I figured out that you let the disk pull you up instead of sitting on it. I had skied about four runs and was actually getting the hang of it when I took a nasty fall. This was the classic yard sale fall where everything falls off: the hat, gloves, poles, skis, and in my case, my waist belt broke and the prosthesis that was still connected to the ski. The ski with the leg still attached slid down the hill on its side until it encountered a mogul and popped upright. The leg began to accelerate and I yelled down the mountain for someone to stop that leg. Just below me was an Iranian woman dressed in the height of ski fashion, standing on a mogul admiring the beautiful vista in front of her. As she glanced behind her to see what all of the yelling was about, a leg came skiing past her and she grabbed at her heart in disbelief. I eventually retrieved my leg, but I had really injured my stump when the leg was wrenched off during the fall.

I was on crutches for the trip back to Cairo with the team. We arrived at the Tehran Airport and began to board the plane. I was in my 3-piece suit, trying to look old and one of my wrestlers was carrying my leg in his arms. I cleared the security desk and was about to board the bus that takes us to our plane when I heard a commotion behind me. I looked back to see my wrestler having a tug-of-war with one of the Iranian guards with my prosthesis. A second guard was sticking a submachine gun into my wrestler's face but he wouldn't let go of my leg. I crutched back and began to argue with the security guards, who wanted to cut my leg in half to make sure that there were no drugs in it. Since this was the only leg I had in the Eastern hemisphere, I did not take kindly to this. After whapping the guard in the face with my empty pants leg to illustrate that I needed the prosthesis, they finally allowed the leg through. I have had many awkward moments in airport security but this was the worst one.

Back in Egypt, the year was winding down and I was looking forward to returning to the United States to begin construction on my house. I received a letter from Aaron who had been in Israel for the past 9 months, asking me to be the best man at his wedding in Paris. He explained that he was living on a kibbutz and met a French girl and they were to be married in a month. Since I was the only friend that he had in this hemisphere, I decided to go. My whirlwind Parisian experience began with a rehearsal, which neither of us understood, and then a late night of heavy drinking. At one point, after two bottles of wine, Aaron told me that the girl he was marrying was 18 years old and pregnant. I had the opportunity to whack him on the head with the wine bottle and get him out of France but I did not, much to his future demise.

The next day we shakily made it to the marriage ceremony, which again, neither of us could comprehend, especially when the justice of the peace started crying and babbling. At the reception I made friends with the maid of honor, Brigitte, who was quite attractive, but after meeting the bride, I had a bad feeling about the future of Aaron's marriage. At 2:00 in the morning I got a nighttime tour of Paris and managed to get a few hours sleep before returning to Cairo the next day. Brigitte and I had a romantic evening. I agreed to keep in touch with her and possibly visit on my way back to the States in a couple of months.

My last night in Cairo was truly a night to remember. One of my best buddies, Ian, kept me up all night long partying at his apartment. About 4:00 in the morning, he beckoned me to join him on some mysterious excursion so we took off in his black Mercedes. We arrived at Giza in the darkness and I was surprised when we parked in front of the Great Pyramid of Cheops. Ian told me that we are going to climb to the top to watch the sunrise over Cairo and since I am basically stupid, I agreed. As we began to climb, an armed guard showed up and told us that it is prohibited to climb the pyramid but after Ian slipped him some "baksheesh," which is a little bribe, the guard became our guide. It took almost an hour to make it to the top in the dark, and it was probably best that I couldn't see well or I would have never done it. We made it just as the sun was lighting the eastern horizon and did yoga as the sun blazed over the desert. This was truly a mystical experience. The climb down with no sleep was harrowing but we made it and I left for the airport and home.

My flight home had a layover in Paris and New York. I met Brigitte in Paris and stayed up all night with her. The next morning, after only a few hours sleep, she took me to the airport. As she dropped me at my gate, she asked if she could visit me in America. I said of course, but didn't really expect a visit. Boy, was I wrong. Six months later as I was living in the middle of the woods in Georgia building a house, she showed up and wanted to marry me. The big lesson there was to be careful what you promise.

This portion of my story does not relate precisely to the topic of prosthetic prescription, but I felt it was important to illustrate some of the things that I went through with my prosthesis. I definitely did not have the right prosthetic prescription for the activity level that I was engaging in as well as access to prosthetic services to compensate for my changes. My point is to demonstrate the importance of understanding the hopes and aspirations of the prosthetic wearer, whether that is bicycling the Alps or going fishing. The choice of prosthetic components and systems is directly related to the prosthetic wearer. If you are a prosthetist or doctor, get to know your patients. If you are an amputee, make sure that your doctor or prosthetist is aware of what your expectations are so that an adequate prescription can be determined. Communication is critical.

The Prescription

Before a prosthetist can legally make and bill for a prosthesis, a doctor must write a prescription for the limb. Generally, prescriptions are either written or suggested by the prosthetist and then copied by the physician. Good prosthetists will spend time with their clients discussing the various options of the suspension, foot, and cosmesis prior to submitting the prescription to the doctor. In my private practice, we were very specific as to the exact billable components and systems that we were going to use and insisted that the physician duplicate our prescription, complete with L-codes. What are L-codes?

Prosthetic L-Codes

1. Medicare lists most prosthetic components or systems in a publication that is the standard billing reference for our industry. The codes that pertain to prosthetics have an L before the number to designate that it is a prosthetic device.
2. Most components and types of systems are represented by a code and a standard fee for service that represents the amount Medicare will reimburse the facility for that service.
3. Not all prosthetic services and components are on the L-code list. New technology and components that are not in wide use may not have a code and, therefore, will be difficult to bill.
4. To ensure that your prosthetist will be paid for your prosthesis, it is important that the prescription have all of the L-codes listed. This minimizes confusion by the third-party payee as to what is necessary for the prosthesis.

Prosthetic facilities make their money by making prostheses, not on repairs or adjustments. Therefore, there is generally a push to make a new prosthesis or at the least a new socket. The most common justification for the making of a new prosthesis is to be able to demonstrate an anatomical change in the residual limb. This is done by measuring the circumference of the stump and comparing it to previous measurements, showing that there has been "anatomical change," the catch phrase that most insurance companies will need as the justification. Another important feature of the prescription is the reference to the amputee's activity level, which is expressed as a K-level. This is Medicare's designation that describes the type of activities that the amputee will likely be engaged in. There are 4 levels (described on p. 110) and Medicare will not pay for components that are not within the amputee's K-level. For example, an amputee has a K2 activity level, which describes the community ambulator. Medicare will not pay for a shock absorbing foot that is designed more for the athletic amputee. It is important that the prescription is consistent with the description of the amputee.

What is a Good Prosthetic Prescription?

1. A good prescription needs to have a paragraph that justifies the need to have a new prosthesis. The catch phrase "anatomical change" should appear in the justification paragraph and should be backed up by measurements showing the amount of change.
2. There should be a reference to the amputee's activity level that is generally expressed by means of a K-level. This K-level is a system that was developed by Medicare to classify amputees and their activities. A list of the K-levels follows.
3. Next on the prescription should be a complete list of the types of components and their corresponding L-codes, which are the Medicare-accepted descriptions of the various prosthetic systems.
4. The prescription needs to be dated and signed by the attending physician. This will give it the maximum advantage when it is received by the third-party payment office.

K-Level Activity Ratings

1. K-level 1: Patient has the ability or potential to use a prosthesis for transfers or ambulation on level surfaces at a fixed cadence. Typical of the limited and unlimited household ambulator.
2. K-level 2: Patient has the ability or potential for ambulation with the ability to transverse low-level environmental barriers such as curbs, stairs, or uneven surfaces. Typical of the limited community ambulator.
3. K-level 3: Patient has the ability or potential for ambulation with variable cadence. Typical of the community ambulator who has the ability to transverse most environmental barriers and may have vocational, therapeutic, or exercise activity that demands prosthetic utilization beyond simple locomotion.
4. K-level 4: Patient has the ability or potential for prosthetic ambulation that exceeds basic ambulation skills, exhibiting high impact, stress, or energy levels. Typical of the prosthetic demands of the child, active adult, or athlete.

Who Pays for Prostheses?

Most prostheses in the United States are paid through Medicare, the Veterans Administration, or private insurance. If you are insured by one of these entities, you should be able to receive a decent prosthesis with minimal out of pocket expenses. The process of obtaining a prosthesis and getting it paid for usually begins with the evaluation where you spend time with your prosthetist and/or doctor discussing the options that are suitable for your lifestyle expectations. Once you have determined the prosthetic prescription and it has been signed by your physician, then the prosthetist can begin the process of obtaining approval by the third-party payee as well as an agreement on the billing.

Generally, the facility will call your insurance provider with your billing information to verify your eligibility for the service. Once your eligibility has been confirmed, the prosthetic facility can have some confidence that the prosthesis will be paid for. However, remember that verification of coverage is not an absolute guarantee that the insurance company will pay.

Here is the hard reality of the prosthetic industry from the facility point of view. Prosthetists are not supposed to send in the bill for the prosthesis until the work is completed and the patient has accepted the prosthesis. What constitutes acceptance? The minute that you take home the prosthesis and wear it. Legally, you have accepted the limb and the prosthetist can then send in the bill. You need to bear in mind that the prosthetic facility has had to pay for all of the work, the cost of the components, and the time that it takes to educate you on the function of the prosthesis. This value was literally fronted to the client in the hopes of reimbursement with nothing more than a verification of coverage as a guarantee of payment. This is quite the risk for the business. If you have a good trusting relationship with your prosthetist, then helping them out by accepting the prosthesis is an acceptable strategy. If there is some doubt that everything is right, insist that you be able to take the prosthesis home on a temporary basis for a fixed amount of time before you actually accept it. **The only leverage that you have in regards to the prosthesis is whether there will be any payment for** the limb. Only agree to payment when you are confident that the prosthesis will serve your needs.

Today, there is generally a copay for most types of insurance or Medicare. The standard amount of copay is 20% for private insurance and Medicare, so be prepared to pay for the balance of the bill. The copay may be collected up-front once the bill is submitted. Prosthetic facilities are bound by law to collect the copayments and can be prosecuted for insurance fraud if they fail to account for them. Only conditions of documented financial hardship will create a situation in which the copay does not have to be paid. Guidelines for financial hardship are outlined by Medicare and your prosthetic facility should have all of the paperwork to justify that condition.

The Veterans Administration will generally pay 100% for all service-connected injuries resulting in the need for prostheses. You will need to check with your local VA to determine your level of benefits. In the past the VA made its own prosthetic devices but has since contracted out to the private sector. There are generally clinics sponsored by the VA to determine the optimal prosthetic prescription as well as any other services needed by the amputee. The VA also is one of the few agencies that will pay for ancillary prostheses such as water legs or specific sports prostheses, but this is not something that they advertise. The VA will also pay to provide their amputees with a backup prosthesis, usually a refurbished old limb, but at least they recognize the need for a spare prosthesis.

I have had the honor of working with many veterans in my years as a prosthetist and their contribution to the field of prosthetics cannot be overestimated. Vietnam veterans started and continue to run most of the sports programs for amputees in this nation, and it was their need that stimulated the explosion of components that occurred over the last 25 years. The gatherings of amputees that began to occur in the '80s created a pressure in the prosthetic industry to innovate and experiment with new designs and materials. This may not have occurred had there been no sporting events that brought together numbers of amputees.

The other option for payment is to pay for it yourself. If you are going to pay cash for the limb, then you will probably be able to work out some type of discount with your prosthetist.

Another agency that has had a history of paying for prostheses is your local state vocational rehabilitation agency. The job of voc rehab is to get people who have suffered some type of incapacitation back to work. They will help with prostheses and education if you are deemed someone who has the desire as well as capability to return to work. The agencies all receive money depending on how many of their clients return to gainful employment so keep this in mind before approaching them for help. If you need a new prosthesis to be able to go back to work or continue the job that you are currently working at, they may be able to help.

Types of Legs

There are 2 basic types of prostheses. Endoskeletal (Figure 4-1), which is like the human body (ie, a structural support on the inside with a soft outer covering), or exoskeletal, which has a hard outer shell and requires no internal structure. The majority of prostheses today are endoskeletal with a pipe or tube on the inside that connects the socket to the foot. Most manufacturers sell endoskeletal systems that

Figure 4-1. A nicely finished endoskeletal prosthesis. (Photo courtesy of Ossur.)

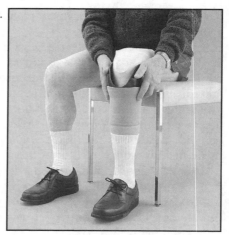

allow for lots of adjustability as well as interchangeable parts. This gives the prosthetist many options for designing or trying different components and the adjustability to fine tune the prosthesis as time requires.

The exoskeletal prosthesis is how all of my initial prostheses were made and it does have its advantages. The hard outer shell of the limb is laminated with an extremely durable acrylic or epoxy resin and if it is reinforced with layers of carbon graphite, then it can be nearly indestructible. The disadvantage of the exoskeletal prosthesis is its lack of adjustability. If the prosthesis is too long, then it is difficult to lengthen. If the alignment is not correct, then the leg should really be cut in half and moved then relaminated in order to correct it properly.

Endoskeletal systems (Figure 4-2) provide the prosthetist with the most complete and adjustable method of constructing a prosthesis. Most manufacturers have their own complete line of components and adapters and most systems are interchangeable with one another. Utilizing these systems has given the prosthetist an important tool to improve the gait of amputees by allowing for changes over time. **In my experience, the alignment of a prosthesis can change over a couple of days, a week, or even months. This is particularly true if a new foot is being used or there has been a change in the medical condition of the amputee.**

Types of Feet

As I mentioned previously, there were only 2 types of manufactured feet available to me when I lost my leg in 1974: the SACH foot and the Griesinger foot. Today, there are literally hundreds of feet to choose from and new ones coming out every year. All of them have advantages and disadvantages depending on their design. The only perfect foot was the one that you were born with, which combines motion, energy, and shock absorption. The trick in choosing the right foot is to talk with whoever is making your prosthesis and find out his or her recommendation. You will obtain the best prosthesis by using a foot that your prosthetist is either familiar with or is excited about trying. Each foot has its own optimal alignment and if your prosthetist is familiar with that foot, then he or she will be able to give you the best gait pattern. If your

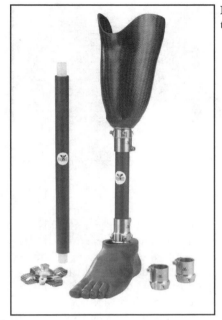

Figure 4-2. A typical endoskeletal system. (Photo courtesy of Ohio Willow Wood.)

prosthetist is trying a new foot, you should be aware that it may take a bit more time to arrive at an optimal alignment so be prepared to be patient.

Most feet fall into 5 categories: SACH, single axis, multiple axis, flexible keel, and dynamic response. All feet have a little of each of these qualities about them but for lack of better designation I will use these 5 divisions to try and describe what is available today. Please keep in mind that most feet were designed to accomplish a particular task and are generally very good at that task but may not be well suited for tasks that they were not designed for. I will list each category of foot and give some examples of each along with a photo or drawing to illustrate the function.

SACH Type Feet

The SACH style foot is the simplest, lightest foot that is available today (Figure 4-3). SACH stands for single axis cushion heel and is basically a lightweight rubber foot that has a soft cushion heel and a springy toe. It is designed for walking on even, smooth surfaces but does not perform well on rough ground. Most manufacturers of prosthetic feet produce a version of this foot; some have cosmetic toes and others have a rounded forefoot. They come in a variety of heel densities based on the weight of the patient. The SACH foot walks smoothly as long as the surface is flat; however, if the terrain becomes uneven, the foot tends to transfer the torque to the residual limb, which can cause pain in the socket. The spring off of the toe is minimal compared to other feet and tends to diminish over time as the rubber breaks down. The foot is easy to replace since it is attached by a screw that goes through the bottom of the foot and into the shank.

Figure 4-3. SACH (single axis cushion heel) foot. (Photo courtesy of Otto Bock Health Care.)

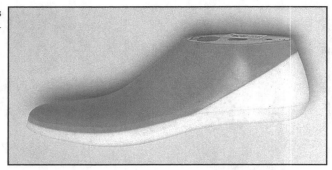

Single Axis Feet

The single axis foot is a mechanical foot that is hinged in the heel portion. This single axis of rotation that passes through the foot allows the heel to collapse quickly, giving the amputee a flatter foot during the rollover phase of gait. The amount that the heel compresses is regulated by a rubber bumper located inside the heel of the foot. This bumper cushions the heel and absorbs the impact of heel strike. There is also a bumper in the front of the axis that gives the foot some spring during the toe off portion of gait. These bumpers come in various densities that allow the foot to be adjusted for the amputee's weight or gait pattern.

The single axis foot works well on even ground and has advantages on incline surfaces such as walking up and down ramps. It is easy to walk on but does not provide any advantage on rough or uneven surfaces such as broken pavement, gravel, or trails. The torque that is generated by the uneven surface is transferred to the stump and can cause imbalance. This mechanical foot is one of the only feet that allows the amputee to move his or her toe up or down by pressing on the heel of the prosthesis. I knew a bilateral amputee who drove using these feet to press on the gas and brake. He also operated the toe levers of his small plane utilizing the same action. If you utilize a single axis foot, it is the only foot that can be used on the leg since part of the mechanism is inside the shank.

Multi-Axial Feet

The next category is the multi-axial foot (Figure 4-4), which as the name suggests, has motion in more than one plane. This foot was designed to try and simulate the motion of the ankle joint in the human leg. Multi-axial feet accomplish this with mechanical bumpers or springs and there are other classes of feet that use a flexible keel or split in the axis of the foot to simulate ankle motion. The purpose of this foot is to reduce some of the stresses that are usually transferred to the stump when the amputee is walking on rough terrain.

Most multi-axial feet use a single attachment point on the foot and then place springs or bumpers around that attachment point to simulate a moveable ankle. This allows the ankle to move in all directions, and the strength of the spring or bumper determines the movement of the foot in any particular direction. Springs or bumpers come in various densities to allow for different weights and activity levels.

The disadvantage of the multi-axial foot is the weight and maintenance issues that are associated with any mechanical foot. Springs and bumpers need maintenance and

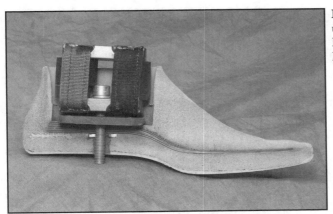

Figure 4-4. A multi-axial foot utilizing dual springs. (Photo by Dale Horkey; foot provided by DAS foot.)

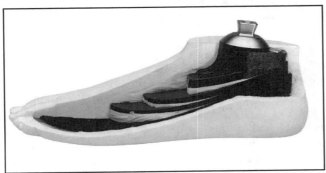

Figure 4-5. Cutaway of a flexible keel foot. (Photo courtesy of Ohio Willow Wood.)

replacement as well as the issue of dirt getting into the mechanisms due to the need to have a separate foot shell. The lip where the foot meets the shank allows dirt and dust as well as moisture to get into the mechanism.

Flexible Keel Feet

The flexible keel foot (Figure 4-5) uses the motion of the inside of the foot, the keel, to accomplish the same thing that the springs and bumpers do in the multi-axial foot. The keel of the foot is the hard, interior part of the foot that gives it structure and creates the place on the foot where the toe bends. Flexible keel feet use a bendable material inside the foot that allows for motion side to side as well as some spring off of the toe. In some feet there are bands that go from heel to toe that create more spring as they are stretched.

The big advantage of flexible keel feet are not only that they simulate ankle motion but they have no mechanical parts that need maintenance or replacement. They generally just screw onto the bottom of the shank of the leg like a SACH foot does and there is no protruding lip that can catch dirt or moisture. This is particularly advantageous when trying to finish the leg in a more cosmetic style. Covering a leg with either a premade skin or a direct bonding skin is much easier with the flexible keel foot since the seam at the ankle can be completely hidden.

Figure 4-6. A dynamic response foot that can adjust for high heels. (Photo courtesy of Freedom Innovations.)

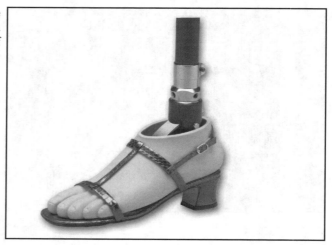

Dynamic Response Feet

The fifth class of foot is the energy storing type that is designed for aggressive activity, regardless of age. These feet generally utilize some type of carbon graphite material that acts like the leaf spring in an automobile. When the amputee puts weight on the prosthesis, the leaf spring is bent, storing the energy of compression. At the point of unweighting, the spring releases this stored energy and gives a push to the prosthesis that simulates the muscles of the leg pushing off of the toe. There are numerous designs for this category of feet (Figure 4-6), and most manufacturers have a version of the dynamic response foot. Some are better suited for high activity and others can be used on moderate activity amputees.

This type of foot became widely used in the last 10 years due to its light weight and the ability of the foot to put the spring back in the step of the amputee. The popularity of the foot increased with the combining of the energy storage with a multi-axial capability that gives the amputee the spring and torque absorption to optimize the comfort of the socket. This unique design was a radical departure from other prosthetic feet that had always bolted to the bottom of the shank. The dynamic response foot can be attached to the bottom of the socket therefore allowing the spring to be longer, which generates more push off of the toe. There are several different designs for the eversion and inversion (sideways ankle motion), but some of the most ingenious designs simply split the leaf spring into 2 parts, allowing the forefoot to move from side to side. Other designs utilize mechanical means to achieve this motion and one design just uses the motion of the foot inside the foot shell as a simulated ankle.

This type of foot is not for everyone. They are usually the most expensive type of foot and Medicare guidelines require a K-level of 3 or 4 in order to justify this foot. If the amputee is timid in his or her gait pattern, then there will not be enough loading of the prosthesis to get much of an energy return. In worse case scenarios, the amputee will actually fight the spring as he or she tries to roll over the toe, which can cause fatigue and torque to the socket. There are many different versions of this foot. Some can be screwed onto the bottom of the shank while others are attached at the socket. Dynamic response feet can be the lightest feeling since some of the weight of the foot

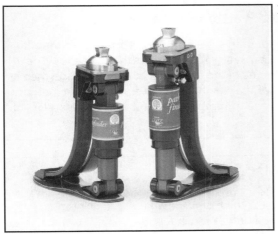

Figure 4-7. A shock absorber attached to a dynamic response foot. (Photo courtesy of Ohio Willow Wood.)

Figure 4-8. Another hybrid foot incorporating dynamic response, shock absorption, and multi-axial capability. (Photo courtesy of Ossur.)

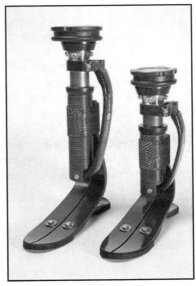

is distributed along the shank of the prosthesis instead of concentrated at the end. Cosmetically, this foot generally finishes very nicely either with premade skin covering or a custom skin, since there is no ankle joint there are no seams to cover.

These feet have also been mated with shock absorbers (Figure 4-7) that really diminish the impact on the residual limb under heavy loading. Shock absorbers can be separate components or part of a dynamic response foot (Figure 4-8). If you are routinely jumping off of heights, then this component can make a lot of difference in the comfort of the socket.

A Note About the Weight of the Foot

Keep in mind that the perceived weight of the foot is more important than the actual weight. A foot that gives spring back generally will feel lighter than one that is dead feeling. If the weight of the foot is distributed along the shank of the prosthesis, then it will feel lighter than one that concentrates the weight at the end of the leg. Remember the farther the weight is from the end of the stump, the heavier it will feel regardless of the actual weight.

Choosing the Right Foot

1.   Take the time to write down what type of activities that you want to participate in and how much of the time you expect to be engaged in these activities.
2.   Spend time with your prosthetist to find out which feet he or she is comfortable working with or is excited about trying.
3.   Talk to other amputees about the type of feet that they are wearing and get the pros and cons associated with wearing them. Try to find an amputee with similar interests or activities. Your local amputee support group is a great place to get this kind of information.
4.   Most likely you will only have one foot that needs to be able to function under all of the circumstances of your life. Make sure that the one you choose is suited for the majority of the time that you wear a prosthesis.
5.   Be aware of the manufacturer's warranty. Most of the manufacturers have a limited warranty that allows your prosthetist to return the foot at no cost. Make sure your prosthetist will work with you if you do not like the foot.
6.   Selling feet is big business. All of the manufacturers will tell you that they have the right foot for you. Treat manufacturers' information as sales literature not fact.

Connector Components

When you have a modular prosthesis (ie, one that generally has a pipe that connects the socket to the foot), it is important that each connector is of the highest quality. Even if you have the best foot in the world, if the piece that connects it to the socket is poorly made, then this weak link can cause catastrophic failure. All of the big manufacturers have a line of endoskeletal components with an array of connectors and adapters. They all prefer that the prosthetist use just their components, which are designed to fit together and have a warranted weight rating. Some systems have color-coded components that are designed for a particular weight or activity level. If you weigh 250 lbs and are fitted with components that are weight rated for 175 lbs, the manufacturer will not honor the warranty. Not only is the component unwarranted by the manufacturer, but there is the risk of the prosthesis breaking under stress.

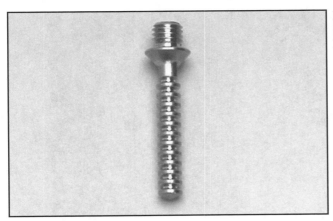

Figure 4-9. Shuttle lock system. (Photo courtesy of Otto Bock Health Care.)

Locking Liners and Shuttle Locks

One of the most popular means of suspending a prosthesis is to use the shuttle lock system (Figure 4-9) incorporating a locking liner (Figures 4-10 and 4-11). As I have explained previously, this system uses a roll-on liner that has some type of pin attached to the end of it. When your residual limb is inserted into the socket, the pin engages a shuttle lock mechanism that is fabricated into the bottom of the socket. The roll-on liner is designed to be form fitting with no gaps on your skin so it holds onto your stump because no air can get inside the liner. This system has 2 parts, the locking liner and the shuttle lock mechanism.

Locking mechanisms come in a wide variety of styles and materials. Some are all plastic, even the locking pins, while others use metal casings to increase durability. Each prosthetist has his or her own favorite type of locking mechanism that he or she likes to use for his or her clients, generally based upon previous success. All of them have pros and cons, but they all are not designed to get wet since they all have some type of metal mechanism that tends to rust or clog when submersed in water. These systems are not indicated for any water prostheses.

Suspension Sleeves

I have worn some type of suspension sleeve on my prosthesis for over 20 years and have tried most of the varieties and styles that are available. The first suspension sleeves were made from latex rubber. They were delicate and tore my skin up all of the time. Still, they were an improvement over the strap or wedge suspension. When the suspension sleeve did not have a hole in it, my prosthesis never felt more like a part of me. Suspension sleeves are designed to basically prevent any air from entering the socket, which creates a sort of suction environment inside the socket. If no air can enter the socket, your leg cannot come off because there is nothing to take the place of your stump. This type of suspension is very positive feeling and will significantly reduce the perceived weight of a prosthesis. **A leg always feels lighter when it is sucked onto you than if it is hanging off of you.**

Today, suspension sleeves come in a variety of shapes, colors, and materials. The most popular materials to use for a suspension sleeve are the same as for locking lin-

Figure 4-10. Silicone liners. (Photo courtesy of Ossur.)

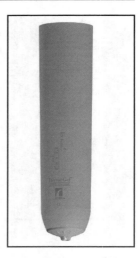

Figure 4-11. Gel liners. (Photo courtesy of Silipos.)

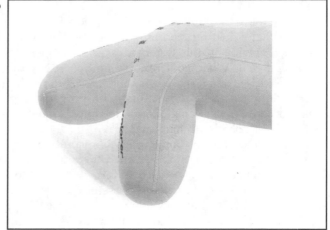

ers with the same advantages and disadvantages. Durability is a big issue if the suspension sleeve is the only suspension for the prosthesis. When a suspension sleeve gets a hole in it, the leg is no longer suspended by suction but by the structure of the fabric of the sleeve itself. You may not feel an immediate difference in the suspension but what occurs is that the friction of the material on the skin increases immensely, often causing damage. This damage looks like a rash and causes itching. What is going on is that the friction of the sleeve against the skin pulls the outer layer of skin off, exposing the delicate inner layer of skin. Combine that with the warm, dark, moist environment inside of a suspension sleeve and you have the perfect set-up for infection of the skin. If this is left untreated, it can get really ugly with complete skin breakdown and the inability to use the suspension sleeve until the skin heels.

There is also quite a difference in an individual amputee's ability to tolerate friction and containment of the skin. Some people can wear neoprene or latex next to their skin and have no reaction or abrasion as a result. Others cannot tolerate anything on the skin so it is important to judge the ability of each amputee as to his or her skin toughness. A few quick questions about his or her skin history will give all the information needed to make a decision as to which material will be most suitable.

Suspension Sleeve Advice

1. Choose a suspension sleeve based upon your skin tolerance and durability needs.
2. Rashes are common beneath suspension sleeves. **DO NOT SCRATCH!** Your fingernails are some of the dirtiest places on the human body and scratching a rash beneath your suspension sleeve will be sure to set up an infection.
3. Use hydrocortisone, an over-the-counter anti-itch cream, to take away the itch and provide a little lubricant to the friction of the sleeve.
4. If you start to get a rash, it means that you are either wearing a material that is irritating your skin or you have a hole in your suspension sleeve. Check for a hole in your suspension sleeve first. Usually the hole will be where the sleeve rubs against the top edge of the socket.
5. To minimize holes developing in your suspension sleeve, you need to soften the top edge of your socket. Your prosthetist can glue a piece of soft fabric over the edge or if you have a thin sock or nylon sheath, wear it as the last layer of whatever else you use in your socket and fold the top over the outside of the edge of the socket. This way when the sleeve rubs against the top edge of the socket, it will be buffered by the sock. This can improve the durability of the suspension sleeve by more than double.
6. Suspension sleeves can become very uncomfortable when sitting for long periods of time such as in a movie theater or an airplane where the knee is bent to 90 degrees. You may want to roll the sleeve down while seated for long periods of time.

Suction Devices and Air Bladders

There are several devices that can alter the shape or pressure within the socket. Suction suspension is a matter of preventing outside air from entering the prosthetic socket or eliminating air in the socket that allows motion of the residual limb inside the container. When there is little air in the socket, the stump only has friction when there is anatomical motion of the underlying muscle or articulation of the knee. The advantages of suction suspension are reduced friction and the highest sensation of the leg being part of the amputee. The prosthetic industry has come up with 2 devices designed to increase the suction in the socket by removing the air from the socket when using a suspension sleeve.

The first device is an expulsion valve that is part of the prosthetic socket. This type of valve has been in use in above-knee prostheses for many years. Today, several manufacturers produce valves especially for below-knee prostheses. When they function properly they are great, keeping a constant negative air pressure inside the socket. Many varieties are prone to clogging or need constant repair to keep them working on a daily basis. There are some simple designs that just screw into the socket and function without maintenance for years. My advice is if it looks complex, it probably is complex. The great thing about them is that if they quit functioning, you can just put a piece of tape over the valve intake in the socket and it is as if it wasn't there. There is also a company that has a one-way suction valve embedded in the suspension sleeve. If you want to get an idea of how suction with an expulsion valve feels, you can try one of these to see if you would like to have a valve placed in the socket.

There is another device that actually pumps air out of the socket using a small electric pump. The theory here is to stabilize the tissue inside the socket in order to accomplish the maximum benefits of the suction suspension. Like any auxiliary device, it depends on how much stuff you want to put up with and how heavy of a leg you are willing to wear.

Air bladders are inflatable nylon or plastic pouches that can be pumped up to accommodate changes inside the socket. They are great if the amputee is experiencing volume changes on a frequent basis. This is a great device if you are willing to deal with the added responsibility of managing your bladder. OK, I know that sounds bad and this does not indicate that I have poor bladder control despite all of the rumors and the inscriptions on bathroom walls. It comes down to what you are willing to work with on your prosthesis and how much stuff you can keep up with. Like the suction valve, if you get tired of the air bladder or it ceases to function, it is generally easy to remove.

Belts, Cuff Straps, and Thigh Lacers

Although these 3 components are being used less and less in the United States, there is still a place for them in prosthetics. There are many people who cannot wear suction type suspension because of skin problems, lack of hand strength, or excessive perspiration. Other than the supercondylar suspension that clamps above the knee of the amputee, these 3 suspension techniques can offer adequate holding even if there are compromises in comfort and cosmesis.

The waist belt with a Y-strap attachment is a very positive means of holding a prosthesis onto the body. If the belt is padded and lined with leather, then it is as comfortable as it can be. The problem is that the belt pulls on the pelvis and is prone to causing back discomfort. It also provides some extension assist at the knee, meaning that it helps the leg swing forward when you step, which causes the muscles that provide that action to weaken. I use a waist belt on several prostheses when I engage in sports to make sure that my leg does not slip or come off inadvertently. I have a removable waist belt with a Velcro inverted Y-strap that I can put on over top of my suspension sleeve when I play handball, climb ladders, or engage in any activity where my leg better not come off.

The cuff strap is another suspension system that is still used frequently, especially in warmer climates where perspiration creates problems with suction suspension. It is still the most widely used method of suspending a prosthesis worldwide. The big advantage of the cuff is that it is inexpensive and it allows for air to circulate throughout the socket, keeping the residual limb cooler than a suction system. These 2 factors are very important in warmer climates, especially in developing nations where the cost of suction suspension devices is prohibitive.

Thigh lacers is another method of suspension that is not seen very often anymore. The knee joints that connect the lacer to the prosthesis are typically made from metal although there are nylon hinges available as well. There is excessive movement of the stump inside the socket when the only suspension is the knee joint and thigh lacer. Most thigh lacer wearers also utilize a waist belt to help hold the prosthesis on since these types of legs end up weighing alot. I have a removable thigh lacer with nylon polycentric hinges that I can put over top of my suspension sleeve when I ski with a prosthesis. This allows substantial unweighting of the prosthesis as well as added control of my ski. One condition that may require a thigh lacer and knee joints is if the residual limb is very short or the knee is very unstable. The added stability of a thigh lacer can be the only way some amputees can wear a prosthesis.

Cosmetics

There are few advances in prosthetics that have made so dramatic an effect on the life of an amputee than those made in the finishing cover of a prosthesis. Some amputees do not care what their prostheses look like and leave them uncovered, allowing access to components or to minimize any added weight that a cover adds to the limb. There are some types of components that do not cover well, such as shock absorbers, and some dynamic response feet have protruding mechanisms that make covering difficult if not impossible.

If, however, you do care about how your leg looks, then you are living in a golden time of the art of prosthetics. Today, there are a variety of covers and skins that have a very lifelike appearance and are adequately durable to make them practical. Before a leg can have a cosmetic skin applied, it needs to be shaped to match the other leg. This is one of the skills of a prosthetist or technician that I still consider an art form. The shaper must know the type of foam that he or she is using and how much it compresses beneath the skin and whether it changes shape over time. I have seen beautifully shaped legs that left the lab and when the amputee came back 2 months later, the leg looked like it had been on a diet.

No one can make a prosthesis that looks exactly like the other leg. I say that because what a prosthesis cannot do is give and move like real tissue; therefore, shadows and contours that naturally occur on the real leg will not be duplicated on the prosthesis. What I learned through years of experience is that the human eye can be tricked into not noticing a prosthesis. As long as the amputee does not draw undue attention to his or her leg, the eye has no reason to scrutinize the cover. Even the most expensive cover cannot duplicate human skin, so the art of distraction from the prosthesis is very effective.

Prosthetic skin coverings have really come a long way in the past decade. Many manufacturers produce premade skin coverings that come in a variety of colors and shades that are designed to match as many skin colors as is economically feasible. These covers are made primarily from silicone, urethane, and fabric. The least skin-like material is fabric, which is just a nylon stocking that has a skin tone color to it. These are the least expensive and least durable, but they are easily replaced by just pulling the old one off and putting another one on, much like putting on hose (Figure 4-12). The other, more lifelike skins are much more difficult to apply and generally need to be put on by the prosthetist. There are off-of-the-shelf skins that are all one color; they are also not too expensive and will actually be reimbursed by insurance or Medicare. In addition to the off-of-the-shelf skins, there is a liquid skin that can be applied to the outer cover of a prosthesis that requires many hours of application. These custom applied skins are more cosmetic since the coloring can be changed to give a more lifelike appearance as well as hair, toenails, and veins. This type of skin takes days to apply and is not generally reimbursable by insurance although the finish is superior to a pull on cover.

Figure 4-12. Pull on cosmetic skin covering. (Photo courtesy of Alps South.)

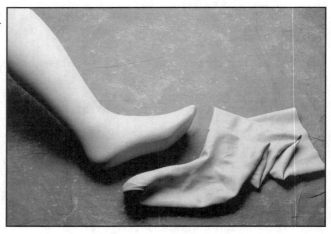

Figure 4-13. A custom silicone skin covering. (Photo courtesy of Artech.)

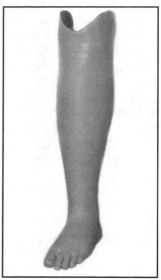

There are several companies here in the United States and around the world that specialize in cosmetic restoration. They usually use silicone as their skin material, which makes a tough, durable covering that is the most cosmetic type of skin available today. This type of skin has to be applied either at the company that makes it or by your prosthetist and these are also the most expensive type of skin coverings available. The prosthetist usually takes numerous pictures of the existing leg and sends them off to the manufacturer who fabricates the skin and ships it back. The silicone custom skins (Figure 4-13) look extremely lifelike but suffer from the same fate as all other skins: they cannot change to adapt to color differences or shading, so in some lighting the color ceases to match. The people who make these skins are real artists and most back up their product if the color is off.

CHAPTER 5

Other Types of Prostheses

My Story

I returned from my 2 years in Cairo, Egypt in the summer of 1978. I was determined to build a house on some land that I had purchased in rural Georgia, fulfilling a longstanding dream of mine. I had contacted my best college buddy, Eddy, who had volunteered to come to Georgia for the summer to help me with the construction for room and board. Room consisted of a tent in the woods and board was often what we could buy at the little country store at the crossroads. I bought a set of plans from the local lumberyard that turned out to be very similar to the plans that I had drawn while recovering from my neuroma surgery in the hospital in Greece. Eddy had worked in the construction industry so he had a little experience, but I really didn't have any idea what I was doing. Fortunately, my parents lived about 25 miles away and provided a lot of help as well as moral support for my ambition.

The lot that we were building on was located on a reservoir about 45 miles south of Atlanta in what was supposed to be a country club development but had gone bust. There was a clubhouse and a pool that provided us with a convenient place to wash up from time to time, but the rest of the infrastructure was crumbling. We went to work clearing the lot and preparing the footers for concrete. My prosthesis did not fit well and was beginning to give me problems, so I applied to the Georgia State Vocational Rehabilitation Program for assistance in getting a new prosthesis. I did not have a job at the time, and the agency bought a new leg for me that enabled me to work on the house as well as find a job with a nearby elementary school.

The land where we built the house was covered with poison ivy, ticks, and chiggers, making it a wonderful place to camp out each night. With help from my father and other professionals that owed my dad some favors, we made good progress and actually had the basement done and some walls put up by the end of July. Remember when I met the French girl, Brigette, in Paris during my friend Aaron's wedding? When I had last seen her on my way back home from Egypt, she had asked me if she could come visit me in America and of course I said yes. Well, she showed up at the end of July determined to marry me. Brigette was unprepared for life in the Georgia woods. There was no bidet (a toilet device that is very common in Europe) and she could not stand the instant coffee that was all we could make at our camp. Although she was very fit in all the right places, she was not much help on the construction.

One day we were working on the roof of the house, putting up the rafters. We would build each rafter on the second story loft, then walk them out along the 4 inch wide top plate to nail them in place. Brigette's job was to hold onto a piece of wood that stabilized the 180-kg (400-lb) rafter as we tight rope walked the narrow board with a 12 meter (40-ft) drop off to the ground below. As I mentioned before, I was wearing a supercondylar suspension leg that just clamped above my knee with no auxiliary waist belt. Right in the middle of walking along the top plate I caught my toe on a board and the next thing I know I am standing on one foot, 12 meters (40 ft) off of the ground, balancing on a 10 cm (4 in) wide board, and my leg is in a ditch beside the house. "Whoa," I called to Eddy and Brigette. I had to stand there and balance on the top-plate until Brigette could go down, find my leg, and bring it back up to me. From then on, I used my waist belt and strap to do any roof work. After a month of complaining about everything, I told Brigette that I was not going to marry her and she left. She came back a couple of months later, but I was still not going to marry her so she went off in search of some other American who would.

The summer ended and I got a job at a rural elementary school teaching fourth grade and science for the whole school. I really enjoyed my job working with the kids, but the same problem that plagued my scholastic career also followed me as a teacher. I spent a lot of time in the principal's office. I was a controversial teacher because I did controversial stuff with the kids. We went outside and took nature walks and I read them the *Lord of the Rings*. One afternoon I was called into the principal's office and confronted by one of the mothers of one of my 8-year-old students. She was making thinly veiled accusations about my sexuality because her son had sat on my knee during story time. I knew right then that teaching was not going to be a viable long-term job for me.

Eddy and I continued to work on the house, and I discovered that I could do just as much manual labor as anyone else—even with an artificial leg. I was sore and my stump would get blisters and abrasions on it, but it was nothing that I hadn't dealt with before. The satisfaction of watching a house take shape that I had built with my own hands was immeasurable and it gave me even more self-confidence. Eddy got a job working in a cabinet shop so we were able to go in and make all of the cabinets and a floor to ceiling bookcase at night when the shop was closed. The house was completed by the following spring, so I decided to get away from the project and go bicycling for a couple of months in Oregon and Washington. Eddy had lived there for a couple of years and knew people in Eugene, Oregon so off we went to see the West Coast and have some adventures.

Prior to the trip I had been into Atlanta Prosthetics for some adjustments and I asked Grant if he still was looking for an apprentice in prosthetics. He expressed surprise because when he had first asked me if I was interested, I said that it was the last thing I could think of doing. However, after working with my hands for a year on the house, I decided that I did have the hand skills necessary to make prostheses and saw it as a career that was very wide open. He agreed to take me on as an apprentice when I returned from my bicycle trip to the Northwest.

We arrived in Portland, Oregon at the beginning of June 1979, during the height of the oil embargo imposed by OPEC. The great thing about this fact was that there were very few recreational vehicles on the road and even the logging trucks were sparse. We bicycled along the coast of Oregon until we crossed the mountains into Eugene. At that time, it was like walking back in time to the '60s. We had a rather good time there, staying with friends of Eddy's and taking in all of the counter culture fun.

Eddy and I parted company, and I headed north to Seattle where I had several high school buddies who were living in the area. One day while bicycling along the eastern slope of the Cascade Mountains, I covered over 120 miles in 1 day, ending up on Mount Hood at the ski area. I was exhausted and could not find a place to stay. Again, I was lucky and met a young lady who offered to let me stay at her house for the night. One night turned into three and the break was badly needed as my stump was sore and had several ugly open areas on it. After I healed, I took off for Seattle and was able to hook up with my friends for a grand reunion.

At a cocktail party one evening at my friend's house, I met someone who told me about the Seattle Prosthetics Research Institute, which I had never heard of. I called them and arranged to go and visit the facility. There I met Dr. Ernest Burgess, one of the persons who motivated and encouraged my career in prosthetics, even offering to help me through school if I needed it. During my tour of the institute, I was shown a film of an amputee who had climbed Mt. Rainer. I said if he can do this thing, then I should be able to do it also. The prosthetist at the institute and the other professionals all agreed that I could not climb the mountain on the leg that I was wearing and that they would like to make me a sports prosthesis. I had never had any kind of specialized prosthesis before and really had no idea what it would be like. I got to spend a lot of time with the prosthetist and help him build the prosthesis, which was endoskeletal in design (I had only had exoskeletal or hard shell prostheses in the past). The foot was a Griesinger multiaxial foot with a rotator on the pylon that allowed 40 degrees of rotation in either direction with a friction adjustment. The socket had a partial silicone gel liner and a supercondylar socket design with the wedge above my knee. There was also metal knee hinges and a thigh lacer to take some of the pressure on my thigh, and this was all held on by a waist belt and inverted Y-strap. The leg weighed nearly 12 pounds but it had so much cushion and impact absorption, thanks to the thigh lacer, that I could jump directly onto the prosthesis without any discomfort.

With all of the wisdom of a lemming, I decided to make the climb the day after I received the new leg. One of my high school buddies, Joe, who is an experienced climber would escort me on my journey and make sure I got back in at least two pieces. Joe had lived out in the Seattle area for 3 years and had moved out with another good buddy of ours from high school named Mark. He and Mark did a lot of climbing in the Cascades. One day, they were making a particularly difficult climb when Mark, who was leading the pitch, told Joe to find another way around a rock outcropping. When Joe looked back to check on Mark, he was gone. Mark fell over 1500 feet into jagged rocks below. He never called out or made a sound; he just fell to his death. It took Joe hours to climb back down and get a search party where they found Mark's body the next morning. Joe had still not gotten over the trauma of the event and may never.

The ascent up Rainier went smoothly and we reached base camp at Camp Muir and I lay down exhausted. The camp was crowded with people waiting to make a summit attempt the next morning, so we found the only flat spot left and unrolled our sleeping bags. I took off my leg and much to my chagrin I find a small but growing blister on the tip of my stump in addition to a very large ugly blister on the heel of my good foot. I knew that tomorrow would require a lot of grit to get to the top. We were awakened at about 4:00 am by the crunch of crampons only inches from our faces as groups of climbers began the ascent to the top of the 14,000-ft mountain. We waited until sunup to begin our ascent, but as we packed our gear we were met by several groups of climbers coming down already. They had not made it to the top due to avalanche danger and said that park rangers were turning back any teams that were attempting to summit. I must admit that I was more than a little relieved at not being able to summit since putting on my leg was not a happy event and the blister on my good foot was killing me. Still, we had made it to the 10,000-ft camp and this was a major accomplishment for me.

Joe and I began our descent of Rainier, which was much more fun than the agonizing uphill climbs. Joe taught me how to do a standing glissade, which is when you stand up and slide down the slope. It's almost like skiing without the skis. We reached Paradise lodge where his car was parked and had an enormous breakfast, having regained our appetites, which had diminished with the altitude. I didn't know it but I had suffered my first case of altitude sickness: nausea, headache, and exhaustion. I could barely move for the next 3 days because my thigh muscles were so sore from hiking. I thought that I was in good shape after bicycling over 1500 miles in the mountains, but climbing muscles and bicycling muscles are totally different. After 3 days, the blisters had healed and the muscles had calmed down enough that I could get off of the crutches. Only because I was young and more than a little stupid would I engage in an activity where I had to be on crutches for 3 days to recover. Even with the specialized sports prosthesis I paid a high price for the activity, but I realized that this could be done and that with the proper equipment the price didn't have to be crutches.

The summer of 1979 had been magical, but it was time to return to Atlanta and begin my apprenticeship as a prosthetist. I had to commute for 80 km (50 miles) one-way until I found a room in a house with 5 Georgia Tech Engineering students. Even though I was the most educated person in the prosthetic facility, I still had to do all of the crummy jobs that no one else wanted to do. After all I was the "new guy" and I had to show that I was not above the dirty work. I learned a lot from all of the old guys, even how to make an articulating foot from wood and leather. The health considerations in the facility left a lot to be desired. There were 5 prosthetists working in one room, each with a bench where we laminated polyester and acrylic resins as well as using glues and solvents. It got to the point where I could not smell the stuff anymore. That's when I knew it was bad.

I had been working there for about 3 months when one of the prosthetists set me up on a blind date with a friend of his wife. We went on a hike with our dogs and discovered that we had a great deal in common. We each had a house, car, dog, steady job, as well as we had both attended Miami University of Ohio but did not know each other there. Our fathers had even both worked for the BF Goodrich Company for their entire careers. This just seemed too coincidental and 6 months later we were married. Jane had a great job as a systems programmer for the telephone company and her house was in a nice suburb of Atlanta. I liked married life and thought that we could raise a nice family and live happily ever after. I went off to prosthetics school the following fall. Jane came along and we got an apartment on the north end of Chicago.

School was tough for me, as it had always been. I got a job working in the research department at Northwestern and worked there after classes. Jane got a job with the computer department at Loyola University and suffered through my struggles with school. I met some very significant people in my prosthetic class, which only had 20 people in it. My best buddy was another amputee named Greg who was equally as crazy as I was and we managed to conjure up a bit of trouble from time to time. One night after we had been sampling a lot of the local brew, we returned to the old dorms where Greg was staying to partake of the ancient steam room in the basement. Greg and I hopped into the long narrow room that is completely tiled and plopped down on the bench. After a little drunken conversation, Greg got this look on his face and all of a sudden hopped up and took about 3 giant leaps before landing on his belly to slide the length of the steam room on his stomach. He did a perfect slide, crashing into the wall at the far end of the room. He hopped up to my triumphant calls only to find that he had hit his chin on impact and had split it wide open. Blood was everywhere. Several stitches later, he was OK. Greg saved me from injury because I was going to be next on the steam room slip and slide.

There was a really different guy who was in our class named Dan. Dan had lost his leg below the knee in a boating accident and was apprenticing in a facility in Michigan. He would ride to class using a large above-knee stump sock as a stocking cap and pretty much kept to himself. He was very spiritual, but it was agreed that Dan was really out there. Out there he was, because Dan is credited with inventing the Flexfoot (Ossur, USA), which revolutionized prosthetic feet. He saw something that the rest of us did not. To me, a foot was something that you screwed onto the bottom of the shank of the leg. Dan made the leap by attaching the foot to the bottom of the socket. This innovation changed our profession and it really demonstrates someone thinking out of the box.

At that time there were 3 instructors for the class. The head of the prosthetic training was Axel, a man who immigrated to the United States and had been trained in the German system. In Germany, the education for a prosthetist is quite a bit more involved than here in the United States. A prosthetist must receive his or her education and then serve a 4-year residency program. The entire education can take as long as 8 years. Axel was a real inspiration to the class. He was very strict and demanding but had a great sense of humor. I learned a great deal about patient evaluation and care from him. Our other 2 instructors were Colin and Jack, who had very different teaching styles. Colin, who has since gone on to be an outstanding contributor to our profession, had a very academic style based on research and study. Jack was his antithesis—long hair and a kind of counter culture style, a very laid-back way of teaching. I felt that we got the most information that was available in this country between the 3 instructors.

We had to make legs in class so the school used professional amputees who would spend all day getting casted and fitted for us students. These professional amputees were hardly the cream of Chicago society since they were paid a stipend of $15 per day, which averaged about $2 an hour plus a free lunch. Needless to say, these people had nothing better to do. One day my patient did not show up so I had to double up on one of the other patients. The next morning, the no-show patient was waiting at the school entry on crutches. When I saw him, I asked why he hadn't been there the day before and where was his leg? He told me that he had been in his favorite bar the previous evening and after having way too much whiskey he began to brag about his leg. Apparently, he told the bartender in a too loud voice how he kept his money hidden in his prosthesis. This must have been overheard by a couple of enterprising young criminals who were waiting for him in the alley outside of the bar. As he staggered down the alley, they tackled him and stole his leg, leaving him bruised and battered in a trashcan. When he came to, he hopped to the bar and they sent him home in a cab. We actually made our first functional leg that day. The lesson here is if you are going to hide things in your leg, don't get really drunk and tell everyone in the bar about it.

I started playing handball again in Chicago. Both of the guys that I worked with in the research department were avid handball players, so we would sneak over to the courts and get in a few games from time to time. I discovered that even though I seldom won, I could hold my own, even against Carl who was a very good player. Mark, who was the head of the research department, was very sympathetic to my school situation. When there wasn't anything pressing for me to work on, Mark would let me study. I am very grateful for his support. I was having a lot of trouble with my prosthesis not holding up to the rigors of the sport. My feet were constantly breaking under the stress of high activity. I got to try 2 feet that were in the early stages of development at that time. The first was a prototype SAFE foot, which is a flexible keel, multiaxial foot with no moving parts. I loved the way it performed for the entire 3 days it lasted before the keel shattered. The second one was the prototype SEATTLE foot that only lasted 1 day on the handball court before the carbon graphite keel shattered. It was fun being a guinea pig for new stuff, but I was a bit dismayed at the durability of these feet. My feedback caused both feet to have different materials in their eventual production versions.

After more than 5 months at school, we had completed our certificate program and were eligible to sit for our written exam. Since the information was very fresh in my mind, I had no trouble with the exam; however, the words of Axel proved to be prophetic. On my final evaluation he told me that I would be a fine prosthetist but that I may have trouble passing my exam. I bid farewell to Chicago, and Jane and I returned to Georgia for Christmas.

I returned to my job at Atlanta Prosthetics after completing my certificate program. I still had to apprentice for another year before I would be eligible to sit for my oral and written parts, which upon passing would make me a Certified Prosthetist. In my work in Atlanta I had met a physical therapist named Jenny who worked for Emory University. I offered to teach an amputee yoga class for her patients so we started to get together once a week for yoga. The group had about 10 people and we started a routine of going out for a beer after class. This was so much fun that we decided to do some other activities as well. The first was tennis since Jenny was an avid tennis player. One afternoon while we were playing tennis on the Emory courts, I went after a side shot and all of a sudden I heard a loud crack. I felt as if I had stepped into a deep hole. When I looked down, my leg was in two pieces. The tennis shoe was still on the foot but it was 3 ft away from the rest of me. The tennis players on the court next to me were in shock at the guy whose leg broke in half and he was laughing. I could see that if I was to continue to engage in sports, I was going to have to come up with a more sturdy design. Only a prosthetist could maintain this kind of active lifestyle and afford to keep himself in legs.

The after yoga class activities became so much fun that we decided to organize ourselves into a club of some sorts. I had heard of the National Handicapped Sports Association while I was in school so I contacted them. We became a chapter of this organization in the spring of 1982. Since the national organization primarily promoted skiing, we decided to attempt a skiing program of our own at Beech Mountain in North Carolina. We raised money by having cookouts and solicited funds from various charitable organizations in the area. The club attracted persons with many different disabilities and we learned that **it's not what you have that matters, its what you do with what you have that makes life rich.** We played something all year around. In the summer we had a disabled softball team. This was really a blast because the blind guys were always the umpires and some of the adaptations we had to make made the game very interesting. Bottom line on these activities was that they were just regular softball or bowling or whatever else we did. People laughed, they argued about the calls, they swore, they cried, they told stories, and some of them drank a little too much. Just like normal people. That was the point and I think all of us grew from the experience. I feel privileged to have gotten to know such inspiring persons such as Al, Reggie, Eugene, Dee Dee, Joe, Jenny, Dave, David, Debra, and all of the others that my old memory cannot remember. My life is all the more rich for the experience.

During the summer of 1982, I experienced a problem at work. I was continually coming into conflict with one of the owners at Atlanta Prosthetics. After one such confrontation, I decided that the personality mix was just not going to work and they were not likely to side with me over the owner so I left Atlanta Prosthetics. I was able to work with another local firm named Georgia Prosthetics who allowed me to basically do contract work for them. This gave me the responsibility of my own patient load as well as the freedom to continue to organize the Atlanta Handicapped Sports Association.

My oral and practical prosthetic exams were in the fall and I went to Chicago to take them, full of confidence and maybe a bit cocky. I breezed through my oral with no problem because talking in front of people has always come easily for me. The practical exam at that time consisted of walking into a prosthetic lab and drawing a number out of a hat. That number corresponded to a bench with a patient sitting at it. By the end of the day, you had to make that person a prosthesis that functioned. I drew the only arm out of 20 amputees and since I had plenty of experience with arms, I was not too concerned. I was done early and even had the opportunity to put a final lamination on the arm. When the evaluators came to ask me questions about the arm and my client, I thought I answered them well but I was probably a little arrogant. I left the exam believing that I had aced it and returned to Atlanta to resume my work.

Axel was right. I had flunked my practical exam, something that was unimaginable to me. I had said all the right things, but I believe my attitude was cocky and the evaluators just didn't like my style. The exam was to be given again in Memphis, Tenn in 6 months so I steeled myself to return and do better. Meanwhile, I dove into my work with my clients and the Handicapped Sports Association. Six months later I returned to the exam and against all probability, I drew the one arm out of 20 again. This time I actually didn't do as good of a job as I did the first time, but I took my time and was terribly humble. I passed. Big lesson here. Sometimes it is not what you know but how you come across that makes the difference between communication and lack of understanding.

That winter I attended the big handicapped winter festival at Winter Park, Colorado. I competed in the downhill events and was talked into trying cross-country skiing. I met hundreds of amputees, many of whom were doing much more than I. Up until this point I had thought that I was one of the most accomplished amputee athletes out there. Boy was I wrong. I didn't do well in the downhill events, but I actually won a medal in the Nordic event, primarily due to the fact that there were only 4 competitors in my class. I was in good shape but I had no clue how to ski on these skinny, long skis that seemed to just slip everywhere. I must have fallen 20 times in the little 1.5 km (1 mile) course. There was only 1 bump, barely a meter (3 ft) tall, that I just could not seem to get over. A paraplegic in a pulk who was poling with his arms only passed me. This was humiliating and as I crossed the finish line, I stumbled, fell, and had to crawl the rest of the way. I found myself leaning over a split-rail fence barfing and hacking from the exertion at 10,000 feet altitude. I looked up and saw this skinny guy with a big grin on his face shoving a bottle of champagne at me. I took a drink that immediately came back up, but I had found a friend for life. Tommy had been cross-country skiing for years and was quite good even then. He is a congenital amputee who has a stump about the size of my thumb and until I started making his legs, I never knew what held his legs on.

I returned from the ski event with great enthusiasm to continue with the disabled sports programs and to pursue my career as a prosthetist. I began to work with amputees from other parts of the United States due to my exposure at ski events. This was an important step for me since it was at this time that I developed many of the strategies for making prostheses that helped to make my business strong. This was also about the time that I made a tremendous leap in my professionalism. After coming out of school and especially after becoming certified, I had the mistaken impression that I knew something. I told amputees what they needed and they believed me. One day, I can't remember exactly when, I realized that I didn't know anything. **There is only one person who knows about his or her amputation and that is the client. I had been ignoring the most important source of information that existed. The amputee him- or herself knew more about what he or she wanted and needed than I ever would.** I now embarked on developing strategies that would elicit information from my clients using my skills as a teacher. Most clients do not have a sophisticated strategy or vocabulary to describe what they need or what is happening to them, so I felt that it was my job to help them communicate. The more that I worked at getting information from my clients, the easier it got until I had a series of questions that permitted the amputee to focus on his or her problems and describe it in a way that would clue me in on how to solve them.

My personal life was busy with work, the Handicapped Sports Organization, and shuffling each weekend to my house in the woods. Jane and I had a typically dysfunctional relationship. I still had lots of pain due to my activity level and tended to take it out on her when I got home. She would endure it in silence since she was the type of person who internalized things. I would rage at the world and at her whenever I got frustrated at things. Even if I wasn't directly angry with her, she got the fallout if she was in the vicinity. It was not a healthy way for me to behave, and I had developed complex mechanisms to defend myself against any dissonant feedback that caused me to take responsibility for my actions. This caused us to begin to emotionally distance ourselves from one another, and I began to seek affection outside of my marriage. Again, I justified this in my own mind because of my amputation. I deserved lots of breaks, if not physically than emotionally. This was a mental trap that I was stuck in for many years of my life. I behaved poorly and expected people around me to "deal with it" since I was a "poor amputee." I had forgotten what my prosthetics instructor had told me about the psychology of the amputee, and I was certainly being a jerk.

I was also making a huge mistake with my marriage by allowing all sorts of friends who were in need to live in our house with us. My motivation for this was generosity but what happened was that it set up a circumstance in which Jane and I never dealt with our own problems. We were always dealing with the problems of others. This was an easy dodge since the people staying with me were always in crisis and I am good in a crisis, something that I discovered when my leg was cut off. What I didn't realize was that I was creating crises so that I would not have to deal with my marriage or myself. I don't know if this was due to being an amputee, but I know that these mechanisms for selfishness were justified by my disability and I used them without regard for who got hurt. This was the same justification I had used when I was single and would hurt women who loved me without any thought for their feelings. I share these thoughts in the hopes that someone will recognize similar patterns in their lives and make fewer mistakes than I made.

The Atlanta Handicapped Sports Association began as just a couple of us disabled people getting together to have fun. Within a year, we had grown to a full-blown organization with programs all year long. Our membership was over 100 persons with all types of disability. I had never spent any time with people in wheelchairs or the blind and was astounded at the zest for life that most of them displayed. Not only did they not feel sorry for themselves, they lived and loved life more than most. It was hard for me to fall back on feeling sorry for myself when I was surrounded by inspiring people who took the time to still be thoughtful and courteous. We had all kinds of strategies for fundraising. One was to sell tickets to professional sporting events in Atlanta and then have a sports demonstration prior to the event. We first did this with the Atlanta Braves back when they could not give away tickets to the games. Our group would get a block of tickets to a Braves game and have a disabled softball exhibition prior to the game. It was really fun and exciting to get to play on the professional field.

Another activity that we participated in was basketball. There was already a wheelchair basketball organization, but we played stand up ball for amputees. This was very rough on amputees since all of us were leg amputees and running up and down the court was brutal. Our team was quite good, mainly due to the skills of 2 of our players, Al and Reggie. They are both African American guys and really had a feel for the game. I was a point guard since I could run faster than anyone else on our team. Unfortunately, I am a terrible basketball player. I was a wrestler and had fundamental problems with a sport where I couldn't grab someone. It was baffling to me. I would get a clean takedown on a guy and they would give him 2 points. Al and Reggie were always passing me the ball without looking at me. I don't know how many times I got smacked in the face by passes that I didn't know were coming. They later explained that the point of the game was to not telegraph your moves. Nonetheless, we won the national championship in the U.S. Amputee Athletic Association 2 years in a row. This sounds impressive until you realize that there were only 3 other amputee basketball teams in the United States. We did get to have fundraisers with the Atlanta Hawks where we sold tickets to the Hawks games. Prior to the games we would put on an exhibition against some local radio station teams who were really good. It did however impress some of the pros and on several occasions we had celebrities such as Larry Bird and Danny Ainge show up at our after game parties. We even got to meet the famous singer James Brown once as he was preparing to sing the national anthem prior to a game.

Our biggest program was our ski program that we held at Beech Mountain in North Carolina, about a 6 hour drive from Atlanta. Our second season we had the honor of hosting the first Handicapped Ski Clinic sponsored by the National Handicapped Sports and Recreation Association, our parent organization. Eight clinicians showed up to teach us how to ski. I didn't know it at the time but some of these people would become lifelong friends.

I was skiing with my prosthesis using an auxiliary waist belt to help hold it on and carry some of the weight of the heavy ski equipment. I thought that I was pretty hot, having picked up the skill of skiing quickly. One day, halfway through a run, I decided to try getting air by flying over a little bump at the end of the run. I got airborne alright; it was the landing that I did not do well on. As I crashed, I heard a loud crack and felt a blindingly sharp pain in my stump. I was sure that I had broken my stump. I laid in the snow for a few moments until the pain diminished to a tolerable level and when I took off my prosthesis, I found that it had broken and not my stump. The side-wall of the socket was broken all the way across so that the leg could not suspend without the auxiliary waist belt. For the rest of the time, I 3-track skied with outriggers that were actually easier to use than the prosthesis. I realized that in order to comfortably ski with a prosthesis I was going to have to come up with something more innovative than my old supercondylar suspension leg with a multiaxial foot. At that time, there just wasn't the technology available nor did I possess the skills to create a viable ski leg, which was years in the future.

Another significant event that occurred at this ski event was more psychological than physical. Like I mentioned earlier, I had developed a powerful internal mechanism that allowed me to ignore negative feedback about myself because of what had happened to me. Whenever people would express their displeasure at some of my more unpleasant personality traits, I would say that they did not know what it was like to be an amputee and even if I didn't say it out loud, I would think it. One night when I was ordering people around and generally being abusive, one of the clinicians named Doug turned and said to me, "Riley, you are really a *&^*%^ sometimes." I immediately prepared to come back with my standard reply when I realized that not only did he know what it was like to be an amputee, being a Vietnam vet he had actually been through a lot more than I. **Something clicked in my brain. For the first time in a long time, I realized that I was responsible for how I treated people and my disability was no excuse to treat people poorly.**

The winter National games in 1983 were held in Squaw Valley, California and I attended along with several other members of the Atlanta group. I had recently been elected to be the East Coast Vice President of the National organization so in addition to competing in the Nordic events, I attended the board meeting where I learned more of how the organization worked. Again, due to the lack of competition, I won medals in the cross-country races and was chosen to be a member of the first Nordic Ski team that the United States had ever sent to the Olympics. The Olympics would be in Austria the following year and we would have to raise our own money, but this was a great honor for me. This was also the first time that I had ever been to California or the Sierra Nevada mountains, little realizing that in the future I would call this place home.

I am telling my story in the hopes that it will reveal the human side of amputation. If you are an amputee or even if you're not, you may recognize character traits that you may share or recognize in others. My journey through life has been full of mistakes, mostly through ignorance as opposed to outright maliciousness, but the results are the same. I still struggle with emotions that I can't quite explain and I still manifest frustration as well as anger when it is not warranted. I get down on myself for my failings, but I can still muster the strength to pick myself back up and keep trying to be the best that I can be. I think that this comes from a deep sense of underlying faith in God and my fellow man, which if you have it, you know what I mean. Well, enough of this serious psychological stuff. I don't pretend to be a psychologist or a counselor, but I thought it was important to share the evolution of my perceptions of my disability.

Backup Prostheses

Not every amputee has a backup prosthesis. I would like to argue that the backup prosthesis is as essential to an amputee's life as the spare tire is to your car. You rarely think about it until you need it, but if you have a flat in the middle of nowhere, you are awfully glad that you have a spare tire that functions. Most backup prostheses are made from the leftover components of old prostheses and are put together to allow the amputee to have a functional prosthesis when something happens to the regular limb.

There are a few agencies that recognize the necessity of the amputee having a backup prosthesis, but most insurances and Medicare make no provision for any type of other prosthetic device. The Veterans Administration is the only federal agency that will pay for a backup prosthesis but they rarely offer this to their amputees due to their budgetary constraints. It is up to the amputee to request the backup limb and then usually fight the system to get it. In the '90s, some state agencies such as vocational rehabilitation or state-funded rehabilitation would pay for backup prostheses but this has also diminished.

Shower, Swim, and Scuba Prostheses

The most dangerous daily activity that any amputee does each day is deal with the shower or tub. Showers are slippery and when you slip on a prosthesis, you often cannot feel it until it has already slipped out from under you. Most amputees either use a shower stool or hop on one foot in the shower, probably one of the most dangerous actions that amputees engage in aside from javelin catching.

I've got to tell you my shower stories. While I was hopping to the toilet one night, I encountered the slip rug on the linoleum floor. My foot went out from under me and I immediately stepped out to stop my fall. Unfortunately, there was no foot on the end of that leg and I came down hard on the end of my stump. This really hurt so I vowed to never do that again. It was several years later that I was in my apartment in college, again hopping in the shower and leaning over too much to grab the shampoo. I began to slip on the slick tub floor but this time I remembered to sling my leg backwards so as to not hit the end of my stump as I came down. Unfortunately, I had my back to the shower and as I slung my stump back to avoid the tub impact the end of my stump cracked against the protruding faucet. Wow! That pain floored me. I must have lain in the tub for an hour moaning. What is the answer? Never take a shower?

For many amputees, the answer is the shower stool or to take a bath. If there is a rail beside the tub, then it is safest to sit on the side of the tub, take off the prosthesis, then scoot over onto the shower stool and wash one's self. After drying one's self, the prosthesis can be put back on and the danger of falling is minimum. What do you do if there is no tub, nothing to hold onto, just a shower stall? Again, the shower stool can be used to sit down and take off the leg and then when you are dry you can put the prosthesis back on. There are problems with the whole shower stool method. One is that if the rest of the shower is not laid out for the amputee, it may be difficult to reach the soap, shampoo, or your rubber ducky. Also, every shower stool that I have ever found is made with 4 aluminum legs and a plastic seat. All shower stalls have floors that are uneven, which is necessary to have the water drain, the result being that at any given time one of the shower stool legs is not on the floor. This stresses the rest

Figure 5-1. Swimming prosthesis with swim/walk ankle. (Photo courtesy of Rampro.)

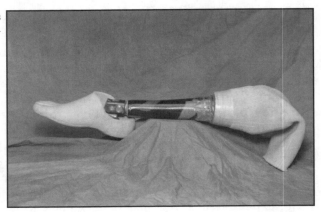

of the legs that are screwed into the plastic and eventually the legs will give out and break away from the stool. This usually occurs when you plop down on the stool or, in my case, when I rested my knee on it. Bathtubs are more conducive to shower stools since the legs of the stool tend to rest more evenly on the floor. Rails are really essential for any amputee in the bathroom. I have them by the toilet and in the shower. One of the most effective rails I have ever used has been the overhead rail, which will keep you from falling even if both feet have slipped out from under you.

What do you do when you travel? If you are staying at a hotel or motel, they will often have handicapped accessible rooms that have extra large showers to accommodate a wheelchair and even some rails to hold onto. What do you do if the place you are staying doesn't have an accessible room or you are staying with relatives or friends? For me, the answer has been to have a shower leg. A shower leg is a simple prosthesis that is designed to receive minimal damage when it gets wet. I have made many shower limbs, using either an existing socket or a new one fabricated specifically for this function. I like to have a pelite (soft white foam) insert inside so that it can be worn with no sock or liner if necessary. I use a SAFE II waterproof foot (Foresee Orthopedic Products, Oakdale, CA) that gives good traction on slick surfaces. Sometimes I even melt a tread pattern onto the bottom with a hot knife and this gives the best traction. I use a suspension sleeve that is as waterproof as possible, and I find that if I hang the leg upside down after use, the suspension sleeve dries rapidly.

The shower leg allows an amputee to stand in the shower, freeing up both hands. What a concept! For the first time since I had become an amputee, I was able to wash my hair with both hands. This may not sound important but if you are an amputee this frees you to be able to travel anywhere secure in the knowledge that you will be able to negotiate any bathroom with a minimum of danger. The shower prosthesis also comes in handy when you want to walk to the hot tub or pool. If there are no metal parts in the leg, then it can be submerged into water either in a pool, lake, or sea.

There are specific prosthetic devices made for swimming or diving. The main one is the swim/walk ankle that with the push of a button or turn of a switch will allow the foot to completely plantar flex (straighten out so that the foot will have a kick to it) (Figure 5-1). I have done a lot of swimming without a prosthesis but find that I have to swim a bit harder to compensate for the lack of kick on the amputated side. I also pull a little harder with the opposite arm to correct single kick stroke. This is OK for swimming laps or just playing around in the pool; however, when I dive I find that I need the kick from the other leg. What happens to me without the scuba leg is that I have to kick twice as hard as the next guy and that I use up my air much faster. The ability to kick evenly with both legs makes diving much more enjoyable and getting in and out of the boat much safer. Another adaptation that I make to any leg that I want to submerge into water is that I wear a double suspension sleeve. The deeper that I go, the more pressure there is to force water beneath the sleeve. By wearing two I have dove to over 100 ft with no leakage under the sleeve. I used to duct tape the suspension sleeve to my thigh but this is very painful when you removed it. Underwater diving is one of the coolest things I have ever done, and with the right equipment there is no disadvantage to having 1 leg. I describe the experience as being on another planet and being able to fly.

Swim/walk ankles are available from at least 2 companies with which I am familiar and any prosthetist can obtain them. They are expensive and generally not reimbursable so be prepared to pay for this item if it is something you will use a lot. If you can't afford to have a specific leg just for diving but have a water leg, there is an adaptation that is easy and inexpensive. All you need is a foot bolt wrench and some duct tape. Unscrew the foot from the end of the prosthesis and remove the foot bolt from the foot. Screw the bolt back into the shank of the leg and tape around it as best as possible to prevent water from getting up inside the bolthole. Take the flipper and slide it onto the shank of the prosthesis until it is snug against the end of the leg. Tape the flipper to the shank of the leg, being generous with the tape to make sure that your flipper doesn't come off when you are over top of a 1000-meter (3000-ft) trench. This works great for the diving part but of course is worthless for climbing back into the boat after your dive. Still, this adaptation will function well and allow you to enjoy the incredible sport of diving. If this becomes a passion, then it justifies the expense of a specific prosthesis.

Running Prostheses

One of the most popular types of sports prostheses available is running limbs (Figure 5-2). These legs are designed specifically to run or sprint on and are not suitable for walking since there is no heel portion to the leg. There is a completely different dynamic of the leg when a normal person runs. As the speed of a person's gait increases, the feet start to come together with each stride. At a full run, the human foot tracks right on top of the other foot so that the distance between the feet moves to nothing, meaning that when you run, your feet track one on top of another instead of a walking gait in which there is space between the feet. The normal human foot compensates for this by turning the toe out more to accommodate the narrowness of the foot position. Unfortunately, the prosthetic foot cannot change the angle of toe-out, so if you run on a leg that was set up and aligned for walking, your toe will point inward as you pick up speed. This is alright if you are just jogging or if you have to run across the street or something. It is not acceptable if you plan on running for exercise or competitively.

Running is a tough activity while wearing a prosthesis even if you have a specific limb just for that purpose. Conditioning of the rest of the body is essential. Do not expect to pick up running as an amputee if you never did it when you had 2 legs. This

Figure 5-2. Sprinters with running prostheses. (Photo courtesy of Ossur.)

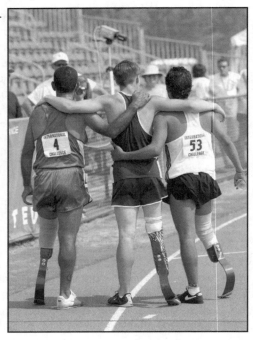

is advice that I did not follow so I'll tell the story. It was the summer of 1983 and I was in training for the U.S. Nordic Ski Team, so I was in excellent physical condition. I had a leg that used a SACH foot with a latex suspension sleeve and an auxiliary waist belt to provide suspension when perspiration caused the sleeve to slip. I was experimenting with liner materials and had just come across this stuff called Sorbithane that was supposed to absorb impact. As I began to jog, I noticed that the end of my stump would get sore and then would burn as if it was on fire. I had committed to running a 10K (6.25 mile) race in Atlanta called the Peachtree Road Race in the summer of 1983 as a way of getting in shape for the 1984 Olympics, in which I was to compete. I had been running up to 8K or 9K at a time and although it really made my stump sore, it was bearable.

On the day of the race, I was pumped up and ready to go along with the 30,000 other people. The previous evening's local news program had aired an interview of myself as well as some other special people running that year. The first part of the race was easy since I couldn't run very fast because of all of the people. By the ninth kilometer (fifth mile), I was hurting and wondered if this was really such a good idea. Just then we rounded the corner into the park where the last kilometer wound past cheering crowds of people, some of whom recognized me from the TV interview the night before. As people started to cheer and call to me by name, the pain ceased and I started to pick up my pace. I sprinted the last half of a kilometer (third of a mile), passing a hundred people and feeling no pain. I crossed the finish line at a gallop and as I slowed, the pain returned to my stump, a burn that I had never experienced before. I knew I was in trouble. I sat down as close to the beer tents as possible and talked someone into getting me a couple of beers. I took off my leg. To my dismay, the entire end of my stump was a giant blister.

I could not wear my leg at all and spent the next couple of days on crutches. I gave a lecture at a local hospital and while I was there I ran into a doctor friend of mine who noticing my severe limp, offered to take a look at my stump. He cringed as he saw the huge blister that was the end of my stump and took a culture of the drainage that oozed out from the skin. The next day he called me personally and demanded that I come and see him in his office immediately. When I arrived, he told me that I had a nasty staph infection in the fluid and he cut the huge blister from the end of my stump. I couldn't believe the thickness of the callous that he cut off; it was at least 0.5 cm (0.25 in) thick and very rigid. The skin beneath the callous was dark and very weepy and was beyond belief painful to the touch. I then began the task of healing this open wound at the end of my stump. I could not wear my leg for over 3 months while the skin healed. The physical therapy that I went through was pure hell as they debrided the wound 4 times a week then applied a pressure dressing to promote skin healing.

I tell this story to illustrate the importance of having a prosthesis that is designed to protect your residual limb during the intense activity of running. In the early '80s, there were no shock absorbing feet or special running legs. I can run on any of my energy storing legs or my dynamic response prostheses without damage to my stump. The rest of me complains, but the stump is fine. This is a great achievement to our profession; technology has come this far to allow such a difficult activity to become a routine part of some amputee's lives. Top runners utilize energy storing feet that are specifically designed for the sport. The graphite pylon that extends from the socket has no heal component since in sprinting the runner is always on his or her toe. There are commercially available running feet from several manufacturers, but this is generally an item that is not covered by insurance. Shock absorbers are a natural component to consider when designing a leg for running

Suspension for running limbs runs the full range from custom double cuff straps to suspension sleeve and suction devices. Most runners use some type of gel, urethane, or silicone liner to reduce friction to the skin. It is my experience that the length of stump is a factor in successful long-term enjoyment of running. If the residual limb is short or scarred, it does not present much room to absorb impact or sheer forces. This does not mean that running is not possible or recommended for amputees with short or difficult stumps; it just means that it will be more difficult. An option for amputees with less than optimal residual limbs is to add a removable thigh lacer that will reduce the impact forces on the end of the stump and transfer them to the thigh.

Golf Prostheses

It is not necessary to have a specific prosthesis to enjoy the game of golf. I have many clients who play golf on their regular limbs with only minor adaptations. If you are an avid golfer and plan on golfing several times a week, then you may consider a limb specially designed for the sport (Figure 5-3).

A comfortable socket is essential to playing 18 holes and being on your feet for up to 4 hours. Whatever system keeps you comfortable in your regular walking leg should suffice with the possible addition of an insert if you don't have one in the socket already. The added cushion and adjustability that the insert provides can increase the long-term comfort of the amputee, especially if he or she is determined to carry his or her own clubs. Suspension should be positive. If the leg uses a locking mechanism

Figure 5-3. Amputee golfers. (Photo courtesy of Ossur.)

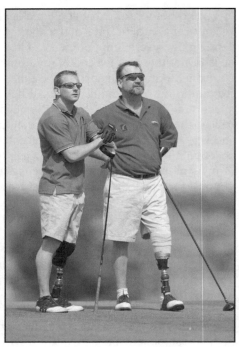

only, it might be a good idea to add an auxiliary suspension sleeve to provide added security. Golf generates a lot of twisting motion inside of the socket so make sure that the prosthesis takes this into account.

The motion of the ankle as it twists to the inside during the golf swing is difficult to duplicate with just a foot. There are several types of rotators available commercially, both endoskeletal (pylon style) and exoskeletal (hard outer shell). The endoskeletal style has the ability to adjust the amount of friction on the rotation and gives a little better control over the movement. The adjustment is inside of the rotator and requires some disassembly of the leg in order to adjust the friction on the device. Both types of rotators require some maintenance over time, so keep this in mind when deciding to use a rotator. Many types of feet have some rotational capability built into them. Generally, multiaxial feet or dynamic response feet have rotation.

One of the best ways to find what you may need for a golf prosthesis is to go out and get dirty. Play some golf and test your swing. If you are a novice, find some professional help. If you played golf prior to amputation, you may need to adjust your swing to accommodate the new balance of your body. I recommend using a cart at first because lugging around the heavy bag of clubs may be more than your stump can handle. There are many amputee golf organizations that have regular events and tournaments, which are listed in Chapter 12. I have never been to these events, but from talking to others that have they are a really good time!

Backpacking, Hiking, and Heavy Duty Prostheses

I love to backpack and hike in the beautiful Sierra Nevada Mountains. When I first lost my leg, I thought that hiking was going to be one of those activities that I just would not be able to do anymore. When I took my first hike into the woods 6 months postamputation, I was able to do it but the pain was nearly unbearable. I had to find a better solution for continued enjoyment of this activity because the woods and mountains were where I had always found peace and serenity.

The problem with using my regular walking prosthesis for hiking was that the added weight of the pack combined with the stress of the uneven terrain placed unacceptable stresses on my stump. First, I used an auxiliary waist belt to help with suspension and this did lessen the amount of pistoning that occurred as I tripped over roots and ruts. Unfortunately, this also increased the torque to the stump even though I was using a multiaxial foot. When I returned from my bicycle trip to the Northwest, I had the sports prosthesis that had been made for me by the Seattle Prosthetics Research Study. I found that the thigh lacer took enough pressure off of my stump to allow me to carry a 22-kg (50 lb) pack around for 4 or 5 hours with minimal damage to my stump. The knee joints and lacer were heavy, weighing over 5 kg (12 lbs), but at least I could backpack. I used my 5 ft tall walking staff to assist me and as long as I continually watched where I was going, I could hike for 20 to 24 k (12 to 15 miles) a day and still be able to hike the next day.

The weight and constriction of having such a heavy prosthesis to use the entire time I was backpacking created a barrier to my enjoyment of my beloved activity. I had to come up with something better. The first big breakthrough came as I got involved in cross-country skiing. In the off-season I would train with cross-country ski poles when I went for long hikes. I realized that with ski poles in both hands using them in tandem with the opposite foot made a huge difference in my stability on the trail. I could actually hike without having to constantly look at my feet. What a concept! I was able to see the scenery and if I did catch the leg on a root or a rut, I would stumble but not fall. This was great.

Momentum and Hiking

When a person loses a leg or both legs, he or she must compensate for the lack of muscle by using momentum to provide forward thrust. The problem in hiking is that the ground is not even; there are roots, holes, bumps, ruts, and the occasional small animal to contend with. Every time an amputee has to accommodate the uneven terrain with an adjustment to his or her gait, he or she loses momentum. This means that a simple hike through the woods can be exhausting since every third step is an adjustment. The solution that I found is to hike with cross-country ski poles. The strap on the pole should circle the wrist with the thumb and fingers lightly holding the pole. You should feel the pull on the back of your upper arm, not your hand. The poles will provide stability as well as continued momentum even when the prosthesis catches on a root.

The use of poles when I hike revolutionized my enjoyment of the outdoors and allowed me to hike without tripping or falling. I have also used crutches to negotiate down steep hills, which allow me to take much of the impact of landing on the prosthesis on my arms instead of my stump. I have old cross-country poles as well as a pair of collapsible poles designed for hiking.

Figure 5-4. A removable thigh lacer. (Photo by Dale Horkey, 2004.)

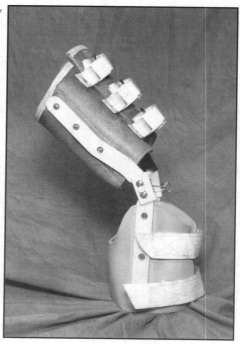

My current hiking leg uses a dynamic response foot that also provides some sideways motion to absorb the torque of the uneven terrain. I use sleeve suspension as well as an auxiliary waist belt and a removable thigh lacer to take some of the weight off of my stump. The leg has a soft-liner made from PPT foam that also minimizes stress to my stump. This system works better than my old hiking leg. I can remove the thigh lacer and wear it just like my regular walking prosthesis when I am in camp (Figure 5-4). The thigh lacer and waist belt are not particularly comfortable items to wear and when you are on the trail for 6 or 8 hours, it is a real pain to have to keep wearing all that stuff when you don't need it. I continue to enjoy hiking and have found that with the proper equipment it is an activity that amputees manage with minimal discomfort (Figure 5-5).

I am not particularly fond of heavy-duty manual labor. I can always find something that I prefer to do when things like hauling wood, digging holes, or pushing a wheelbarrow have to be done. However, there are times when these things need to be done and I can't get someone else to do them. The removable thigh lacer provides the added stability as well as impact absorption that allow me to push a wheelbarrow or be on a ladder for hours without damage to my residual limb. If you are going to engage in work where your leg can't come off, it is best to have some type of secondary suspension like a waist belt or suspension sleeve.

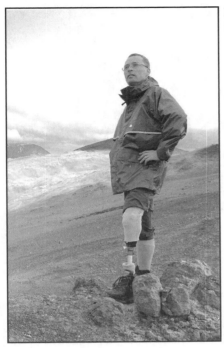

Figure 5-5. An amputee enjoying a hike. (Photo courtesy of Ossur.)

Skiing Prostheses

After nearly breaking my stump when I fell downhill while skiing, I decided to three-track for a while. This was much easier since I was not trying to control a large heavy board with my short stump. The only problem was that as I got older and less in shape, I could not really enjoy downhill skiing due to the fatigue in my thigh. My left thigh would start to burn after the first run and I could only ski for a couple of hundred meters (yards) before I had to stop and rest my thigh. I had seen some trick skiing prostheses at ski competitions so I decided to make one of my own.

My first consideration was for my stump so I used a high walled socket that contained my entire knee for protection. I have a PPT foam insert and an expulsion valve to give me a good solid feel inside the socket. Two suspension sleeves hold the prosthesis on as well as an auxiliary waist belt with removable Y-strap and I attach my removable thigh lacer over top of the suspension sleeves. This seems like a lot of stuff but I found that if I wanted to ski all day, I needed to have this much to protect my stump. The foot is an energy-storing pylon with no sideways motion capability. I want to have as much control of the ski as possible so instead of wearing a ski boot, I have a Delron plate that we fabricated to bolt to the bottom of the foot. The plate attaches to the ski binding just like a boot except there is not the added weight or the motion that wearing a boot would create. The spring action of the foot allows me to unweight my turns with both feet as long as I have the rhythm of the hill. I only run into trouble when my rhythm gets off.

My version of the ski prosthesis is not the only one. Many competitors use a different type of foot and have success with it. If the residual limb is longer and in better

Figure 5-6. Downhill skiing feet that attach directly to the skis. (Photo courtesy of Freedom Innovations.)

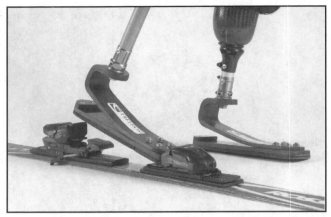

shape, then the auxiliary thigh lacer is not necessary. I have heard of people placing warming devices inside of their sockets to keep their stumps from getting cold. Keep in mind that the forces placed on your stump during downhill skiing are tremendous and that you need to do everything possible to prevent injury when and if you fall.

My competitive sport was cross-country or Nordic skiing. As a member of the U.S. team for 8 years, I needed a leg that was specifically designed for the sport. My first leg was an endoskeletal design with a SACH foot and was designed to give me as much control of the ski as possible. Cross-country skis are not near as heavy as downhill skis so suspension is not as critical but control is vital. My current Nordic leg has double suspension sleeves and an expulsion valve like my downhill leg, but it doesn't require the waist belt and thigh lacer. I also use a dynamic response foot with no sideways motion (inversion and eversion) to give me as much control over the edges of my skis as possible. With this leg I can even skate on the skis, which is similar to ice-skating but requires minute control over the edge of the ski. I also have modified my ski boots to bolt directly to the foot, giving me as much control of the ski edges as possible (Figure 5-6).

Both alpine and Nordic skiing (Figure 5-7) are well suited to the below-knee amputee since they have little impact on the stump. There are numerous programs around the United States to instruct and adapt the sport. I always recommend that a person try the sport with their regular walking prosthesis before investing in a specialized leg. Most programs have staff members who can assist the amputee in adapting his or her prosthesis to try the sport. With cross-country skiing the only adaptation for the prosthesis is to put a 0.6- to 1.2-cm (0.25 to 0.5-in) wedge beneath the heel of the prosthesis. This will get the center of gravity forward enough to get a good push off of the ski. A list of organizations that provide assistance in these sports is contained in Chapter 12.

The Peg Leg

Yes, I have a peg leg (Figure 5-8). I use mine primarily for my pirate costume that I love to wear at Halloween. This is one of the few times that being an amputee really has its advantages. My costume has gotten pretty elaborate over the years, even

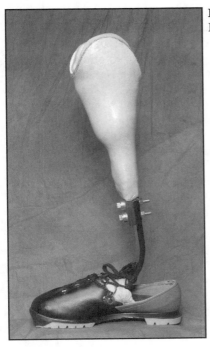

Figure 5-7. A Nordic skiing prosthesis. (Photo by Dale Horkey, 2004.)

Figure 5-8. My pirate peg leg. (Photo by Dale Horkey, 2004.)

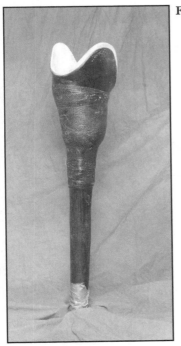

down to the talking parrot. I can always tell how good the Halloween party is by what time it is when some drunk comes up to me and comments on my costume. It usually goes something like this, "Hey buddy, that is a great costume. How do you do that with your leg?" I reply, "I use mirrors," which causes him or her to circle me several times to try and find the trick. I am a great dancer on my peg leg because I can spin at least 3 times before falling over and stumbling into people.

Outside of costume parties, how often would one use a peg leg? You would be surprised at how many amputees use pegs. The big advantage of the peg is that there isn't any forefoot to catch on things. I know a gardener who wears nothing but a peg, and a sailor (no kidding) who always wears it when on his boat. He claims that it keeps his prosthesis from getting caught in the ropes, but I think he just likes his image as a pirate. There is a specific component made for the peg leg called the Trowbridge foot, which is a soft crepe soled peg bottom that has a complete multiaxial joint at the ankle. It is great for hunters or working around the house when you don't want to have to worry if your foot is getting tangled up.

CHAPTER 6

Integrating the Prosthesis With Your Body

Stories

My Story

I worked at Georgia Prosthetics designing and making prostheses for 2 years, catering to disabled athletes and amputees who were well off. I learned a lot from Aaron, my boss, and began to learn from my patients as to how to ask the right questions in order to get accurate information. I continued to be involved with the Handicapped Sports Organization, but I also saw that I needed to involve some people who could take over when I wanted to move on. I also decided to devote myself to training for the 1984 Olympic games in Austria and to compete on the Disabled Nordic Team.

The summer of 1983 was significant in that as part of my training for the team I took up running. This is a sport that I thoroughly disliked when I had 2 legs so why I decided to use this as part of my training regime baffles me. I do not have a runner's physique. I am more suited to running into immovable objects than to running with any grace and speed. I have already related the story of my participation in the Peachtree Road Race, in which I had a decent placing but spent the next 3 months on crutches as a result. I didn't heal until the end of September and only had 5 months to get into shape before the Olympics in February. I swam, rode my bicycle, lifted weights, and played handball at least 3 times a week. On weekends, I would cut firewood at the cabin and take long hikes in the woods. In those months, I lost 30 lbs and got into the best shape of my life. Unfortunately, I was living in Georgia where the opportunity to cross-country ski was nonexistent.

I went to the first training camp prior to the games in Austria in January of that year at Kirkwood in the Sierra Nevada Mountains of California. I flew into Reno, Nevada and thought that it was the most dismal place that I had ever seen, never suspecting that one day I would call it home and feel totally different about the desert. The camp at Kirkwood was held at a nearby Nordic center, but we stayed at an old fishing lodge that was never designed to be used in the winter. I had never seen so much snow in my life. It must have snowed over a meter (3 ft) while we were there for a week of skiing. I did improve my technique, but nothing was going to make me a world-class competitor in the few weeks before the competition. I did, however, learn from some of my teammates how to avoid those long ski-training sessions our coach sent us on. Joe is a partially blind skier who had to ski with a guide and they would go out for the 10K (6.25 miles) training loop and always come back late with suspicious smiles on their faces. One afternoon my ski partner and I decided to follow them on their long distance training route. We tailed them through the woods in the big loop around the valley. At the far end of the valley was the base lodge for the alpine ski area and instead of going up into the hills where they were supposed to go, they headed straight for the local pub. When we caught up to them, they were already into a couple of steaming hot toddies and were quite surprised to see us come into the bar. We promised not to tell on them if they bought drinks for us. That day there were 4 late incoming skiers with big grins on their faces.

It was an incredible experience to get to be a part of the team and travel to Austria. We had one more training camp in New England just prior to our departure. We then went to New York and were treated to a reception at the United Nations building where we met various dignitaries. After a long trip, we arrived in Innsbruck where we were quartered in a nice hotel in the middle of the oldest part of town. We trained every day in preparation for the events that were to come and in the evening, after preparing our skis, we would take in a little of the local scenery. My best buddy on the team was Tommy and he was my savior as well as the coach's nightmare. We enjoyed going out at night and exploring the local pubs where I could practice my bad German. I was the only one on the team who spoke any German so whenever we went to a restaurant I would have to order for everyone. One evening I was just picking things off of the menu for various team members. I could pronounce German but had no idea what it meant so I ordered something for my partially blind friend Joe. To the whole table's horror, there was an entire fried pig's head staring up at him when he received his plate. We have never let him live that down.

Finally, the day of the Olympics arrived and in my first event I discovered what world class really meant. We all got our butts kicked by the rest of the world, with the U.S. team bringing up the last 3 of 5 places. There was only one other competitor worse than I and I don't think he had ever skied before. The rest of the races were not much better, and my best placing was 19th out of 21st. I realized that if I expected to become a world-class athlete, I would have to find a way to live somewhere that had snow.

The last race was over on Thursday and the Alpine skiers still had one more day of competition so all of the Nordic skiers met in a little town outside of Innsbruck to celebrate our triumphs. The pub was full of skiers from Britain, Australia, Canada, the United States, and Poland. None of the Poles spoke much English, but they sure were friendly. We all proceeded to get very inebriated and began to sing filthy English songs that the Brits were all too willing to teach us. When we finally left, we were standing outside of the pub waiting for our taxi when 3 very drunk British blind skiers came singing out of the door. They all had their arms around each other's shoulders and were singing the refrain from one of their filthy songs. They were totally blind but still managed to stumble out the door and weave their way across the street till the skier on the end ran into the houses on the other side of the street. Then they wove their way back across the street till they ran into the houses there, then stumbled on in a zigzag fashion until they reached their hotel a block or so away. That was a real example of adaptation, if you ask me.

Our taxi finally arrived and as we left town, I noticed one of the colorful Olympic banners that were all over the place. I asked the taxi driver to stop and George, the 50-year-old father figure of us all, got out with me to help me take the flag down as a souvenir. We struggled with the flag for about 10 minutes before giving up, since the banner was not strung up on the pole but wired through the guide holes to keep treasure hunters like ourselves from making off with the souvenirs. The taxi left the little town and as it entered the highway that would take us to Innsbruck, there was another flag. Again, I made the driver stop while George and I attempted to take it down. This flag was also well protected against the likes of me. I kicked in frustration at the wooden wedge that held the 13 meter (40 ft) shaved pine pole in its metal collar. To my surprise, it popped right out and the pole was now loose. In my state of inebriation I thought that I could just pick the pole right up and then it would be easier to remove the flag. Sure enough, I was able to lift the pole but when it cleared the collar I was unprepared for the staggering weight of the pine tree. I quickly lost control and was very fortunate that when it fell it missed the back of an oncoming car by only centimeters (inches). The flag was mine and today it hangs in my shop as the only trophy of my participation in the 1984 Olympics.

I returned to Georgia full of pride at having participated on the U.S. team but also very full of myself. My narcissistic attitude did very little to improve my relationship with my wife and I began to grow weary of the life I had. I actively pursued a career move to work in a prosthetic facility somewhere nearer to snow and with the responsibilities that I thought I was ready for. None of my friends or family particularly liked my idea of moving away from the south, but I felt that I needed a change.

Frank

Frank was born in 1930 in a small town in Arizona. He was a rough and tumble kid who always put himself in the front of whatever was going on. In high school he got involved in rodeo, becoming the state champion roper of Arizona. He had belonged to the ROTC program and naturally joined the Army upon completing his studies. The year was 1953 and he was sent to Korea as head of a tank platoon. Frank was not afraid to get into the front lines with his fellow tankers and experienced numerous battles up until that fateful day that changed his life forever.

His platoon had just occupied a hill that dominated the line that the American and Korean forces were struggling to hold. They had set up a command post in a bunker that had been dug by someone in the seesaw actions that permeated this section of the line. He and the other tank commanders were having a briefing in the bunker when artillery rounds penetrated the roof and exploded amidst them. Frank was thrown against the wall and knocked semiconscious by the blast but was otherwise unhurt. Like most brave men, he quickly got his wits about him and looked for his comrades. Half of the soldiers were badly injured and he and the other half of the uninjured men carried the wounded out of the bunker and into a trench in the rear. Experience had shown that the Chinese artillery generally would continue to bombard a target over and over to insure that the bunker was knocked out. When they stopped to catch their breath, they realized that there was a soldier missing. One of the men said he thought that the radio operator was dead and that it was no use going back to get him. Frank got up without thinking about the imminent danger he was in and ran back to find the radio operator. He found the man buried under rubble in the bombed out bunker and picked him up. He couldn't tell if he was alive or not, but he hefted him on his shoulders. As he was stepping toward the communications trench, he heard the whine of another shell coming.

Frank awoke in the Army MASH hospital with burning pain in his right foot and shrapnel imbedded in his back and arms. The foot was still there but it had nearly been ripped off from the blast. He was soon shipped to Japan where they did numerous surgeries to try and rebuild his foot. A colonel presented him with the Silver Star for bravery and a Purple Heart, but Frank felt that the rest of his men deserved this more than he did. Still, it gave him a great deal of pride to return to Arizona as a war hero. The wound got better but never completely healed. It would drain all the time and he never could put full weight on it.

While convalescing at the Veteran's Hospital in Phoenix, he was visited by Joan, a friend of one of his buddies. Frank was immediately taken with her striking good looks and her firm but gentle manner. By her second visit, he told her that he was going to marry her. Three months later he did. He was discharged from the hospital but was relegated to using crutches since the wounded foot never would heal. Frank entered law school at the University of Arizona on crutches at a time when there were no handicapped parking or accessible buildings. He wore a brace that allowed him to partial weight bear but his mobility was limited and the constant pain wore him down.

After dealing with the brace for a year, he decided that the best thing he could do for his future mobility was to undergo amputation below the knee. This was not an easy decision since Joan was expecting their first child and he still had not finished law school. Nonetheless, he went in for the surgery but just to make sure there were no mistakes, he tied a note around his good leg that said, "Do not cut this one." In 1955, the state of the art of prosthetics was still primitive compared to what it is today. He wore a wooden socket with large heavy metal braces beside his knee with a leather corset that wrapped around his thigh. A waist belt held on the leg, and he wore numerous wool socks that were hot in the summer and smelly all the time. The adjustment was difficult for a former state champion rodeo competitor, but his positive attitude got him through and helped his family cope with the trauma.

Frank finished law school and went into private practice in Arizona until 1969. Joan and he had another 3 children that are the pride of their lives. He specialized in business law and helped several California companies acquire property in Arizona that led to his next business venture. After one of the larger deals that he helped broker, he was offered a partnership and management job with a large engineering firm out of San Diego. The family moved to California where Frank eventually became the CEO of one of the largest engineering firms on the West Coast. His prostheses were getting better as the years passed; plastics replaced wood, pelite inserts replaced the numerous wool socks, and a cuff strap replaced the waist belt. Frank worked very hard, putting in 10 to 12 hour days managing a growing business that eventually employed over 1000 workers.

Frank and Joan have remained friends and lovers for over 50 years and have weathered more than their share of traumas. One of their daughters was killed in a car accident, which is a trauma no parent should have to live through. They have 10 grandchildren and a close-knit family even in today's world.

I had the honor and privilege of working with Frank several years ago. He inspired me with his tales of war and recovery. Most of all he influenced me with his reverence for his wife, Joan. Every time he talked about her he would almost get teary eyed, and

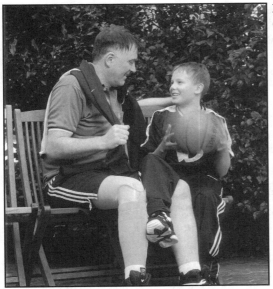

Figure 6-1. Time with your kids. (Photo courtesy of Ossur.)

you could see at once that he loves her as much today as he did when they first met. I once asked Frank what was his secret of success in business. I was expecting to hear some quote out of Forbes, but his reply floored me. He said that his secret to business success was that he loved people and he built relationships. He said that he couldn't turn on the computer in his office if his life depended on it but that if someone wanted a project done on time and within the budget that they stipulated, he could be trusted to make sure that occurred. This man inspired me to work on my own business and I strove to embody those ideals with my employees and clients.

The Emotional Impact

I was only 20 years old when I became an amputee (Figure 6-1), but it shocked me into a frame of mind for which I was not prepared. This is a uniquely personal experience for all who go through it, but experts have outlined 5 stages of grief that most people go through.

The Stages of Grieving

1. Denial and isolation: "This is impossible. It's not really happening! I feel nothing at all."
2. Anger: "Why is this happening to me? I'm enraged! God is unjust!"
3. Bargaining: "If I promise to do such-and-such, then maybe I'll get my old life back."
4. Depression: "I feel hopeless. Everything is beyond my control. Why bother trying? I give up."
5. Acceptance: "I don't like it, but the amputation is a reality. I'll find ways to make the best of it and go on."

Reprinted with permission from Winchell E. *Coping With Limb Loss*. Garden City, NJ: Avery Publishing Group; 1995: 105.

My personal progression through these phases was uneven and sporadic, and there were times when I regressed backward due to my inability to cope with life situations. I did not spend much time in denial. My amputation was immediate and I witnessed the entire event and interacted with it. Even when I woke up in postop, I knew what had happened and was shocked but not surprised that my right foot was gone. I have been a bit of an angry person my whole life, often times venting frustration by yelling or acting out. The loss of my leg finally gave me the excuse I needed to use my anger in all types of social and intimate settings. My justification of, "You don't know what it's like," was finally blown when another amputee confronted me. I still manifest my anger in unhealthy ways, but I no longer blame my amputation for my lack of control. Sometimes I'm just a jerk, just like any other person.

The bargaining phase was another part of grieving that I didn't spend much time in. The accident was not my fault, but it happened nonetheless and I was grounded in the reality that I was not going to be able to change the situation, only make the best out of it. I also did not spend much of my time in depression. I was scared and frightened of the pain that I knew was an inevitable part of my present and future, frightened of how people would treat me, and particularly terrified of what women would think of me as "half a man." I did have some depressing days, especially when there were setbacks in my healing or when I would have visitors and then they would leave. The worst of these was when I split my stump open in 3 places while wearing my postoperative cast. I spent 6 weeks without a prosthesis, and I had incredible pain as the tissue had to heal from the inside out. It was one of the few times of my life when I actually marked off the days on a calendar, wishing the time to go by.

I moved rapidly into the acceptance phase of being an amputee; however, I did regress back into anger and depression frequently. I took great pride in my ability to overcome the amputation and live with the pain. I kept my game face on whenever I was in public but would often resort to anger when I was home amongst people who would love me no matter how much of a jerk I was. One of the things that impressed me most happened about 2 weeks after the amputation; I had a dream that I was running. I was an amputee and I was wearing a prosthesis but I could run with it in my dream. This indicated to me that my brain had accepted the amputation deeply into my subconscious.

One of the things that is evident from losing a leg is that it changes the image of your body. This can have a variety of impacts on the amputee dependent upon gender, age, and how the person perceived his or her body prior to amputation. If you are a woman, generally the impact of losing part of the body is more difficult to deal with than if you are a man. This is not always the case but is generally so. The older you are the more difficult it is to get used to looking down and seeing part of your body gone since you have had more time to get used to what you look like with 2 legs.

Some people recommend that the new amputee should visualize the leg as still there, while others claim to still feel the energy or aura from the missing limb. I don't know much about visualizing something that is gone. I am under the opinion that an amputee needs to face the fact that the leg is gone and get on with things. Life is about living, not about holding onto something that is gone and cannot come back. This is my personal philosophy and other professionals as well as amputees have different perspectives that are gentler on the psyche.

I have always felt that attitude is everything. For many amputees, the loss of a limb is a catalyst to experiencing a richer, more rewarding life. Many who have come near to death as a result of disease or trauma have a greater appreciation of the life they have and use the experience to find a deeper spiritual understanding. So much of life is how one perceives it. If you look at the world and see barriers, then you will be halt-ed in the realization of your dreams. If, by the same token, you see opportunities instead of barriers, then you will find ways around the seemingly impossible adver-saries. I know that this sounds a bit hard-core, but it has been the truth in my life and it was the transmission of this attitude to my prosthetic clients that made my business successful.

Not everyone can project a positive attitude toward the world, even after process-ing the grief of limb loss. There are some things that will help though. One of the best tricks that I learned personally and passed onto my clients was the skill of eye contact. If you can make eye contact with people, then they can see that the basic person has-n't changed. It is very frightening to be lying in bed with your leg cut off, excruciating pain filling your head with red lightning, and friends or loved ones coming to visit. It is also terrifying to the friends or loved ones who are coming to visit with you. Most people who encounter a new amputee who is in obvious distress have no idea what to do or think. What they generally think is how it would feel if the amputation happened to them. Imagining what it is like to have your leg cut off is like a trip into the abyss; a journey into a hell that most people don't willingly take. I have always felt that amputees have a duty to try and minimize the fear of people who care about them. Not only does this have the effect of putting friends or relatives at ease, it allows them to see the amputee as a person rather than some image of their fear.

Tricks to Help Calm Friends and Family

1. Make eye contact with everyone who visits with you. This will help them see that even though you are obviously in distress, the same person is still inside of you.
2. Smile. Yes, even if you have to fake it, you need to smile. Nothing will help put your loved ones at ease more than seeing you smile again.
3. Make a joke or two. This may seem difficult but it really works to minimize the tragic effects of your experience. It will also make you feel better to joke around a bit. If you can't think of any jokes, ask someone to tell you one and then memorize it. After all, what else do you have to do?
4. Find some other amputees to talk to, preferably ones that have a similar level of amputation. This will not only help you but your family will see that there is some degree of normalcy that they have to look forward to.
5. It is important to keep in mind that these are the people that you will be leaning on in the future as you become rehabilitated. Keep your abuse of them to a mini-mum and they will be far more willing to help when you need it.

Physical Integration

The goal of integrating the loss of a leg into your body may be the easiest part of the whole process. If you have mastered the mental integration, then the physical will follow, but there are some things that definitely help. If there are no other physical complications, then exercise will be one of your best friends in the quest for wholeness. Your body will have to compensate for the missing part through strength and balance. It is possible to do just about anything that you did prior to amputation, but there will have to be adaptations as well as increased strength needed to make up for what is missing.

Exercise is very important once you have recovered from surgery and should become a part of your daily routine. If your prosthesis permits, walking is an excellent form of exercise that will keep you fit and is gentle on your stump. I also recommend bicycling as a great, nonimpact form of exercise to give you the workout you need but no pounding of the prosthesis. Make sure that if you bicycle, you have made any adaptations to the prosthesis or bicycle prior to making it a routine. Another great form of exercise is swimming, which can be done with or without the prosthesis. Swimming is an excellent form of cardiovascular exercise and produces no stress or impact to the residual limb. The only downside to swimming is accessibility to a pool and getting in and out of it. A swim leg is ideal since you can use it to climb up and down the ladder or walk up and down the steps. I began swimming soon after I lost my leg and found that the only adaptation that I had to make was to swim a bit faster because without the two-foot kick, I tended to sink a little in the water. I discovered later that a small flotation device clamped between my legs leveled out my body and allowed me to swim at a comfortable pace with ease.

Stretching and Yoga

I was never into stretching while I participated in sports during high school or college. I hated the mandatory stretches that the coach put us through prior to games or matches, but I did recognize the importance of being limber and its contribution to performance. After I lost my leg, I still didn't like stretching but found that the months of relative inactivity had left me tight and unable to touch my toes. Back in college all my friends were new age kind of people and they had gotten into yoga in a big way. My best buddy had convinced me to try it because their yoga sessions had lots of girls who attended. I thought this could be a great place to meet girls so I started going to the classes. To my surprise, I actually liked doing yoga and even though I didn't really meet any girls, I did become quite limber. I had to adapt many of the postures since my prosthesis hurt too badly to be able to accomplish the standing positions. I would take off my prosthesis and perform the postures on my knees, which enabled me to participate in nearly all of the yoga positions.

Yoga is one of the best rehabilitation techniques for amputees that I ever personally experienced. I taught a yoga class for the disabled at Emory University Rehabilitation Clinic for 2 years and found that nearly any level of amputation could participate with minor adaptations. The key to yoga is that the focus is on breathing and awareness of your body. The postures have no particular goal; the important concept is to stretch the body until it resists then allow it to relax by breathing in order to achieve greater flexibility. This slow motion stretching with a focus on breathing is perfect for the amputee who needs to learn how to balance all over again. There are yoga techniques out there that are more power oriented and these are not so well suited to the amputee. The most effective technique is to slowly move into a posture using your breath as a natural way of relaxing your muscles. The awareness of your balance and the body's integration of the new way in which it must perform are the keys to using yoga as a rehabilitative tool.

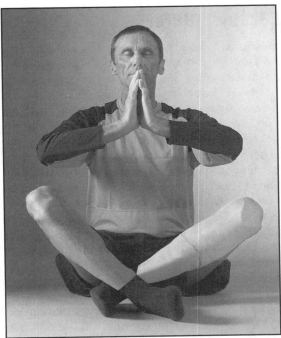

Figure 6-2. Yoga is a great way to stretch and relax. (Photo courtesy of Ossur.)

Yoga may not be for you, but stretching of any sort is very beneficial to a new amputee. Even people who have been amputees for many years will benefit greatly from stretching or yoga since as an amputee, the body is being stressed in an unnatural way. The human body was designed as a bilaterally equal mechanism and that balance is disturbed when you lose a limb. Muscles have to compensate for lack of balance and musculature on the amputated side so after years of this, the body can get out of whack. I highly recommend some form of stretching or yoga to assist the body in attaining some equilibrium that if left untreated will result in musculature and even structural problems later in life (Figure 6-2).

Another method of achieving body equilibrium is massage. I discovered massage back in college. Yes, I was trying to meet girls. I found that the relaxation that I received from a real body massage went a long way in relieving the stresses of body abuse associated with the amputation. I now try to get a weekly massage in order to balance out the muscles in my body and remove the buildup of waste products in my good leg. I also tend to store stress in my back and shoulders, and the massage gets me back to neutral at least once a week. I don't stretch and do yoga like I should so the massage keeps me from getting so tight that I can't enjoy exercise. There are some great books and videos that illustrate yoga techniques as well as legitimate massage. **The point here is that the body is put out of alignment when amputation occurs and the more the amputee can do to maintain proper body alignment through stretching, yoga, or massage, the damage to the compensating parts of the body will be minimized.**

Spiritual Integration

Losing one's leg is often the single most tragic thing that happens to someone in his or her lifetime. I think that there are worse things in life and even though that is my personal perspective, it is what allowed me to put my amputation in its proper place. In my experience, losing my younger brother 1 year after losing my leg was far worse than my amputation because I was powerless to do anything about it. At least with my leg I could fight and overcome the disability. I never even got to say goodbye to my brother or tell him that I loved him. Possibly this experience galvanized my spirit, allowing me to rise above the grief and sorrow that was also a part of how I felt.

Becoming an amputee is generally something that one does not consider will happen to him or her in his or her life. When it does, it is a shock whether it is immediate and traumatic or a result of some disease where there is too much time to think about it. How someone copes with amputation is as varied as there are people. Some put it behind them and move on, while others get stuck in one of the phases of grief over their loss. Having a strong spiritual belief is, in my experience, one of the more important factors in the acceptance of one's circumstance. People who are truly spiritual, not just religious, often have an easier time accepting what has occurred than people who have no faith. Religion can play a part in this but it seems to me that a personal relationship with God, or a higher power, is the only place where one can get an answer to the question, "Why me?" I think that all amputees ask that question at least once in their quest to come to terms with what has happened. I know I asked it but for me the answer was simple and yet logically inconclusive. It happened and that was that. I could not undo the event; I could only take what life had dealt me and move on from there. Other people wrestle with this question and allow it to influence their lives for many years if not for the rest of their lives. For me it just wasn't an issue.

I worked with one older woman who had to be in her seventies when she lost her leg. She was a very well dressed and proper lady who had been to several prosthetists with limited success. She constantly complained of pain in her prosthesis and was very focused on how it had ruined her active church and social life. Her son always came to her appointments with her, and she was often verbally abusive to him. We made her a prosthesis that solved most of her pain problems, but it didn't really have the effect of returning her to her previous lifestyle. During one of her adjustment sessions I was trying to determine the reason that she didn't wear the prosthesis or go out like she used to. Prosthetically, there was no reason that she couldn't walk to the store or go to church on Sundays, which constituted her primary activities. When I pressured her as to what was wrong, her son offered encouragement to her and she snapped at him, "Shut up, you don't know what it is like." Of course I didn't appreciate the abuse of her son and bluntly asked her what her problem was. She replied in a disgusted voice that she wished that she had died instead of having lost her leg. I looked her in the eye and told her that she should be ashamed of herself. She looked me back in the eye with disbelief and shock. I told her that it was God's choice that she lost her leg and that she should be grateful for this time in which she was able to see her grandchildren grow. She started crying and her son took her and they left my office. I knew that I had told her the truth but thought that because of my bluntness I would probably never see them again. An hour later her son called. I was nervous as I went to get the phone because he was a lawyer. He thanked me profusely for talking to his mother, saying that no one had ever confronted her before and that my words had profoundly changed her. From then on until she passed away several years later she attended church every Sunday and treated those around her more like people than pincushions.

Another client of mine was a very successful real estate developer and multimillionaire who at the age of 45 developed a staph infection that his body couldn't fight. He went into the hospital and when he finally came out of his coma he had lost both of his legs below the knee and most of his fingertips. The shock was profound and he felt as if his life was over. No more 16K (10 mile) runs in the mountains, no more playing of his 12-string guitar that both his wife and children loved so much. His initial days were spent in excruciating pain as his stumps and fingers healed from the numerous skin grafts. How was he going to go to the bathroom or take care of himself? All of the things he had taken for granted were now changed. He slipped into a deep depression from which he thought he would never recover.

The feelings that this man experienced are not that unusual. He was not a particularly religious person, he rarely went to church and yet in the end he found the strength to not only carry on but to return to most of his former life. He endured the humiliating experience of not being able to care for himself, not an easy thing for a man or woman, while his family provided empathetic care. He was grateful but frustrated at having to be watched after and catered to. I saw him in the hospital where he was not a happy person but still asked relevant questions that showed he understood what it would take to recover. The preparatory prostheses that we made were not what he had hoped for and when he got home he threw them across the room. Still, the next day he put them on and managed to get around on his walker. The next day was better and the next even a little better than that.

What he discovered was that deep inside of himself was the will to live and the faith that tomorrow would be a better day. His family was supportive and he didn't take his frustrations out on them, which allowed them to be there for him and enabled them to let him go when he had become rehabilitated. He now enjoys a very active lifestyle in which he runs his business and plays golf whenever he wishes. He has numerous grandchildren that he spends as much time with as he can. He never looks back and longs for the day that he had 2 legs because he has his life to keep him busy.

The Good Foot

When you first lose a limb the stump is what consumes your entire focus. This is only natural since you have to heal it and mature it in order to wear a prosthesis. However, after many years of wearing a prosthesis, the good foot can start to cause problems. With most of the focus on the amputated side it is easy to overlook the sound, or intact, side. Remember that if you have one good foot it is taking the abuse of two feet. When the body seeks balance, one uses both feet to give subtle and generally unconscious signals to the brain that tell it where the ground is and what the terrain is like. This kinesthetic sense combined with visual and auditory clues is how humans judge how to move across the ground beneath them. When you have only 1 leg, the remaining foot has to provide all of that feedback to the brain so it rocks side to side, simulating what would occur if you had 2 feet. The feedback to the brain is not as good as with 2 feet, but it suffices to provide adequate ambulation, even over rough terrain.

The added stress on the remaining foot is generally well tolerated for the first 8 or 10 years but then problems can arise. In my case I started getting fatigue and pain on the outside edge of my foot. At first I didn't pay much attention. I just figured that since I was on my feet all day, usually on a hard surface, that I should expect it. After several months though, the pain became so intense that I couldn't walk without limping. I was dating a physical therapist at the time and she immediately diagnosed me as having a definite overload on the outside edge of my foot. She said that it was evident in the callusing of the outside edge of my heel and forefoot. She immediately put me in a simple shoe insert that within a few days had taken away all of the discomfort I had been experiencing. I still wear a shoe insert in all of my shoes and have to adjust them from time to time to keep my foot in a neutral position. A podiatrist, physical therapist, or orthotist can provide a shoe insert that can correct most deviations of the good foot, and I highly recommend it for any amputee who has had a leg off for over 10 years.

Not everyone manifests their problems in their foot or ankle. Some amputees start to experience discomfort in their knee or pelvis due to the undue stress placed upon them as an amputee. The first course of treatment should be the same (ie, a simple shoe insert that puts the sound side foot in a more neutral position). If this is the source of the pain, then it should improve in a very short period of time. If this does not solve the problem, you should consult your physician and explore other options.

Clothing and Shoes

Wearing a prosthesis and trying to be fashionable can be a real test for a fashion designer. Many prostheses are bulky at the knee and do not hide well beneath even moderately tight clothes. Short skirts can be a real dilemma, not that I have ever worn a lot of short skirts. One solution is to stay with looser fitting pants that allow room for the prosthesis to move freely. I was fortunate to have lost my leg in the '70s when pants had bellbottoms and at times were baggy enough to be used as parachutes if the necessity arose. Today, fashion has once again blessed male amputees as men's pants have gotten extremely baggy and the crotch often times comes down to the knees. This provides more than adequate room to wear a prosthesis without it being obvious. Women have a more difficult time with maintaining a fashionable presence but with a little creativity and shopping around, suitable clothing can be found.

When I wore the superpatellar style of prosthesis that clamped above my knee, I always tried to take my leg off whenever I was sitting for a long period of time. This was impossible when I was wearing tight jeans or dress pants since I would have had to remove the pants to take off the leg, not a particularly appropriate gesture in most social situations. Today there are some really cool designs that seem as if they were made for the amputee. There is a style of pants that can unzip into shorts, allowing the wearer to easily access the prosthesis for removal or adjustment without having to remove the pants. There are also many types of sweatpants that have zippers along the entire outside edge that allow easy access to the prosthesis. They come in enough styles and choices to allow some degree of fashion acceptance. Still, if you want to wear shorts or short skirts that show off the prosthesis, then you either need to not care what people think or obtain a custom finished cover that looks lifelike.

Shoes are another one of those areas that most amputees don't consider important. They figure that now that they only have one foot they can wear any old shoe or slipper. Wrong. Good shoes are critical for the proper function of the prosthesis as well as the health of the good foot. I always recommend that the new amputee purchase lightweight shoes that have a good, firm heel support. Cheap shoes that allow the heel of the prosthetic foot to move from side to side will cause undue stress to the residual limb inside of the prosthesis as well as unnatural forces on the sound side foot. I do not recommend boots or high heels for the first prosthesis since these are either heavy or unstable. Motivation is the only time I will vary from this recommendation. If the amputee is adamant about wearing heavy motorcycle boots, then as long as they are aware of the consequences then so be it. The same with high-heeled shoes; there are not many feet that are designed to be worn with high heels and in the initial prosthesis I do not think that it is in the amputee's best interest. However, if the woman insists on wearing high heels and the motivation is enough to have her actually wear the prosthesis, then as long as she is aware of the difficulties then more power to her. I told the story of Laura in Chapter 1. When I met her, she was already in her 70s and would wear nothing but 3-in high heels. She always claimed that they gave her balance but she was definitely an exception to the norm.

Once an amputee has progressed past the preparatory phase of his or her rehabilitation, there are not many types of shoes that can't be worn. There are specific feet to accommodate everything from cowboy boots to spike heels. Your prosthetist can acquaint you with the different feet that are available and their pros and cons. I personally have gravitated toward low heel shoes that are lightweight and well made. It is not in the amputee's best interest to skimp on shoes since it is important not only for the stability of the good foot but also the proper function of the prosthetic foot.

Once you have worn a prosthesis for a while you can do a little experiment that will show you how much difference the weight of the shoe makes to the feel of the prosthesis. This is particularly effective if you have a short stump. Take the shoe off of your prosthetic foot and walk around barefooted for a while. It may feel a bit off balanced but it is striking how much lighter the leg feels with the shoe off then with it on. My shower leg is set up and aligned for walking with no shoe and I find myself wearing it around the house much of the time.

Shoes and the Amputee

1. New amputees should use a new pair of shoes, preferably with a low heel and stiff reinforcing around the heel of the foot.
2. Avoid slippers, high heels, work boots, or cowboy boots on the initial prosthesis unless you won't wear the leg without them. It is better to suffer through the imbalance and discomfort of inappropriate shoes than not to wear a prosthesis.
3. Once the preparatory phase is over, it is time to experiment with different types and styles of shoes. Ask your prosthetist to explain the pros and cons of the different feet that can accommodate greater heel heights.
4. Good shoes are important for the rest of your life as an amputee, not only for the function of your prosthetic foot but for the health of the sound side foot.

Ambulatory Aids

In the initial stages of recovery from amputation, some sort of ambulatory aid is necessary. Many amputees utilize walkers or crutches for the rest of their lives if strength and stability continue to be issues for them. A cane will often provide the added confidence to allow the amputee to be mobile in most community settings. I will talk briefly about each of these devices and offer the pros and cons of their use.

Prior to being fit with a prosthesis or if there has been some type of postoperative device applied the amputee will require an ambulatory aid. Usually these take the shape of either a walker or crutches. It is ideal if the amputee can get some physical therapy in order to determine which device is best suited for him or her as well as training in their use. This is not a long and involved process in most cases as these are simple devices and their use can be taught in a session or two. Probably the most common initial device is the walker that has either wheels or prongs on the front. The wheels make it easier to slide the walker across the floor, but care needs to be taken that enough weight is placed on the front to prevent the walker from slipping on the wheels. The standard walker does not have wheels and needs to be lifted with each step. Choices of which device to use should be determined by the environment in which they will be used and the strength of the amputee. If the amputee lives in a nursing home environment that is well monitored and free of barriers, the wheeled walker is suitable. Walkers are great and enable many amputees who otherwise would be relegated to a wheelchair to ambulate throughout our communities. They do, however, promote a gait pattern that is not the best. When using a walker, the hands are placed forward of the rest of the body, causing the amputee to have a hunched forward walking pattern. Any gait pattern that is repeated many times for weeks or months becomes the body's normal mode of operation. If the amputee has the potential to progress to other ambulatory aids or shed their use altogether, then it is important to keep the process moving.

Amputees who have the strength and balance to stand on their sound leg can use crutches as their initial ambulatory aid. Crutches can also be the second step for an amputee that has improved his or her strength and stability on a walker and has demonstrated the competence to progress to the next step. Crutches come in many forms, from underarm style to custom designs. Which style will work for any particular amputee is up to the individual and his or her health care assistants, physical therapist, doctor, or prosthetist. The most common type of crutch is the underarm crutch, which has a padded bar that should be adjusted to fit just beneath the armpit and a handgrip that should leave the arm slightly bent at the elbow. The fit of the crutch is very important because if it is set too high, then the amputee will be unstable and vault over with each step in addition to cutting off circulation beneath the arm. If the crutch is set too low, the amputee will have a hunched over gait similar to the walker.

Another crutch style that is better for ambulation but requires more strength and balance is the forearm or Lofstrand crutch. This style has a cuff that clamps around the forearm and does not come up beneath the armpit. The cuff holds onto the forearm and allows more freedom of motion with the hands. If the cuff is adjusted properly, this style promotes the most upright gait pattern. There are many new crutch designs that some amputees swear by that have a combination of the two styles or a redesigned structure. I have always kept a pair of crutches around for those times when I cannot wear a leg. It is not a bad idea for most amputees to do the same even after they have progressed beyond their needs.

Here are the pros and cons of crutches and a few stories to illustrate the point. The underarm crutches are easier to use because you can lean your body into them and be supported by the padded bar beneath the armpits. You can even clamp the crutch under your armpit and carry things although this is risky and dangerous if you slip. The downside to the underarm crutch is what do you do with the crutch when you want to use your hands? They have an uncanny ability to fall over no matter where you place or lean them. If you place them on the floor, they will invariably trip the next person who comes by. Walking through a roomful of amputees on crutches is like trying to negotiate a minefield. The forearm crutches will clamp onto your forearm, allowing you to use your hands to pick up things without having to set the crutches down or lean them against something. The problem is that you cannot carry anything except a bag or a crumpled piece of paper. I still have the same crutches that I obtained when I first lost my leg over 30 years ago. There is a noticeable bend in the left one due to my early attempt at carrying a cup of coffee with them. I discovered that carrying coffee was not an option as I managed to spill it all over the floor and myself. I threw the crutch across the room in my frustration and it struck the kitchen cabinet, breaking the door off and putting a good bend in the crutch. After repairing the door, I tried to straighten my crutch but to no avail. I finally took it out into the driveway and placed it beneath the wheel of my car and drove over it several times until it straightened out somewhat. To this day my crutch reminds me of my lack of tolerance and frustration at my inability to function as I had hoped.

The third type of ambulatory aid is the cane. Canes come in many styles and designs from ones that have 4 prongs on the floor to hand carved ones that have swords inside of them. As with all ambulatory devices, it is important to fit the cane to the correct height to provide the amputee with as normal of a gait as possible. If the cane is too short, then the amputee will bend forward and if it is too long, he or she will not get much support from it. There is some confusion as to which hand the cane should be held in. I am married to a physical therapist who swears that all canes should be held in the opposite hand as the amputation. Most of the amputees that I know hold their cane in the same side as their amputation unless they are in therapy and don't want to be yelled at by their PT.

I never used a cane, but I did use a walking stick that I made myself. I liked the feel of holding onto my ambulatory device at shoulder level with my elbow bent; this seemed to give me more stability. I had also carved the walking stick, which I thought was cool. Plus, it made a good defensive weapon that actually came in handy one night on the beach in Mombassa, Kenya. One important safety aspect of any cane or crutch is to make sure that the rubber tip on either device is in good working condition. If the rubber pad is worn or is poking through, it seriously increases your chances of the crutch slipping out from under you.

Integrating Sex

Certainly one of the big problems facing most amputees, regardless of age, is the question of sex. Can I still have sex? Will the opposite sex still find me attractive? Will my sexual parts still work? Is there sex after death? OK, that is not one of the questions that people have but it sounded good. The answer to all of these questions is that it is up to you. Sex is a relationship. It starts with yourself; if you have a decent relationship with yourself, then generally you will enjoy sex. You may start by having sex with yourself and if that is successful, then you can move on to partners. I am not a sex counselor and have no degrees in the subject, but I know from experience and honest feedback from friends that the key to a rewarding sex life begins with yourself.

I was 20 years old when I lost my leg and was only beginning to enjoy the fruits of being a youth in the '70s. I had a girlfriend but she was living a thousand miles away and I barely remember her visit shortly after my accident. I was very nervous about the whole sex thing; after all, I was now only half a man and seriously wondered whether women would still find me attractive. I was still in the hospital when I experimented with masturbation to make sure that everything still worked. It did, but the morphine made it take a lot longer than normal. I later discovered that any pain medication inhibits ejaculation to some degree so if you are on medication, you may have to be patient. It is also an excellent reason to get off of pain medication since performance will suffer as long as you are routinely taking painkillers. I had always been a somewhat bold male, having the philosophy that I needed to be persistent because I was not that good looking. Now though I was very nervous about approaching women, imagining that they would be disgusted with my disability. I was also living with my parents so there was not much opportunity to meet girls. When I visited my girlfriend, I was relieved to find that I was still very interested in sex. We spent a couple of nights together and although we had sex as much as she would allow, it was not quite the same as before. She was tentative and nervous that she would hurt me, which was not helped by my falling in her bathroom and nearly busting my stump open.

I returned to college in the winter of 1975 and began my classes, often on crutches. My girlfriend was in a different college so I only saw her a couple of times per month. It was at this time that I discovered something very important about my sexuality. **People treat you like you treat yourself.** I projected a positive attitude about what had happened to me and found that women were attracted by my attitude. I am sure that some of my sexual encounters were due to what amputees call "sympathy sex" but most of my relations were honest desire. My girlfriend broke up with me in the spring of that year and I always felt that it was due to the fact that she only saw me during the recovery period when I was in a lot of pain and on crutches all of the time. I was pretty crushed by the event but like my amputation, it didn't keep me down for long. I was then free to experience the full potential of a time when there were few deadly sexually transmitted diseases and people were open to experimentation. I have always been grateful that I got to experience that time. The last 2 years of college were full of many relations with women that had the effect of supporting my self-esteem and giving me the confidence to be bold with women. Unfortunately, there was a downside to this also. I am an over-compensator and my desire to experience all types of women did not allow me to develop what I now know to be good relationships.

Other than having an amputated leg, the rest of me was in good shape. I was bicycling and playing handball so I had an athletic body and because I was doing yoga I was very limber for an athletic guy. At no time did any woman project revulsion at my amputation and generally they weren't even that curious. Again, I think that it was my attitude that made the difference; if it didn't bother me, I don't think that it bothered them.

When I took my first job in Egypt, I was in a place where there were very few Western women and I didn't have many choices as to sexual partners. Egyptian women were beautiful, but the Islamic culture has different rules regarding sexual conduct and sex out of wedlock was a major violation. After a long stretch of enforced celibacy, I began to have affairs with married women whose husbands were largely absent. This did satisfy my sexual urges but placed me in great danger and did nothing for the relationships that the women were in.

Some of the most provocative sexual stories that I have ever heard from either men or women occurred while they were in the hospital. I have several buddies who have told me of delicious encounters with nurses while they were in the hospital recovering from their amputation. In nearly all cases this experience caused them to have greater self-esteem and added to their confidence when they returned to the real world.

Wherever and whenever you have sex for the first time after your amputation, it is likely that you will experience doubt, fear, and possibly shame. This is normal, and the trick is not to let it stop you from finding a way to make it satisfying for yourself and your partner. It is just like learning to walk; it was tough at first but you figured it out. My insecurity manifested itself in a desire to please my partner. I figured that since I was at a disadvantage as an amputee, I needed to be able to be better than the next guy at the technical aspects of performance. I studied books and asked my buddies (who often lied about their exploits and techniques) but it wasn't until I met a Swedish woman on New Years Eve of 1977 that I really met a partner who took the time to instruct me as to what pleased her. What a concept! Actually talking about sex and showing each other how to get the maximum pleasure from one another. This served me well and I am eternally grateful to Eva for the information, but I was still a long way from attaining a wholesome sexual relationship.

My first marriage lasted 8 years and we had no children. I lost my monogamy in the first year and used extramarital affairs as a way of compensating for my insatiable desires. It took a long time to realize that this desire or lack of self-esteem was a bottomless pit that no amount of sex was going to fill. The only thing that my affairs did was to ruin my marriage and divert me from real relationship issues. This was a tough lesson and the temptation to revert back to old patterns never quite dies.

The evolution of my personal sexual experience as an amputee is still happening but I feel that I have finally reached a stage of healthy balance. I am married and have two wonderful boys, and my commitment to my family takes precedence over my urges or desires. I still have those urges and desires, but I realize that I will not fill them by looking outside of my marriage. Our sex life is really good. For me it's never enough but maybe that's just me. I know many other male amputees who feel the same way about their sex lives but then again most of the able-bodied guys I know have the same feelings. I guess that means that I have reached a degree of normalcy, since my problems are the same as everyone else's.

The experience of amputation can be far more difficult for a woman in regards to her sexuality than to a man. I am not a woman and cannot begin to appreciate what it must feel like to be in their shoes. Yet, as an amputee who has worked with many women amputees, I know that the women who have the most satisfying sexual relationships share the same attitude that men have—self-confidence in their own sexuality and in the knowledge that the men who are turned off by their amputation are losers anyway. A very good friend of mine who is a bilateral amputee claims that her amputations are the perfect screening process for shallow men. They just don't come around and the ones that are attracted to her have some depth.

There are men who are attracted to female amputees because of their amputation. There is even an organization that holds conventions where female amputees are invited to participate with all expenses paid where these men are in hopes of having sex with amputee women. Here the object is the female amputee. These are not relationships beyond sex and I caution female amputees about this organization since the solicitors are not always honest about their motives. Many amputees go through a process to reach a healthy sexual perspective, and gratuitous sex may be one of the phases. Please be forewarned that organizations that promote sex for its own sake are not about relationships and you will be used. There are also organizations devoted to women who seek male amputees. I was solicited through the Internet by one such organization. Ostensibly, this organization was trying to match women, who are either devotees or fetishists, with male amputees. They claim to be honest and not just sexually oriented, but I found that the chat room was full of a lot of needy people.

Marriage and Relationships

Probably one of the toughest situations to be in is when you are in a long-term relationship and you find that your partner no longer finds you attractive after amputation. I recommend counseling since the ramifications of any other choice most likely will not achieve a very satisfying sexual experience. Generally, patience and tenderness will have the best results in an attempt to regain a sexual relationship with a partner. This isn't easy since marriages and long-term relationships always have patterns that the partners have fallen into and breaking patterns is never easy. A good counselor can make all the difference in the world, someone with which both parties are comfortable. The worst thing you can do is to do nothing. The relationship will degenerate into unfulfilled desires and building resentment that will eventually destroy a good relationship if left to fester.

My experience is that trauma within a relationship is often the deciding factor as to what the couple is really made of. If the relationship is based on superficial values and if one of the partners becomes an amputee, then the relationship is likely to fail. However, if the couple is bound by solid values that transcend appearances, then the couple will not only survive the trauma, they will grow in strength and love by it. I have had the pleasure of working with a couple that both were in a motorcycle accident and both lost their right leg. These were some rough people who rode with a gang and from time to time had their altercations with the law. I got to make prostheses for both of them and they had weathered the obvious trauma of the dual amputation by drawing on each other's strength. Their teenage kids were some of the most polite and motivated teenagers that I had ever met. Certainly the trauma of amputation will test the strength of a relationship but in surviving and growing through it, a relationship will come out stronger.

I would also like to address the subject of homosexual relationships. I know plenty of homosexual amputees and have found them to have the exact same problems with relationships as heterosexuals. I was even made an honorary lesbian by 2 technicians that worked with me, which I accepted as an honor. Basically, there isn't an issue here. Whether you are gay, lesbian, black, or from India, the problems of relationships are universally similar. Don't let your sexual preference stand in the way of a healthy relationship with someone you love. Most people are accepting and with a little time will return feelings of affection despite the fact that you are an amputee. If they don't eventually come around, then they are shallow and not worth your effort.

Different Cultures

I have lived in 3 distinct cultures since I have been an amputee. The first is the American culture with its diversity and dynamic nature. The second is the Islamic culture, which has a more ordered style of life that is bound by faith. The third is the Spanish culture, which orients more by family and image. Each of these cultures has a little different perspective on the amputee and I will share what I observed.

The American culture is the one in which I have lived most of my life and the one in which I lost my leg. In the 1970s there was not much of a perception by the general public of disability issues. There wasn't handicapped parking and very few special programs to provide assistance or recreation. These became more prevalent in the 1980s and 1990s with the advent of disability organizations as well as the ADA, or Americans with Disabilities Act. In the United States there were structures set up to assist you if you lost a leg, such as Medicare, vocational rehabilitation, and other private organizations. However, there was and still is an element of self-help to obtain assistance. No one will sign you up or make sure that you go to the right agency; the amputee has to do this him- or herself. The system in the United States provides some help to obtain a prosthesis or to provide training and rehabilitation, but it will not walk you through the process. One of the most refreshing aspects of the system in the United States is society's acceptance of amputees as normal people. Compared with some of the other cultures in which I have lived, the United States has probably one of the most open-minded cultural perspectives anywhere in the world. You will not be taken care of as in European systems, but you have more equal social and employment opportunities.

The Islamic culture does not provide the social acceptance of the American culture. Depending upon the family commitment and social status, an amputee may be accepted within the family and given a place in society. Amputation is often seen as the penalty for some transgression either now or in the past that was the cause for your misfortune. If you become an amputee in this world, it is not acceptable to show or reveal your prosthesis in public. A man or woman must take off their shoes to enter a mosque and this not only reveals the prosthesis but it is not an easy task as there is generally no place to sit in order to remove the shoes. Praying, which is done 5 times a day, requires kneeling, another act that is very difficult if not impossible for a below-knee amputee. These seemingly simple acts can create a circumstance that makes it difficult, if not impossible, to integrate into normal society. At no time was I treated with disdain or derision when I lived in Egypt or traveled in the Middle East; however, I avoided places where I would have to conform to Islamic traditions. On the contrary, the people that I got to know always treated me with hospitality and genuine warmth and I gained a great deal of respect for Islam. The customs and mores of the culture and religion make it difficult for an amputee to fit in with the same degree of comfort that is available in the United States and Europe. There is also very little in the way of support for amputees either emotionally as in support groups or sports organizations.

I had the good fortune of getting to spend 2003 living in southern Spain with my family. We resided in Granada, the capital of Andalusia where Spanish culture is still very strong and there were not many people who spoke English. I chose this place because one of my best friends in the world, Miguel, lives there. We even got a house only a block away from his in the oldest part of town called the Albaicin. This is not only a strikingly beautiful city but it is nestled in the heart of the Sierra Nevada Mountains. At first everyone seemed friendly in the traditional part of town in which we lived. I did notice that very few Spanish men wore shorts even though it got quite hot in the summer. Miguel, who is a bilateral below-knee amputee, never wore shorts in public. I thought that this was strange since he had 2 very nice prostheses that were made for him in Switzerland and he was famous as an Olympic medallist in both Nordic skiing and bicycling. It wasn't until my Spanish improved and I could understand what people were saying as I passed by that I started to get a clue as to the cultural acceptance of amputation. I overheard people who were polite and seemingly friendly to my face make remarks such as, "How dare he show his deformity off in public" and "What is he trying to prove?" This upset me and I asked both Spanish and other Hispanic friends of mine what was going on. Again, it goes back to the ancient perception that what happens to you is the result of some punishment from God. To reveal your disability by wearing shorts as an amputee is not only distasteful but an affront to the traditionally minded people. This perception is changing as it is in the rest of Europe. There are a multitude of nationally funded organizations to support and provide recreation opportunities for amputees. This exposure has helped to change people's perceptions, especially younger people. In time amputees will not have to feel the sting of social rejection, which can be a big inhibitor to participation in the culture that they are born into.

I have traveled and spent a lot of time in the rest of Europe. Due to the age of most of the downtown parts of cities, it is not a particularly handicap-friendly place. An amputee needs to be able to walk and negotiate uneven steps in order to get around. However, great strides are being made in most Western European nations to make their businesses and public buildings accessible. More important is that the social attitude is one of acceptance and understanding, perhaps this is due to the large numbers of amputees. I found it to be an easy place in which to get around and wearing shorts did not attract stares or snide remarks. I have also traveled in sub-Saharan Africa and although it was not a particularly accessible place I never felt social animosity. I am even in contact with an amputee support group in Ghana so there seems to be a movement, not hindered by culture, that provides help for amputees. I have never traveled in Asia (although I hope to someday), but have heard from other amputees that in most places there is not a cultural aversion to amputees. There is, however, a problem with the custom of removing shoes before entering a house as well as a distinct lack of chairs. One problem that amputees will encounter in Asia is that most meals are served on low tables where you have to sit on the floor cross-legged. This is nearly impossible to do comfortably with a prosthesis. There are specific components that were created for above-knee amputees that allow the shank of the prosthesis to rotate in, allowing the amputee to sit normally but there is nothing for the below knee.

My experience in traveling is that as an amputee you must be willing to adapt. No culture likes a whiner in their midst. If things are not necessarily easy, try not to make a big deal out of it. Most people are willing to help you and accommodate your needs if you ask in a polite manner. Demanding assistance will not ingratiate you to the culture and can cause just the opposite. Be flexible and find ways to overcome obstacles, which generally has the effect of attracting admiration instead of hostility. Traveling is a great way to broaden one's experience whether you are an amputee or not and amputation should not be a barrier to travel. However, it may be wise to take a few things with you.

The Amputee Survival Kit

Over the years I have found that every amputee will benefit from carrying with him or her a few simple items in case of emergencies. You never know when something can break or come loose on your leg and if you have the right tool with which to fix it, you can generally carry on. I also include a few specific medical aids that can help get you by if you incur minor damage to your stump.

Imagine that you are on vacation in Hawaii, a dream that you have had your whole life. The first night you are drinking a few too many mai tais and you start to join the hula line. You are having the time of your life until you get back to your hotel and you discover a blister the size of a dime on your stump as you take your leg off. This could ruin the rest of your vacation, as you have to sit with your leg off because you don't have crutches or any kind of mobility aid. Blisters can be very painful and will ruin a vacation in a heartbeat; however, there are ways to treat them that will allow them to heal while you are still active.

Survival Kit

1. The first item in any kit should be specific tools that your prosthesis needs, such as an Allen wrench that tightens the foot or specific wrenches if you have modular parts. Sometimes fittings can come loose and with the right wrench they can be fixed easily and properly.

2. Second Skin (Spenco Medical Corp., Waco, TX) or some other skin protection material that you can put over top of a blister or abrasion which will provide cushion as well as friction relief. In combination with an antibacterial agent or Mercurochrome this can allow you to heal a wound while still wearing the prosthesis. Band-aids are not recommended since they increase pressure on a wound and the adhesive can cause as much damage as the original injury.

3. Some type of antibacterial agent such as Mycitracin (Pharmacia & Upjohn Consumer Healthcare, Kalamazoo, MI) or a triple antibacterial salve that can be obtained at any drug store. Use topically for any type of open wound or abrasion.

4. Vaseline or some other type of topical lubricant. Apply in places where there is undue friction and redness. Hydrocortisone cream is also helpful for rashes.

5. Duct tape or some other kind of strong, reinforced tape to make minor emergency repairs. I have hiked many miles on feet that were duct taped onto my leg when they broke in the middle of the woods. I only got off of Mt. Shasta by duct taping my leg to my thigh when my old latex suspension-sleeve disintegrated on me. One warning: removing duct tape from the skin is not a happy event and you should try to soak it in hot water prior to removal.

6. Waterless hand cleaner is a new item that is great for a quick cleansing of the stump, especially in warm, humid environments. You can purchase small containers of this at most drug stores.

7.   Moleskin or some other self-adhesive thin padding can be used for minor repairs to an insert or to make temporary, minor reliefs to a socket. To make a relief in a socket or preferably on an insert you must make a donut over the effected area. First, cut a piece of moleskin twice as big as the problem area and in a circle. Next, cut out the center the same size as the blister or abrasion. Place on the inside of the socket or on the insert. If this is not enough relief, cut a second donut slightly smaller than the first and put on top of the first one. If this is too much, then it is easy to remove.

8.   A small folding pair of scissors is very handy for cutting second skin, moleskin, or holes in socks. A Swiss Army knife or Leatherman tool that has a variety of items on it, from scissors to knives to pliers, can be real handy.

9.   Carry any medications or pain pills with you in case of emergencies.

10.   Remember to be creative and prepared. Don't let a minor problem ruin a vacation or business trip.

CHAPTER 7

Bilateral Amputees

Stories

Julia

Julia is a beautiful woman who became a bilateral below-knee amputee when she was in her mid-30s. She had gone into the hospital for a minor surgical procedure and when she awoke 2 days later, she had both legs amputated below the knee and most of her fingertips were missing. The doctors told her that she had had a reaction to the anesthesia and her body had cut off circulation to her extremities, necessitating their removal. She went into a deep state of shock and denial.

Julia had always prided herself on her stunning good looks and shapely body. She was well educated with a husband and young son. The thought of what she looked like now was unbearable. At first her husband seemed supportive. She was in the hospital and then rehabilitation for 60 days. The rehabilitation process was extremely painful as the skin grafts on her hands healed. The constant need to manipulate the grafted and scarred skin shot bolts of agony through her but because of her family, she persisted. Her son was deeply disturbed by the trauma and only came out of his shock when he was with his mom. She knew that she had to be strong for him and somehow dragged the inner strength out of her soul. Many days she wanted to give up and die but it was not to be; she had her son to live for.

She received her preparatory prostheses and was able to get around the house on her walker. She just couldn't get used to not being able to go for walks or ride a bicycle. The preparatory legs she had were heavy and had exposed pipes that she was ashamed to be seen with, even to her family.

Her husband seemed to change once she came home. He started working longer hours and was often absent on weekends. He no longer wanted to make love to her, claiming that he didn't want to damage her healing. Julia had been a very sexual woman and needed the affection as well as just the gratification of her natural desires. She began to suspect that he was seeking his affection elsewhere. She had always been a straightforward kind of person and yet it was terrifying to confront him with his adultery. In some ways she couldn't blame him; after all she was not the woman he had married, the thought of which caused her to weep uncontrollably. Julia did have some close friends as well as her mother with whom she had a special relationship. In one of her talks with her mother she finally confessed her fears. After much crying, she decided that she had to confront her husband. That night after their son had gone to bed she waited until they were both in bed and the lights were off. She asked him if there was another woman and his dispassionate reply confirmed her fears. She cried softly, but surprisingly she felt relieved, as if a chapter had closed. Julia awoke the next morning and asked her husband to move out and requested a divorce. She sat down with her son that evening and explained the impossible to him; much to her surprise he was not shocked. Kids usually know what is going on in the house even if they allow their parents to believe they don't.

After her amputations, Julia contacted an attorney to represent her in a lawsuit against the doctors, anesthesiologist, and the hospital where the surgery was performed. She discovered that she had been given the wrong anesthesia and that the mistake should not have been made. She didn't feel particularly vengeful but if she could recover some money, it would help pay for prostheses as well as her son's education. The courts were backed up badly at the time of her suit and it took nearly 4 years for her case to finally come to trial. More painful than her legs was the constant reliving of the experience every time she met with her attorneys as well as the torment of seeing her ex-husband each time. Her son was clearly traumatized by the proceedings as he was a witness and had to give a deposition. One week before the case was to come to trial, the judge that was to hear her case died of a massive heart attack. When her lawyer came to her with the news and informed her that it may be as much as 3 more years before a new trial could be heard, she decided to drop the case. She felt that she could not continue to put her son through the painful process and that she could not fully heal until this thing was behind her. Julia received no money from losing her legs and fingertips in such a senseless way.

Julia got on with her life. She got her first permanent prostheses after 6 months and life got better. She could walk with crutches and after a few months with a cane, which gave her the confidence to begin to be seen in public again. She started swimming at the local pool early in the mornings before many people arrived and really enjoyed the exercise. Financially, she was strapped since the alimony and child support were barely enough to get by. Her son was brilliant and deserved the best education so she decided that she needed to go back to school and get her master's degree, which would enable her to get better employment in her field. She had a degree in business but wanted to branch out into city planning, so back to school she went. It was tough raising her son with little help from her ex-husband and going to school full-time, but she received her Master's Degree in Urban Planning after 2 years. Her son was beginning high school now and it wouldn't be long before he was ready to go to college. He had his sights set on an Ivy League school so she knew that even if he received scholarship help, she would have to support him to some degree. Julia got a job working for one of the local municipalities of the greater Boston area and quickly worked her way up to the Senior Planner's position. This position gave her the salary and benefits necessary to provide a decent education for her son as well as the professional image that she desired.

Like I said, Julia is a beautiful woman and the loss of legs as well as fingertips initially had a devastating effect on her self-image. The divorce from her husband didn't help either, so she imagined that dating was something that was not going to happen for her. Much to her surprise, she was asked out while taking classes at school. She went out some, but was fearful of anything that even remotely felt like a relationship. Her initial sexual experiences were timid at first, but she found that men didn't seem to mind her lack of legs at all if she was aggressive with her desires. Her girlfriends would take her to singles bars where she determined that 8 out of 10 men were just jerks. Once they found out about her legs, the jerks would beat a hasty retreat. After a while she looked at the amputations as a great filtering process. If the guy stuck around after he learned of her disability, then he at least had some depth to him.

Julia is now in her 50s and is fit and healthy since she either walks every day or swims. She has tried all of the new prosthetic technology that has been available but has always returned to the supercondylar suspension although she now uses a urethane gel liner. She tried energy storing feet but felt that they fatigued her more than they energized her so she went back to her multiaxial style of foot. Her son graduated with honors from an Ivy League college and is married with 2 children. She still does some consulting with some of the local municipalities but is looking to retire in a couple of years. Financially, she is not rich but is reasonably well off. She has lived with several men over the years but does not want to remarry. Her sex life is healthy and she says she has no problem finding men, just finding the right one. Julia is one of the most remarkable women I ever met, taking a life that would crush most people and turning it into one that is rich in experience and relationships.

Bret

Bret was 29 years old and a logger by trade. He was married to a wonderful woman named Helen and they had 2 sons. The oldest boy was helping him to clear brush one hot July afternoon. One of the crew of loggers was working on a large tree where they were clear-cutting a stand of second growth fir that grew in the mountains outside of Boise, Idaho. Bret was running the bulldozer and grading a road so they could get the big trucks into the clearing to haul out the logs. The logger working on the large tree had only been logging with the crew since the beginning of the summer and had been trying to prove himself to the rest of the crew. As he cut his back wedge into the tree, he thought he felt it nudge the wrong way. He pulled out his chain saw and looked up at the 90-ft fir tree. It seemed stable enough and he really didn't want to ask any of the rest of the crew for help since they would only give him grief at lunch about not being able to handle the work. He glanced around to make sure that the spot where he intended to fell the tree was clear and continued his cutting. A chain saw makes a lot of noise when you are holding it and he never heard Bret in the bulldozer behind him.

All of a sudden the chain saw stuck and he heard a sickening crack as the tree finally gave up its life and started to fall. Only it wasn't falling where he wanted it, instead the tree fell backward so he ran perpendicular to the fall of the tree with the chain saw still running and stuck in the tree. Bret never heard the tree fall but he felt something vibrate and looked up just in time to see the main trunk of the tree come crashing toward the open cab of the bulldozer. Two seconds later, Bret was crushed beneath tons of tree and trapped in the twisted metal of the bulldozer. He never lost consciousness and never went into shock as he lay there with both feet pinned beneath the log. The pain was like an inferno erupting from his feet and he knew that he was in trouble. His son, who was only 10 at the time, came to his side and Bret went calm despite the pain. Bret was made of tougher stuff then even he imagined and the thought of what his son must be feeling to see his father in such pain gave him a strength and calmness that he never dreamed he could have. It took almost an hour for paramedics and rescuers to free him and load him on the helicopter for the flight to the hospital in Boise. By the time he received medication for the pain, it had been 2 hours and he was beginning to come unglued, but Helen was at the hospital and the sight of her determined strength calmed Bret. When he woke up hours later he looked down to see his right foot gone just below the knee and the left foot missing at the ankle.

Bret had grown up in Idaho living the life of an outdoorsman; hunting, fishing, and logging had been a natural extension of this life. Now it seemed that the outdoors life was over. How could he operate machinery with no feet? How could he heft the 13.5-kg (30-lb) chain saw that was his livelihood? What were his kids going to think of their crippled father? Helen was there with him now but how was she going to take to life with a legless man? These questions plagued him as he lay in the hospital, his mind fogged with morphine.

Bret was not a particularly religious man. He rarely went to church and although Helen was a regular at Trinity Methodist he only went on Christmas and Easter. Bret was not going to give up on the life that he had made for himself and as he wrestled with his demons he found that there was a spirit inside of him that gave him strength. When his 2 boys came to see him, he found himself making jokes about his legs instead of feeling sorry for himself. Where did this come from? He had always been an optimistic person who had a noncomplicated way of looking at things but this inner strength surprised him.

Bret knew nothing about prostheses and didn't know anyone who wore one. After 3 weeks in the hospital, a man who described himself as a prosthetist (which to Bret sounded suspiciously like prostitute) visited him. The man talked with him for several hours about artificial legs and what he was going to be able to do again. When Bret asked him when he could go back to work, the man said that returning to the logging profession was probably not an option. The prosthetist said he would be returning in 3 more weeks to take casts so that he could make Bret a new pair of legs. Bret got angry after the prosthetist left. "What does he mean that I can't return to logging? It's all that I know and I'm not about to give that up. I will show him," he thought to himself. Helen could tell that he was upset and comforted him the best that she could, but she was afraid that the prosthetist was probably correct in his assessment.

After a month in the hospital Bret was released to go home in a wheelchair. He had a hard time getting around in the chair and their house was hardly accessible. He experienced his first real days of intense frustration. When he was alone during the day he would begin to curse the day of the accident and wonder why this had happened to him. His logging buddies came by and they would stay up late having a sip of whiskey, he asked what had happened with the guy who had cut the tree that fell on him. His friends said that the man had quit the next day and had moved to Florida or somewhere, unable to cope with what he had done. Somehow Bret didn't feel any satisfaction from the news. He didn't blame the man for his predicament. As a matter of fact, blame didn't really enter into his thinking. What had happened to him had happened and no amount of revenge or bitterness would ever bring back his feet. Life isn't about what happens to you, it's about what you do with what happens to you.

Most days the pain was bearable. He had pain medication to take the edge off but Bret was leary of becoming addicted to those pills and he didn't like the way it left him fuzzy all of the time. He started to cut them out and only use them if he really needed them. The pain that really drove him crazy though were the "electric shooters" as he called them. They would come out of nowhere and send waves of electric agony through him that caused him to grab the chair and hold on for life. Fortunately, they only lasted a few seconds but there were times when they would come in a series and this was the worst time. That's when he would turn to the whiskey bottle for a quick swig to get him through. Bret knew that if he kept on like this he was eventually going to go crazy and then the prosthetist showed up.

The prosthetist came in and asked how he was doing. Bret didn't particularly like the man but asked him to get on with it so the prosthetist proceeded to wrap plaster bandages around his stumps. He explained to Bret that the longer stump was called a Syme's amputation and the shorter one was a below knee. He said that he would take the casts along with all of the measurements that he had back to the lab and then send him the legs in a couple of weeks. Bret asked what he would do when he got the legs and the man simply answered that he should put them on and walk.

The next 2 weeks went by slowly, but one day a large package arrived from the prosthetic facility. Inside were two shiny plastic legs, one with some type of strap that went over his knee and the other was long with a removable door on the shank. It took Bret a couple of hours to figure out how to put them on and finally he had to call the prosthetist to figure out what to do with all of the socks he had gotten. He finally got them on and stood up with no cane or crutches. It felt good to stand even though there was a lot of pain in both of the legs, something he figured he'd get used to. Now it was time to walk. Helen took his arm and he took his first steps down the narrow hallway. He could do it; it was like walking on stilts, but by God he could do it. That night he walked up and down the hallway holding onto the walls to keep from falling. When he finally took the legs off his stumps were red and sore, but no serious damage had been done. For the first time since the awful accident Bret had hopes that he could return to his life.

Over the next several weeks Bret mastered walking on the prostheses and got himself a cane to use when he went out to the barn. Rough terrain was difficult since the feet were pretty stiff and anytime he stepped on a stone it would pitch him in the opposite direction. He had to call the prosthetist again to learn how to add socks as his stumps shrank. He now understood why they had sent so many. One morning when he had just added some socks and the legs were actually not feeling bad, he went out to the barn to feed the horses. As he looked for the pitchfork he came across his chain saw. The big Stihl with a 91-cm (36-in) cutting bar was like he had left it, worn but not a speck of dirt or grease on it and the chain was sharp enough to shave with. He reached over and picked it up. It started in an instant and he moved over to some logs stacked nearby. He spent the next hour cutting up the logs and actually working up a sweat. It felt good. Bret determined right then and there that he was going to go back to the profession that he loved.

Bret returned to logging after being off the crew for only 6 months. He worked with his brother and several other men and after a week he was pulling his own weight on the job. He even was able to run the bulldozer as well as all of the other heavy equipment that they needed. No one could believe how well Bret had recovered from what to most men would seem like a life-ending tragedy. To Bret it just seemed like a natural thing and wondered what the big deal was. He went on to raise his boys, who chose to go to college, which suited Bret fine. One day when he was visiting another pros-

Figure 7-1. Walking on the beach. (Photo courtesy of Ossur.)

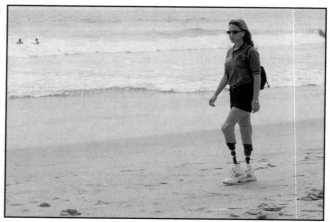

thetist facility, one that didn't mail the legs to you when they were done, he saw a brochure about handicapped skiing. He had always wanted to learn to ski and even though he was 36 years old, he figured he would try it. The local resort was hosting a "learn to ski" clinic and he attended. This was another natural for Bret and after the first day he realized that he loved this sport. He went on to compete in the Nationals in Colorado and won several medals.

I had the honor of making Bret several pair of legs over my career and was continually inspired by his good nature and easy ways. He took the worst that can happen to you and made the best out of it. It was unbelievable to me that his first several pair of legs were mailed to him from the prosthetist with no adjustments or instructions. He exemplified the "can do" spirit that I believe resides within each of us (Figure 7-1).

Prosthetic Considerations

Bilateral amputees have a much different situation then single leg amputees and their prostheses need to be designed to accommodate those needs. Designing prostheses for bilateral amputees is different from unilateral amputees because they have no direct physical contact with the ground. One bilateral friend suggests that it is like living your life on stilts and, in reality, this is exactly what it is like. Components and systems that work for unilateral amputees are not necessarily be what is best for bilateral amputees.

One of the most important issues with bilateral prostheses is height. You may think that this is taken for granted, but the majority of bilateral amputees that I worked with in my private practice had a leg length discrepancy that they had lived with for years. This almost inevitably leads to back and spine problems. It is critical for the prosthetist or physical therapist to check height for some months after the prostheses are fitted in order to ensure that the pelvis is level. Height can change as the amputee adds socks or settles into the socket, creating a leg length difference that has long-term ramifications. I can't emphasize how important this is and if you are a bilateral amputee, then it is important to make sure that your pelvis is level.

Components for bilateral amputees is another area where there seems to be a lot of misunderstanding. I encountered many bilateral amputees who actually had 2 different types of feet on their legs. You can imagine how off-balance this made the amputee feel, with one foot having a different spring or softness than the other. Most of these amputees had adapted but it did not contribute to the ease of body motion. Many types of feet make it difficult for bilateral amputees to stand in a relaxed position. I tried to convert them to energy storing feet that gave them a lot more spring off the toe, but many of the amputees complained of fatigue from wearing them all day. It seems that the feet that store the energy in the pylon of the prosthesis require a constant body motion forward and backward to keep your balance as a bilateral. This is not even noticed as a unilateral since that balance is achieved with the good foot. Many bilateral amputees need what I call a "dead spot" in the feet where they can relax when the balance is just right. This is not the case for all bilateral amputees, but enough of them experienced it that I felt that it needed to be addressed.

Socket stability and suspension are critical for bilateral amputees. There is no good leg to lean on so the sockets need to provide enough side-to-side stability so that the amputee can stand easily without losing his or her balance. I often raised the side walls of the prosthesis in order to gain stability, using a modified supercondylar-style socket to give added medial-lateral control. I also generally aligned bilateral amputees forward of unilateral amputees since the sensation of falling backward when there is no way of catching one's self is very scary. Both of these recommendations are most critical when the stumps are short or one is very short. They are less critical when the residual limbs are midlength or long. Bilateral amputees are one case in which dual suspension may help, usually in the form of pin system bolstered by suspension sleeves.

The comfort of the socket is also critical. Since there is no good leg to limp on when a bilateral amputee has pain or abrasion on his or her stump, he or she may not be mobile. Gel or silicone interfaces definitely increase the comfort level of all amputees but can be most critical to bilateral amputees. It is also important that bilateral amputees have a good concept of how to adjust their legs for shrinkage or swelling since they have to depend upon both prostheses to function.

Mobility

When a unilateral amputee is not wearing his or her leg, he or she can hop or use crutches to get around. When a bilateral amputee is not wearing his or her legs, he or she is either on his or her knees or in a wheelchair. This is a significant difference. Most bilateral amputees that I know have calluses on their knees from walking on them too much. A simple way to minimize the damage of walking on the knees is to wear kneepads such as those used by people who work on floors. They may need some modifications to keep them from slipping off during usage.

Where unilateral amputees need to have a walker or crutches around for the non-ambulatory times, bilaterals have to depend on a wheelchair. It is important to have a chair that is lightweight and can fit through doors in their house. Even though the wheelchair may have infrequent use, it is important to have a house or apartment that is wheelchair friendly. It would be rough to find yourself separated from the kitchen because the chair won't fit through the door.

Figure 7-2. Children are naturally curious. (Photo courtesy of Ossur.)

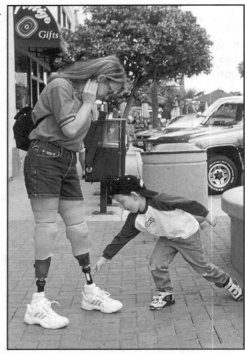

Showers and tubs are particularly challenging for bilateral amputees because they may find that getting into a tub without their legs is a very daunting if not impossible task. One solution is to have a pair of shower legs that allow safe entry into any shower or tub. This is especially critical when traveling because you never know what type of accommodations you may encounter.

In today's world the bilateral amputee can function in most circumstances without any special adaptations. It is important that prosthetists and therapists take the amputee's circumstances into account by making sure the prosthetic components are well suited. A pair of shower legs can give the bilateral the same freedoms that unilateral amputees or able-bodied people take for granted (Figure 7-2) as well as provide back-up legs in case of emergencies.

CHAPTER 8

Syme's and Partial Foot Amputees

Stories

Chip

I was called into the hospital to do an evaluation on a new amputee. As was usually the case, I was given almost no information so I was quite surprised to meet a man in his late 40s who was totally blind. He was so thin that he looked skeletal and his skin was the color of paper. Chip, however, exuded a humor and energy that was infectious, even though my prognosis for his recovery from the amputation was grim.

Chip was a childhood diabetic who, due to his disease, slowly started to go blind by the time he was 35 years old. His circulation was not good and when I met him he had just undergone a Syme's amputation, which is the complete disarticulation (removal) of the foot. A good Syme's amputation removes the foot at the ankle. If there is time, the surgeon can choose to shave the lateral malleoli or anklebone, which makes the prosthetic fitting much easier. This surgeon was quite good and had shaved the bone as well as preserved the heel pad, which is the main justification for a Syme's amputation. The heel pad of the foot has specialized skin that is designed for weight bearing and only the palms of the hands have similar skin. Still, I was not encouraged when I looked at Chip's stump. The skin still showed signs of lack of blood flow and parts of it were turning dark and dead looking. The suture line had not completely healed and my personal opinion (which I kept to myself) was that this was not going to heal, resulting in an eventual below-knee amputation.

I put a shrinker sock onto his residual limb and talked with him for an hour, explaining the process of making a prosthesis. His attitude and composure were almost disarming because he was so positive about the future. I looked down and saw a man who was almost a corpse and yet he looked out from his blindness and saw only the fact that he was alive. I was very impressed with this man and found myself going by to see him for no particular reason other than to be rejuvenated by his exuberance. It must have taken almost 6 weeks for the suture line to heal, but it did and we casted him for his new preparatory prosthesis.

Due to the size of the end of his stump, which was almost like a ball, we built the preparatory leg with a removable door on the inside of the prosthesis. When the door was off, he was able to get the end of his stump down inside of the leg and then Velcro the door back into place. The large size of the ball at the bottom compared to the smaller size of his shin made for great suspension so that there was no need for belts, straps, or even suspension sleeves. The first time Chip put on the prosthesis he walked with his walker and before we were even done with the first fitting he was walking with no aid other than his seeing cane. Everyone at my facility could not help but be struck by Chip's infectious humor and positive attitude.

Chip found out that he had diabetes when he was a teenager and took it in stride as he matured. He was on insulin injections by the age of 16, but this didn't stop him from being a varsity letterman on his high school's cross-country ski team. He graduated and studied engineering at college, completing his studies in 3 years. After graduation he got a job with the state as a surveyor and spent the next 13 years working out of doors surveying projects all over the beautiful Sierra Nevada Mountains. He got married and had a daughter by the time he was 26 years old; life seemed pretty good. Then the diabetes that had (up to that point) been fairly manageable began to affect his sight. At first his vision was just a bit blurry but after only a year he became legally blind. He could no longer perform his duties as a surveyor and he went on disability. The change in Chip's lifestyle was too much for his wife to handle and she asked him for a divorce. The entire physical trauma of his life seemed minor compared to the pain of separation from his daughter and the feeling of abandonment of his wife. It took years but he finally regained his composure to become his old self again. After all, he needed to be strong for his daughter who suffered from the divorce as much as he did.

He was just beginning to regain his dignity when he started having problems with his foot. Since he couldn't see, he was often remiss in simple things like cutting his toenails or making sure that his feet were clean. The diabetes had rendered his feet insensitive so he often couldn't feel them until they got infected when he got small cuts or abrasions. He weathered several such minor abrasions before one that was between his toes went too far. The toe became gangrenous and it had to be removed. Once one toe was gone, things really went downhill. The combination of lack of sensation and the fact that no one was around to check on him created a disintegrating scenario that would eventually lead to his amputation. His surgeon removed a second toe but told Chip that he was afraid that the infection had spread to the rest of his foot and it may require amputation. At first he was absolutely against the idea of losing his foot since he could not figure out how he would be able to function as a one-legged blind person. A couple of weeks went by and even with the lack of feeling in his foot the pain began to be unbearable. He knew that something would have to be done.

This was when I met Chip in the hospital. He was recovering from the amputation and had an intense curiosity about what the prosthesis would be like. After we fit him with his preparatory prosthesis, he entered the guide dog program and obtained a golden retriever named Sally. The next time we saw him he arrived with Sally and it was astounding to see how well she led him around. She was his constant companion and best friend. The glow on Chip's face could not be missed and he embodied one of my favorite sayings. In the movie "Little Big Man," there is a scene at the end of the film where Dustin Hoffman is taking his blind Indian grandfather up to a hilltop burial mound to die. His grandfather, who is a proud old Cheyenne brave, looks to the heavens and utters his death prayer, "Thank you oh Great Spirit for letting me be a human being. Thank you for my eyes and all of the beauty that I have seen. Thank you for my blindness where I have seen even further." This is the spirit of taking what life gives you and finding the blessing in it. It is there; it's only your perspective.

About a year after Chip's amputation, he decided to embark on a new profession. He became a masseur and started working for some of the casinos around Lake Tahoe. He was a very popular masseur and worked as much as he wanted to. Mind you, he didn't need to work since he was on permanent disability in California, which was very generous at that time. He just liked it and it gave him a way to meet new people. This is where he met his new wife Janice. They started to date and despite the obvious physical challenges that she knew she was going to have to live with, Janice found herself falling in love with Chip. She asked him to marry her after dating for a year, which is a little backward of the usual scenario, but Chip was not about to burden anyone with his disability.

Then another tragedy struck. Chip's kidneys failed, an indirect result of the diabetes. He was on dialysis for almost 6 months before he was able to get a transplant, during which time he finally relented and agreed to marry Janice. After his rapid recovery from his transplant, he got married in a small ceremony at Lake Tahoe and then resumed his work as a masseur. Everything went along fine for several years. I had made Chip several legs in that time and he was now using an energy storing Syme's foot. This is a special foot designed to fit on the bottom of a long socket where there is no room for a pylon. He loved the added spring that the foot gave him as well as the better proprioception or feel of the ground beneath him that the foot provided. Due to the fact that his stump had matured and was not so bulbous at the end he could use a different style of socket. Since we were always nervous about any type of abrasion on his stump, we decided to keep using an insert inside of the prosthesis. We fabricated the insert so that when he slid it onto his stump, the outer contour was almost straight with only the slightest dip in the thin area just around his lower shin. When he put that into the socket it provided excellent suspension as well as enough cushion to insure that he would not be dealing with skin breakdown. He liked the ease of donning or putting it on and appreciated the slimmer profile of the finished product. Chip wore shorts all of the time and because of the diabetes he always looked very tan. It never ceased to amaze me how fashion conscious blind people tend to be. Chip was no exception; we had to finish his leg with a natural skin cover so that he would look good on the beach.

Chip received a double blow when Sally, his faithful guide dog, became ill and died and he learned that his transplanted kidney was failing. Janice was a wonderful support for him through this very tough time. He went back on dialysis and waited for another kidney transplant. Dialysis is really a pain to live with. You are hooked up to a dialysis machine, which basically cleans your blood, for 4 hours a day 3 to 4 days a week. This time Chip was luckier, he received a new kidney after only 6 weeks and was back on his foot, as he liked to say it. Still, the loss of Sally and the imminent demise of his new kidney preyed on him. Two years went by and I saw Chip both professionally and socially. He never lost his sense of humor, telling me very bad jokes every time he saw me. I realized that this was one of his best strategies for putting people at ease with his disabilities, telling jokes. He always had a new one for me and invariably they were awful, so awful that they made you laugh anyway.

I was up at Lake Tahoe for a hospital visit and went to see Chip at his home. He had retired from being a masseur after his last kidney transplant, so he was home all of the time. Janice was a piano instructor and worked during the days so Chip and I were alone when I came to visit. We always had an honest relationship and he confided in me that he thought that his 2-year-old kidney was failing. I asked him if he had signed up for a new one and he replied that he had not. I told him that the eventual result of not having a kidney was death and he said that he knew that. He said that he had lived a very good life and that the strain of waking up every morning wondering when his kidney was going to fail was just not worth it. He had decided to pass on and leave the kidney transplant to someone else that had more life to look forward to. I got the sense that Chip was not giving up but had come to some awareness that it was time to move on. He died 3 months later, quietly in his bed, surrounded by the people that he loved. I will never forget him and the outlook that he had on life.

Brenda

Brenda is a 75-year-old woman whom I met in the hospital 10 years ago. She was overweight and had severe diabetes that had resulted in the loss of 3 toes on her right foot. The doctor had called me in to discuss the possibility of a below-knee amputation with her. She was not happy to see me. After I introduced myself and explained why I was there, she told me to get out of her room and that she was not going to let anyone cut her leg off. She was not going to be a cripple and that was that. I left and called the doctor to report her attitude and he revealed that she had not been receptive to the idea of amputation but had hoped that I would have better luck.

When she got out of the hospital she returned to her small home where she had 2 dogs and 6 cats. The house was never clean due to the number of animals everywhere and since the diabetes made her tired she didn't have the energy to tidy up. Brenda didn't have many friends and only 1 daughter who did live nearby. Her daughter cared for her mom but had a job as an accountant and worked long hours, even on the weekends so she did not get much of an opportunity to visit with her. Brenda returned to her bad eating habits and was not very consistent on taking her insulin shots and it wasn't long before a new sore developed on one of the remaining toes on her right foot.

Brenda's daughter came by one Sunday afternoon for a visit and was cleaning up a little when she found some dirty socks under the bed. As she was throwing them into the laundry hamper she noticed that there was dried blood crusted on the toe of the sock. She asked her mom about the blood and Brenda said it was nothing. Her daughter insisted that she take her slipper off immediately and allow her to examine her feet. There was the weeping sore on the big toe of her right foot with the whole toe red and swollen. Her daughter demanded that she go to see her doctor the next day, and Brenda reluctantly agreed.

The doctor examined her toe and said that it was gangrenous which by then was obvious due to the rancid odor that gangrene produces. It is unmistakable. The doctor said that it also would have to come off and that there was a chance that once he removed the toe he might find that the infection had spread into the foot and that part of that may have to be removed as well. Brenda broke into sobbing tears as she asked why this had happened to her and what she had done to deserve this fate. The doctor was silent but said that this needed to be done or eventually the gangrene would enter her blood stream and kill her. She went home in a deep depression. She agreed to the amputation. What else was she going to do? She called her daughter with the news. Her daughter called the doctor who confirmed her mom's story and told her to call me if she wanted more information about prosthetic devices.

That's when I came back into the picture. The call from the daughter began as an apology for the curt way that her mother had treated me on the first meeting. I told her that I understood and that I didn't hold it against her mom. I then explained what the pros and cons of the various levels of amputation were with the worst scenario being to take too little so that her mother would have to undergo multiple surgeries. Her daughter explained all of these things to Brenda but when it came time for the surgery, she begged both her daughter and the surgeon to take as little of the foot as possible. When the surgeon got into the amputation he found that the gangrene had indeed begun to invade the first metatarsals, so he removed the front of her foot up to the second metatarsals. He brought up as much of the intact forefoot skin as he could and created a suture line on the very top of her foot.

When Brenda recovered from the surgery she would not even look at her amputation. I saw her in the hospital and talked to her about partial foot prostheses as well as hygiene and how important it was for her to treat her diabetes. She seemed pretty despondent so I thought that I needed to come back in a couple of days and review all of the information that I had given her. I have learned as a teacher that one of the critical components of imparting information is the timing. If the person is not ready to hear what you have to say, then even your best spiel won't get through. I put a shrinker sock onto her foot and showed her how to use it.

I came back the next week and she was in better spirits, having just watched her favorite soap opera on TV. This time she was much more attentive and I actually got her to don and doff the shrinker by herself. I went over all of the information I had told her the first time and she seemed to be much more receptive. She was discharged the next day and returned home to her house full of animals. The person who had been feeding them had not let the animals out very often so the house was full of feces and urine. The physical therapist that came to her house for the home evaluation nearly gagged as she walked through the door. The physical therapist made arrangements for the house to be cleaned through social services and told Brenda that if she didn't keep things cleaner, she would end up getting another infection or be sent to a nursing home. Brenda promised she would do a better job at housekeeping but found that her foot still hurt her most of the time. Her housekeeping improved at first but soon the house smelled more like a barn than a home.

Brenda's daughter drove her out to my facility where we casted her for a partial foot prosthesis with the goal to supply support without putting pressure on the still tender end of the foot. The wound was healing with only a small amount of redness along the suture line. I instructed her on how to massage and desensitize the skin around the incision but she still had a very difficult time applying any pressure to the area. I emphasized how important it was to continue the massaging, but I would have bet money that when she got home it was not going to happen. I showed her a sample of the partial foot prosthesis that we would fabricate for her and she seemed mildly interested.

We saw Brenda for her fitting appointment 1 week later. She seemed in good spirits and was wearing a spring dress that actually improved her appearance. I could tell immediately that she had not been doing her desensitizing in any kind of routine fashion because she could barely even tolerate the donning of the prosthesis. I used a gel-impregnated sheath that fit over her remaining foot snugly to cushion the still very tender skin and this helped some. When she walked, she actually didn't look too bad. Her gait had suffered from months of sitting and she hunched over when she shuffled, but her stride length was even. We worked several more times on the donning and doffing of the prosthesis until I was comfortable that she knew what she was doing. Her daughter said she would keep tabs on her, so I was comfortable rescheduling her for a follow-up visit in 1 month.

A month went by and Brenda called the day before her follow-up to postpone her appointment. This did not raise any red flags at the time and we really didn't think of her case until during the staff meeting 2 weeks later. She had never rescheduled so I instructed the secretary to call Brenda for a new appointment. Our secretary couldn't reach her on the phone so we sent out a letter. After another week went by with no reply. I called her daughter at work but again had to leave a message. It was tax preparation time and all accountants were up to their necks in IRS forms. Almost another week went by and we finally heard from her daughter. Brenda was in a nursing home and they were trying to get her to agree to a below-knee amputation.

When Brenda had returned to her house after the fitting she had worn the prosthesis all night, even when she went to sleep. I had expressly instructed her to take it off, but she decided it was OK to leave it on. She left it on most of the next day but finally removed it late on the second day. The next morning her foot was very swollen and painful. She crammed her foot into the prosthesis despite the pain but had to leave the gel sheath off, which ended up being a big mistake. The swelling had abated some, which left room in the prosthesis, and without the gel cushion she got a series of blisters across the top of the suture line. She left off the prosthesis and started wearing the filthy slippers that she liked so much. The blisters broke. Since the slippers were crawling with bacteria from the animal hair and feces that were starting to accumulate in the house again, she got another serious infection. This time the infection moved fast and before her daughter could come by it had invaded her ankle. The minute her daughter came by she called the emergency room because Brenda was running a fever and the deep redness at her ankle was ugly. The emergency room doctor told Brenda that she needed an immediate amputation to save her knee but she would have none of it. She stayed in the hospital for a couple of days until the antibiotics had reduced her fever and was then put in a skilled nursing home.

Brenda was one miserable person when I visited her in the nursing home. She was angry at the world and at me for her fate. Her daughter had taken all of Brenda's pets to the Humane Society and she cried as she spat out the tale. I was there at the request of her daughter and doctor to try to convince her that an amputation was in her best interest and without it she would likely die. After a while she calmed down and listened to what I had to say and I left feeling as if she was going to let them finally take off the leg. The infection appeared to be below the knee but there was no guarantee.

Two days later the surgeon performed the amputation. When he got into the tissue below her knee he found that the infection had reached her knee and was actually beginning to invade the muscles above the knee. Brenda's daughter was in the waiting area when the surgeon called her and informed her that he would have to take her mother's leg off above the knee. She agreed but feared that her mother would never forgive her. When Brenda awoke to find her leg off nearly halfway up her thigh she went into a rage. They had to keep her heavily sedated for almost a week. When she did recover enough to be let out of the hospital, she could not cope with the loss. Her daughter tried to help but Brenda always blamed her for the loss of the leg and eventually her daughter quit visiting. Brenda spent the rest of her days in a nursing home where she was verbally abusive to all who had to deal with her. She only lived for another 18 months before she passed away.

I tell Brenda's story not to offer hope; I tell it to illustrate what happens when a person can't accept what life has dealt them. No, losing her toes was not fair. Life often isn't fair. Because she couldn't accept that *her* actions were one of the primary causes of *her* circumstances, she would not follow the recommendations of professionals or the people who loved her. Bitterness and regret are part of the process of loss. Remember that this is a process and needs to pass through the person. Dwelling on the loss and letting it become your life will only drive away the people who care about you the most and can result in the failure of your rehabilitation.

Thousands of people who have partial foot amputations function quite normally and have only the minimal amount of inconvenience. Prosthetic advances in this area are giving the partial foot amputee choices that they have never had before. Graphite springs that provide push off of the toe can return the amputee to a very normal gait pattern. Gel socks and sheaths provide a level of comfort and cushion that minimizes pain as well as the risk of abrasion. Had Brenda been more diligent in her lifestyle and with the care of her limb, she most likely would be taking her dogs for a walk.

Syme's Prostheses

Many prosthetists aren't very excited about working with Syme's prostheses. It is not a particularly common type of amputation nor is it an easy prosthesis to fabricate. The bulbous end of the stump creates difficulties in fabrication for the prosthetist as well as limitations as to the number of feet that can be used. However, for the right person, a Syme's amputation makes an excellent residual limb that can permit end-bearing and actual ambulation without the use of a prosthesis. I am not implying that people with a Syme's amputation can walk around without the aid of a prosthesis. There is generally a 10 cm (4 in) leg length difference and no toe lever. Still, it comes in real handy in the middle of the night when an amputee has to go to the bathroom; the Syme's amputee can hobble into the bathroom without the need to put on the prosthesis.

There are other advantages to having a Syme's amputation. If the surgery is successful, then the amputee still has his or her heel pad intact. The impact-absorbing nature of the skin cells as well as increased vascularity of the heel pad skin makes it nature's perfect body part on which to walk. This minimizes the amount of pressure that any other part of the stump has to take. It is recommended that the Syme's prosthesis come up to just below the knee so that the top edge of the prosthesis is not in the middle of the shin. The reason being that the shin has very little muscle covering and to end the lever of the prosthesis half way up the leg puts undue pressure on the bone. The other big advantage of the Syme's is that there is generally no need for any type of external suspension. A form-fitting socket will hold the leg on due to the larger bottom and smaller middle of the shape. The ball of the ankle is larger than the shin area so without removing the door or displacing the insert the prosthesis cannot come off.

There are also some disadvantages to the Syme's prosthesis. The major one is cosmetic in nature. When there is a ball of ankle tissue at the end, you get a socket shape that is unnaturally large at the ankle. Making this look good in a cosmetic cover is almost impossible. If cosmetics are a main issue for the amputee, then this will generally be a disappointing type of prosthesis. Other disadvantages are if the prosthesis has a door to allow for donning of the leg, the door always uses some type of strap or buckle to keep it closed. Straps show through pants or are very obvious when wearing shorts. If the amputee has lost his or her leg due to poor circulation, then there is always the danger of the Syme's amputation not succeeding due to inadequate blood supply. The shin does not have much muscle coverage, which is where the blood supply is best, so the longer the amputation is the more chance for poor circulation.

I have always thought that the Syme's prosthesis is a very functional limb that allows the amputee to have the greatest mobility with the most direct contact on the ground. The choice to have a Syme's amputation versus a below-knee amputation needs to be made with care since the disadvantages can make acceptance difficult when cosmesis is an overriding factor. It is important for the prosthetist to have skill in fabrication techniques as well as the component options available to the Syme's amputee.

Advantages and Disadvantages of Syme's Prostheses

Advantages

1. Syme's amputations provide the amputee with his or her intact heel pad, which is one of the few body surfaces that was designed for weight bearing.
2. The large ankle ball will generally provide enough suspension for the limb, reducing the need for auxiliary suspension.
3. The socket design of the Syme's prosthesis needs to come up to just below the knee but because there is end bearing, minimal pressures are needed elsewhere.
4. The Syme's amputee can develop the ability to have limited ambulation on the end of his or her stump. This is a big aid to getting around in the house or going to the bathroom in the middle of the night.

Disadvantages

1. Due to the nature of the level of amputation, there is a large ankle ball that is not very cosmetically appealing. It is not possible to finish this type of prosthesis with the same level of cosmetic appeal that a below-knee prosthesis can have.
2. Because of the long residual limb, the number of feet available for the Syme's amputee are limited.
3. Circulation to the end of the stump can be a problem if the cause of amputation was due to poor vascularity.
4. Fabrication of this type of prosthesis is difficult and requires that the prosthetist be familiar with its construction and the various options that are available to the amputee.

Materials and Components

Many foot manufacturers now make special feet just for the Syme's amputee. There are many options ranging from energy storing to multiaxial. There are adapters that can accommodate as little as 7.5 cm (3 in) distance from the end of the stump to the floor. There are waterproof feet for the creation of water legs, but I am not aware of any system that allows for scuba diving and kicking with the prosthesis. Cosmesis has come a long way also even though there is not much that can be done to hide the over-sized ankle. If the anklebones are shaved, then a barely noticeable cosmesis can be achieved but otherwise this seems to be the compromise with this type of amputation.

There are special socks for Syme's amputees that have a larger end portion to accommodate the shape of the stump. Most liner manufacturers also fabricate gel or silicone liners specifically for the Syme's. There are gel socks and sheaths that are also available. Most of the materials that are available for the below-knee amputee are also available for the Syme's.

Partial Foot Prostheses

Partial foot amputees can often function without the use of any type of prosthetic device. This is not necessarily recommended, since normal human gait requires push off of the front of the foot. When that is missing, it will cause an imbalance in the amputee's pattern of walking. If this situation goes on for years, it can cause pain in the back or hips that will degenerate into permanent damage to the skeletal system if left untreated. Many partial foot amputees just obtain a pair of high top shoes or boots and stuff socks into the front of the shoe to give a little cushion. Again, this may enable the person to get around the house but it will not be a serviceable solution if the amputee wishes to be a community ambulator.

The normal human walking pattern (gait) is a complex series of body motions. First, there is heel-strike where the heel of the foot absorbs the shock of impact. Then there is foot-flat where the weight of the body begins to roll over the axis of the ankle and onto the front of the foot. In normal gait, the last part of the process is called toe-off where the front of the foot pushes the body onto the other foot's heel strike and gives forward thrust. In addition the toes give the body balance and the ability to sense the ground beneath them (proprioception), especially the big toe, which provides a large portion of the balance of the foot. When the front portion is missing, not only have you lost the push off of your foot but also the balance that keeps your momentum going forward. What occurs then is that during the roll-over phase instead of weight bearing on the padded forefoot section of the foot the weight concentrates on the end of the cut part of the bones, probably the worst place that it can. In order to minimize the forces on this usually tender part of the foot, the amputee will avoid bearing weight there and shuffle the foot along without rolling over the toe. This makes for a limping, shuffling gait pattern that will suffice to ambulate around the house but can cause damage if left untreated. One of the other major dangers of an untreated forefoot amputation is that the end of the amputated foot is subject to pressures that can cause breakdown of the skin. If poor circulation was the initial cause of amputation, then this can be a set up for further amputation.

It is important to remember that whenever there is an amputation it disrupts the body's ability to maintain blood flow. The flow of blood from arteries to veins is like a plumbing system and when you sever the end of the loop it forces other pipes to compensate for the lack of flow. In the amputee the body compensates with the remaining tiny blood vessels called capillaries but they can never match the original system's ability to maintain a normal volume. This is why there is always a tendency for the remaining limb to want to swell if not contained; it's like a backed-up plumbing system. In children the capillaries can grow and expand to nearly compensate for the lack of a complete system; however, in adults where the vessels are no longer growing, the body's ability to pick up the extra volume of blood is rarely adequate. Therefore, if there is a skin breakdown at the end of the partial foot the body is going to have a tough time healing because there is not enough blood flow to bring the body's natural defenses into play. Preventing skin breakdown in this area is critical and choosing to not wear a prosthetic device is courting danger.

What does a good partial foot prosthesis do? It provides a cushion to the front of the foot where it is most likely to have unacceptable pressures. It also stabilizes the foot inside of the shoe to keep the front of the foot from taking the majority of pressure during the rollover phase of gait. This also has the benefit of reducing the pressure on the top of the foot which, if laced into a high top shoe, will stabilize the foot. The other huge advantage of wearing a prosthesis is the return of the toe-off part of the gait pattern. This is usually accomplished by inserting graphite plates into the shoe beneath the prosthesis that provide spring at the toe. The plates come in different degrees of stiffness that allow the amputee to gradually work up to the desired amount. Another prosthetic design is to fabricate them directly into the prosthesis that then allows the amputee to wear the prosthesis without the shoe.

Partial foot prostheses come in many different designs, from a simple insert into the shoe, to a slip on cosmetic restoration, to a more rigid device that encapsulates the ankle. The design of the prosthesis depends upon how much foot is left and the condition of the skin coverage at the end of the foot. The longer the remaining forefoot and the better the skin, the less need to stabilize the foot. Whereas if the remaining foot is short and/or the skin is in poor shape, then a more rigid confining device is necessary.

One of the greatest advances in prosthetic supplies that has proven to be very important for the partial foot amputee is gel-impregnated socks. These socks have a layer of gel that covers the vulnerable cut end of the foot and provides an impact- and torque-absorbing layer of cushion. This has cut down on the incident of skin breakdown and given the amputee a much greater level of comfort. I always recommend that the amputee wear some type of sock beneath the prosthesis to provide a buffer for the skin and to absorb perspiration. The prosthesis should always come with socks. There is a lot of discrepancy between the number of socks that the prosthetist provides but I think that an amputee should be provided with a week's supply of socks as part of the prosthesis. It is critical to keep the socks clean and unless the amputee washes his or her sock every night, he or she will not be able to keep the foot clean. It is important to have a week's supply of socks especially in the initial first few months of prosthetic usage when the suture line may still drain a little and dead skin is sloughing off.

Partial foot amputees have a huge advantage over the below-knee amputee in that they can carefully ambulate on their residual limb. They can even get by without the use of a prosthesis but as I have mentioned before, this is not recommended and over

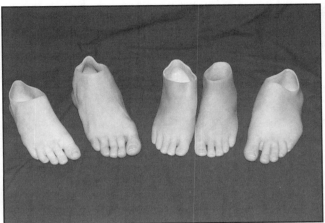

Figure 8-1. Custom silicone partial foot prostheses. (Photo courtesy of Artech.)

time will cause damage to the rest of the skeletal system. It is important to note that when using a partial foot prosthesis (Figure 8-1), the amputee should remove the insole of the shoe to allow more room for the prosthesis. It may even be necessary to add a lift to the other shoe so that the pelvis is level. Having an equal height is important to prevent back problems, so don't ignore the good foot. The good foot will now be taking more than its share of the pressure and it needs to be kept in good shape.

CHAPTER 9

Child Amputees

Stories

Tommy

When Tommy was born with a deformed right foot, the doctors told his mom that it was probably due to the umbilical cord getting wrapped around the foot during the pregnancy. Tommy was the third child in a large family in Wisconsin where the communities are tight and everyone pretty much knows everyone else. The deformed foot really didn't create a problem with development until around 2 years old when Tommy should have been walking. The foot was small and the length of the leg did not match the good leg so he could not learn to walk normally. When Tommy was 4 years old, his local doctor recommended to his parents that they amputate the foot. He felt that providing Tommy with a prosthesis that would enable him to walk would be the best thing they could do. After much heartbreaking discussion, they all agreed and went to Minneapolis where the hospital provided the surgery as well as rehabilitation for young Tommy. When he got home he had a short below-knee amputation with only the main bone, the tibia, remaining.

He doesn't remember much about the amputation or the hospital stay but he definitely remembers his first trip to the limb shop that at that time was also in Minneapolis. The smell of wood and glue still sticks in his mind and the feel of the man with big rough hands who made his first prosthesis. His first leg was made of wood with big metal hinges that came up over his knee and a leather lacer that he tied like shoes to give him support. The leg was very heavy and although Tommy was not a big child, he was strong as well as determined. Before he was 5 years old he was playing with his siblings as well as all the other kids in the tight knit community. His leg clanked as he walked so he had to endure a great deal of chiding and name calling but it only made him want to fit in all the more. He learned to take the teasing with humor. It seemed to be the best way to get the bullies to leave him alone since he was not a big kid.

Family life was not very happy. His dad worked at a factory all day and was an alcoholic. He would beat the kids, including Tommy, when the mood struck him and the children learned to keep out of his way when he was in a nasty mood. His mother had affairs while his father was at work or whenever they would go to Minneapolis to get his leg worked on, which occurred frequently. Tommy remembers many times when he would sit in the hall or the bathroom of a hotel while his mother was in the room with another man. He didn't blame her but he never could quite forgive her either. His older brother was his best friend and protected him from the bullies as well as clueing him in to when to get out of the house to avoid a beating.

It was one of those balmy summer Wisconsin evenings when the sun doesn't set until 9:30 pm and the mosquitoes are buzzing near the water. Eight-year-old Tommy was playing in the backyard experimenting with tree climbing when his brother came out and warned him that the old man was on the rampage. Just then they both heard the sound of breaking dishes and yelling from the kitchen. It was time to disappear. He ducked beneath the thick hedge behind his house and clanked along the alley, his leg warning anyone that he was coming. All of a sudden he was pelted with a shower of dirt. He turned to see 2 of the rougher kids in the neighborhood emerge from behind a garage, laughing at their ambush. He didn't particularly like these kids because they always teased him and embarrassed him in front of others. Still, his brother wasn't around so he had to deal with them. They were making fun of him and finally taunted him by daring him to climb over the fence of the local junkyard a couple of blocks away. He knew this place. It was full of mean mongrel dogs that rabidly barked anytime you got near the fence, and all the kids were afraid to go near it. Tommy wasn't big but he did have guts. He told them he would.

The three boys walked the 2 blocks to the edge of the junkyard, a high wooden fence surrounding the compound with a large oak tree growing near the edge. The branches of the tree grew above the fence and a couple of big ones hung over into the yard itself. The dare was for Tommy to climb the tree and hang down into the junkyard. If he fell or slipped, he would be at the mercy of what sounded like hundreds of viscous rabid dogs that would tear him limb from limb. He climbed the oak tree, which was easier than he had expected since his arms were very strong for his size and age. He looked down to see the two other boys taunting him to go on. He then looked down into the junkyard. The dogs were beginning to notice him and bark. There weren't hundreds of them after all, only 3, but they looked as viscous and mean as he had imagined. They were now all at the fence beneath the tree barking, yelping, and jumping up to try and get at Tommy. He stole a quick look at the house that was at the other end of the yard to make sure no one was coming, but it was supper time so there was no one about.

He knew that he had to decide right now if he was going to do this. Should he back down, or prove to those 2 bullies that he wasn't afraid? His decision was quick. Tommy had guts, so out on the limb he went. When he was just over the fence, he grabbed hold of what he thought was a solid branch and then swung out and down over the now crazed dogs. The branch was not as solid as he thought and allowed him to sink lower then he had judged. He pulled hard to try and get his good leg back up on the branch that he had just been on but he couldn't do it. All of a sudden he felt a large weight on the end of his prosthesis and his grip on the branch began to give way. He looked down and to his horror one of the dogs had actually jumped high enough to grab the shoe that was on his prosthesis so now it was hanging, suspended in air from his leg. He yelled at the other boys to come and help him but all he could see of them was their backs as they ran away. He hung there for what seemed like hours. The dog must have gotten his teeth entangled in the shoe because he wouldn't let go. His arms ached and burned but he knew that he would be torn to shreds if he let go so he just hung on and yelled for help. The next thing he knew he heard a loud voice telling the dogs to shut up. Mr. Bellows, the owner of the junkyard, came walking over. "I guess my dogs have finally caught something," he said with a chuckle. He got the dog disentangled from Tommy's shoe and escorted him to the gate. The dogs weren't mean at all with Mr. Bellows around, and Tommy pleaded with him not to call his father. The man knew about Tommy's father and promised not to tell him if Tommy promised not to pull a stunt like that again.

As Tommy walked out of the gate and back down the alley, the 2 boys came up to him to find out what had happened. They were awestruck when Tommy told them of his encounter with the dogs and how Mr. Bellows had rescued him. From then on he didn't have much trouble with bullies anymore. The word had gotten around that Tommy was not a coward and was not to be messed with. His home life didn't get any easier, but school was not a place that he had to fear anymore. He couldn't play the team sports that all the other kids did but he learned to skate and play pick-up hockey on the numerous frozen lakes around the neighborhood. At first he was only allowed to play goalie but soon his buddies discovered that Tommy could skate as well as anyone and he absolutely had no fear of pain. Soon he was playing all the positions and proving to himself as well as his friends that he could keep up with anyone.

When he was 14 years old he finally got a leg that didn't have a massive thigh lacer and knee joints. On this trip the prosthetist introduced him to the supercondylar style of suspension where the socket comes up over his knee and grabs the area above the condyles. This was heaven for him since now his leg didn't clank every time he took a step and he was finally able to shed the waist belt that had shaped his waist for the past 10 years. It took some getting used to having all the pressure on the inside of his knee but after a couple of weeks, it stopped hurting. He could hop run on this leg as well as skate so he started playing baseball and football with the neighborhood kids after school.

This was also the time of his life when girls started to be important to him. At first he was very shy about asking anyone to a dance, but then one afternoon something very special happened to him. It was only a month after he had gotten his new leg and he was walking home from school. He was walking through the alley behind his house when he heard someone calling his name. He turned to see a pretty girl named Peggy who lived on the other side of the block motioning to him to come over. She was 2 years older then Tommy and was on the cheerleading squad, so way above him on the social ladder. He approached her and she asked him if he wanted to come inside of her house to have a glass of lemonade. He was a little hesitant but followed her anyway. Inside she announced that her parents were still at work as she poured them both a glass of lemonade. She told him of how impressed she was with the way he played baseball and hockey. This was really unnerving for Tommy since this girl had never even spoken to him in the years since he had been in the same school as her. The next thing he knew they were sitting on the couch and she began kissing him. Nature took over where Tommy's mind couldn't, and he had his first sexual encounter. This changed everything for him. He no longer feared approaching girls. Sometimes he would get rejected but most of the time the girls seemed to be impressed with his boldness. He discovered that it was his attitude toward himself that made the impression on women, not how he looked.

Tommy went on to graduate from high school with decent enough grades to be able to get into the local community college. He traveled some during the summers and discovered that there was a big world out there that he wanted to see. He met Susan when he was 24 years old and fell madly in love with her. They were married 2 years later and began a family. He got a job at the factory where his father had worked and had to start at the bottom of the rung in the hierarchy of the union positions. This meant that he was shoveling heavy loads of iron ore from beside the conveyor belts that delivered it to the boats. This was the heaviest of manual labor but Tommy never complained or shirked his job, which earned the respect of his coworkers.

One winter Tommy got involved with the local disabled ski club. He found that not only was he good at the sport, it gave him a self-esteem that he had never experienced before. He started skiing every chance he got and even tried his hand at cross-country skiing. He was good enough to compete in the local races that eventually qualified him for the national championships. He traveled to Colorado and found that this sport could provide him with the traveling experiences that he had always craved. The only trouble was that he and Susan had 2 infants as well as another child on the way, not to mention his full-time job at the plant. However, Tommy was not about to pass up an opportunity like this so he just jumped into all of it "feet first."

Today, he still enjoys skiing although his competitive days are over. His children are grown, 2 live in town and one is in the military, stationed overseas. He and Susan have a good life and still live in the same home where his children grew up. She works at the town hospital and he is retired from the factory but works part-time tending bar at his favorite local tavern. Life hasn't always been kind to Tommy, but he is living proof that it is possible to overcome tremendous odds and live one's dreams.

Ashley

Ashley was 3 years old the day she was playing in the driveway with her Legos. She was always a very focused child who devoted her attention to whatever she was doing, even at the age of 3. Her older brother and a friend were playing on the new riding lawn mower that their father had bought. They were forbidden to play on it but as 11-year-old boys they were getting into mischief. Ashley didn't take much notice of the engine start. She knew that the boys shouldn't be playing on the mower but thought that Mom would soon be out to scold them. Mom unfortunately was in the bathroom and didn't hear the mower so there was no stopping the 2 boys who wanted to just take it for a drive around the house. They did not know how to operate the clutch or throttle so when they managed to accidentally put it into gear they were nearly thrown off the back from the rapid acceleration that occurs when the throttle is pushed to the start position. Ashley's brother tried to steer the machine but it was very responsive and he continually overcorrected the wheels. The lawn mower careened out of the carport and straight at Ashley who was faced away from the oncoming machine. She heard it coming and turned around to see it bearing down upon her. Her natural reaction was to push herself out of the way but unfortunately her brother jerked the wheel at the same time and the front tires ran over Ashley's right leg. The whirring blades caught her tiny foot and turned it into pulp as her screams pierced the air.

Fortunately, her mother was a nurse and did not panic at the sight of her injured daughter. Ashley went into immediate shock and her mother placed a tourniquet on her leg just above the knee. Her brother and friend also went into shock at the sight of what they had done. Her mother treated all 3 of them until paramedics arrived to whisk Ashley and her mom off to the hospital, while neighbors looked after her brother and his friend. It was determined in the operating room that there was no way to save the foot and that amputation was the only viable treatment. Ashley's mom was faced with a terrible dilemma. She had to make the decision about the amputation. Her husband was away on business and was probably on an airplane where he could not be reached for several more hours. Thankful for her medical training she knew that she must make a decision, and she gave the doctors permission to amputate if there was no hope of limb salvage. The memory of these moments haunted her nightmares for years afterward.

When Ashley awoke she was in a lot of pain. Her mom was sitting next to her, holding her hand with a pained look on her face and tears in her eyes. "How are you feeling, honey?" she asked. Ashley replied that her leg hurt and she was really thirsty. Her mother didn't know what to say to her little girl. How do you tell your precious 3-year-old daughter that she had her leg amputated? She had to tell her something though. "Baby doll, you were accidentally run over by the lawn mower and they had to remove your right foot," her mom said in a choking voice. Ashley didn't cry or get upset. She said, "So that's why my foot hurts so much. Will it grow back mommy?" "No darling, it can't grow back but before you know it you will have an artificial foot that will work as well as your old one," replied her mom. "OK," said Ashley and her frank calmness did a great deal to soothe her mom.

Ashley healed quickly and seemed to adapt to the idea of only having one foot rather easily, much to the surprise of everyone. One of the toughest days was when her brother came to visit her in the hospital. He was near panic as he entered her room. He burst into tears the minute he saw her and could hardly speak as he apologized over and over again. Ashley never blamed him for the accident and stroked his head as he cried in her lap. For a 3 year old she displayed a remarkable maturity and resilience that inspired everyone around her. Her father also had a hard time seeing his little girl in such a predicament. He nearly lost his composure the first time he saw her but again her smile and charm gave him the ability to accept what had happened. He was furious with his son though, and the tension between them would take years to heal.

After a week in the hospital, they were able to take out her stitches in her stump and she could go home. The physical therapy staff was excellent and not only taught Ashley how to walk on crutches but worked on massaging and desensitization. Just before she was discharged a man from the prosthetic shop came to visit her. He was a tall, nice-looking man named Dan who talked to her and her parents about prostheses. Dan assured her that she would be able to walk and run in a few short months but at first she would have to get used to the new leg. Just before Dan was to leave he asked Ashley if she had noticed anything unusual about him. She said no she didn't. He pulled up his pants leg to reveal a below-knee prosthesis. He said that he had lost his leg in a motorcycle accident many years ago and that not only could he run but he could ski, as well as ride a bike, doing just about anything he wanted. This brought a big smile to Ashley's face and she was even more upbeat than usual for the rest of the day.

The first week home was not so bad. Her stump still hurt, especially at night before she went to bed, but she found that if she rubbed it like the physical therapist at the hospital had shown her that it would get better so she could fall asleep. She went out to play with the rest of the kids in the neighborhood but couldn't engage in any of the running games that they played. Her brother was still very upset about what had happened and avoided Ashley; he would stay in his room playing video games all day.

At the end of the week her mom took her to go visit Dan at his prosthetic shop in the city. It was a nice place with a big room in the front to wait in. There were books and games for her to play with over in one corner of the room and there were some older people sitting reading magazines also. She crawled over to a man who was reading the paper and pulled up his pants leg to see about his leg. Instead of a real leg there was a shiny silver pipe with lots of screws and things on it. She tugged on his pants leg to get his attention. He was delighted with her curiosity and answered all of her questions. He had lost his leg in a war many years ago, he told her, but he had never missed a day of work as an insurance salesman and he still enjoyed dancing with his wife.

Ashley was taken back into a room that was kind of like a doctor's office. It had a sink and was white all over. There was a big table with paper on it just like at the doctor's office. Dan came in and explained to her that he was going to take a cast of her leg so that he could make her a prosthesis. Ashley couldn't pronounce the word prosthesis so she called it "little leg." He wrapped plaster that was nice and warm around her stump but then slipped it off when it got cool. He showed her the laboratory in the back where there were a bunch of men working at benches. All of them were working on different "little legs" and it sure seemed like a busy place to Ashley. Dan told her that he would have her leg ready in a week and that when she came back she would get to walk.

The week went by quickly and Ashley was back to the prosthetic place. She could hardly contain her excitement and kept telling everyone in the waiting room that she was going to walk today. Dan finally came out and took her to a different room; this one was long and skinny with a set of rails that went all along one side of the room. There was a big mirror at one end of the bars and leaning next to the chair was a tiny "little leg" that she imagined must be hers. Dan came in and began by taking a soft, white insert out of the plastic socket part. He then took a rubbery, sock-looking thing out of a box and held it up to her leg. He cut the thing in half and then rolled it onto her stump. It hurt a little at first but after it was all the way on it kind of felt good. Next, he took the white foamy insert and slipped it onto her "little leg" over top of the sock thing. Then, he put a sock over the whole thing and slipped it into the socket of the prosthesis. He told her to stand up, which she did and to her surprise, she was standing. Her stump was a little tender but not painful. Dan fiddled with the screws and raised the new leg up so that she was even. He asked her to take a step forward and one step backward. Instead, Ashley just took off. She went up and down the parallel bars before he could slow her down. Dan told her that she had to take it slowly at first or else she could cause damage to her new leg. He made some more adjustments to the leg and had her walk again. This went on 3 more times before he was happy with how she walked with her new leg.

Before Ashley left, Dan took her leg back to the workroom to make it look more realistic for her. He used an old cover that was from another prosthesis to temporarily give the leg some shape. Ten minutes at the router and he had a fairly decent looking preparatory prosthesis. He pulled a couple of cosmetic stockings over it and the shape began to take on the appearance of a leg, the stockings even matched her skin tone to some degree. Ashley was delighted with it and gave Dan a big hug for his effort. He set up a follow-up appointment for a week later and she went home wearing her new leg. She said that it looked almost like her real one.

That night Ashley couldn't wait until her father was home to show off her new leg. What was even more significant was that her brother finally began to come out of his withdrawal now that his sister was walking again. He even began to tease her again, which was a sure sign that he was beginning to accept what had happened to Ashley. He would still be plagued by nightmares about the tragic day, but he could finally begin to heal himself because she didn't seem to hold any grudge.

Ashley was able to walk without crutches from the very beginning. Somehow, being only 1 meter (3 ft) tall and fairly new to walking anyway made it easy for her to make the adaptation. She fell a lot, especially at first. It was easy for the toe of the prosthesis to catch on things and for her to go tumbling, but Ashley always got back up with a smile on her face. Over the next 2 years she was able to run for short distances and ride a tricycle that allowed her to keep up with the other kids in the neighborhood. She had to get a new prosthesis every year in order to keep up with her growing stump. Dan saw her at least every 6 months in order to keep the prosthesis the right height since she was growing so fast. He also made her 2 liners every time he made a new socket. One liner was inside the other so the outer one was slightly larger than the inner one. When her stump grew, they could remove the inner liner leaving the outer one. The extra room that this provided allowed the prosthesis to be worn for another couple of months.

Ashley loved the water and would spend hours playing in the shallow freestanding pool that her father had bought. Once a week her mother would take them to the municipal pool where she learned to swim and jump off of the diving board. Ashley would always hop everywhere around the pool or the board, taking no notice of her leg. The only problem was when they went to the beach. It was very difficult to hop in the sand or play in the surf on one leg. When her mother told Dan of the situation, he told her that he could make something special for her that would allow her to go in the water with her prosthesis. He duplicated the last socket and created a waterproof prosthesis that was laminated with a colorful finish. Ashley loved it. She wore it to the pool, the beach, or when she went into the shower. She had taken a nasty fall in the shower and appreciated that now she could use both feet to stand on in the slipperiest place in the house.

Ashley's bubbling personality and self-confidence made her an instant hit in her school when she started. None of the kids seemed to take much notice of her prosthesis unless they were curious. Her matter of fact way of explaining what had happened to her answered their questions and once the mystery was gone, they treated her like any other kid. She could participate in most of the games at recess as well as the activities during physical education with little adaptation. When she took an interest in soccer, they let her play goalie at first but then found that she could move almost as well as the other players. She did have a problem once when she was kicking at the ball and her prosthesis hit another of the children, giving him a nasty bruise on his leg.

It was in second grade that she noticed that the tip of her stump was very sore. No matter how many socks she tried to wear with the prosthesis it continued to stay sore and was red all the time. The skin at the tip looked so thin and stretched that she asked her mother if they could go see Dan about it. He took one look and said that her bone was growing faster than the skin and that they should go to see the surgeon at the hospital. The surgeon explained that this was not uncommon in children who have traumatic amputations. The bone continues to grow and if left untreated could actually grow through the end of the skin. He recommended revision surgery to shorten the bone some and give it a nice bevel that would make it much more comfortable to wear a prosthesis. They agreed and arranged for the surgery to take place. It was the middle of winter and she wouldn't miss too much by being off of her prosthesis for a couple of weeks until it healed. The surgery went smoothly, and Ashley had to use crutches for the next 3 weeks until the end of her stump healed.

After Ashley was completely healed, she and her dad went in to see Dan about a new prosthesis. Usually her mom took her, but this time her dad wanted to see first hand how prostheses were made. After the casting Dan took her dad back into the laboratory to see the process of making artificial legs, which he found fascinating. Dan showed Ashley the new foot that she was going to get. It was black and thin and acted like a spring when it was bent. He explained that instead of screwing onto the bottom of her shin this foot went all the way up to the bottom of the socket. It would give her a lot more spring off of the toe and she may even be able to jump or hop with it. She was very excited about the new leg and couldn't wait until the next week when it would be ready.

The next week finally arrived and her dad took her back to see Dan. The leg was ready for her to try on and after getting used to the springiness of the foot she took off running through the lab. Dan asked her to slow down or she was going to knock something over if she wasn't careful. They went outside and she started to jog around the parking lot as well as the adjacent yard. The foot not only had more spring, it was split into two halves that allowed it to act like an ankle joint, giving and moving as the ground beneath it changed. Ashley was giddy with excitement, as they got ready to leave that day. Dan will never forget the look on her dad's face as her put her in the car. The amputation had been a terrible ordeal for a father; he had felt so helpless in the face of his daughter' suffering. To see her running and hopping like any other child was too much of a joy for him. Her dad had been in some real hell as a combat veteran of Vietnam and to see tears of joy come down his face as he put Ashley in the car was the greatest reward that Dan had ever experienced in his career.

Ashley went through grade school with very little impact on her life due to the prosthesis. Dan always took good care of his star client and was always showing her off to other less motivated amputees. She needed a new leg every 8 to 12 months as she continued to grow like a normal child. He always took time to put a shapely cosmetic cover on the leg, eventually using a latex skin covering that not only looked real but also protected the foot mechanism inside. The leg was held on with suspension sleeves but had a removable belt that had a strap that attached to the leg whenever she wanted to run or play sports. This arrangement ensured that the leg would not fall off during times of high activity. The only thing was that the leg couldn't change colors as her skin tanned in the summer, a small thing now but an issue that would have more impact in her adolescence.

In junior high school, Ashley became a cheerleader for the basketball team. She was a very pretty girl and also popular with the rest of the kids. Her personality made her a natural for the squad and the leg didn't get in the way of most of the cheers. Then came boys. She was beginning to be a young lady by the time she got into high school and the boys were beginning to take notice. At first she was just a little bit shy when boys started to talk to her in "that way," asking her to go to the movies or out for a hamburger. Soon though, her natural enthusiasm for life overwhelmed her shyness and she was one of the most popular girls in her high school. Kids can be cruel sometimes, and some jealous girls would make fun of her prosthesis, especially in the locker room when she had to take a shower in her waterproof leg. At first Ashley was very hurt by these remarks, but after talking with her mom about it, she moved to a position where she felt sorry for the girls who were being cruel. Once they saw that their remarks did not have the intended results, they quit making them. Ashley continued to be on the cheerleading squad throughout high school in addition to being an honor student.

She went on to college where she followed in her mother's footsteps and decided to go into nursing. At nursing school she fell in love with an intern at the hospital where she was doing her residency. A year later they got married. There has never been a father and mother so proud of their daughter as her parents were at her wedding. Ashley went on to have a family of her own and a successful career as a surgical nurse. Her husband is an anesthesiologist at the same hospital and they have two children, 1 boy and 1 girl. Life is not easy as an amputee, but Ashley knows that attitude is 90% of the struggle.

Prosthetic Considerations of the Child Amputee

The greatest prosthetic challenge in working with child amputees is dealing with their constant growth. Many children will need a new prosthesis on an average of once a year. Growth in children is rarely consistent; they don't grow by an inch a year. Instead it comes in spurts, barely growing one year then shooting up 3 inches the next. This makes it difficult to keep up with since it is so unpredictable. It is important for someone, preferably the prosthetist, to check the fit of the prosthesis at least once every 6 months. If the prosthetic facility is too far away for periodic check-ups, then one of the parents has to learn the skill of determining the correct height of the prosthesis. This is not hard to do. It is a matter of putting the fingers on the crest of the pelvis while the child is facing you. Hold the hands out flat and look at them. If they are level, then the leg is the proper height; if they aren't, then place magazines or thin boards beneath the short side until the hands on the hips look level. You can't rely on the feedback of the child because he or she does not experience the sensation of the body gradually getting off balance until it does some damage. Most physical therapists or prosthetists will be glad to teach a parent how to do this. If there is a height discrepancy, then the prosthesis needs to be taken in and lengthened.

Socket problems are different. They need to be diagnosed and treated by a prosthetist, preferably the one that made the leg. The parent may begin to notice continued redness on the stump or the child may complain of a recurring pain that doesn't get better. These are sure signs that an adjustment needs to be made. Children are going to usually push the envelope on activity without much concern for damage until it is too late. Minor blisters, abrasions, and the occasional pimple are not necessarily cause for undue alarm. If these problems persist or come back in the same place time after time, then the prosthetist needs to see the amputee in order to make an adjustment.

One of the techniques that we always use in our lab in order to give a little extra longevity to a child's prosthesis is to use liners within liners. This is merely making 2 soft pelite liners one on top of the other, so that as the child grows out of the first one, it can be removed. The second liner can still provide the cushion that is necessary while allowing room for the growing child. Depending upon the child and whether he or she seems to have more growth at the tip of the stump, I would also add an extra layer of foam between the two liners, which gives even more room at the tip. I could do this wherever I thought growth might be uneven on the stump, based upon my experience with the child.

There is a wide range of components available for the child to use. Most types of foot designs come in children's versions, although due to the short amount of space between the socket and the ground there may be some limitations in very young children. Most of the major manufacturers have a complete line of modular components that are designed specifically for children. Modular, endoskeletal construction makes the heightening and adjustment of a child's prosthesis much more convenient and therefore more frequent then the traditional exoskeletal limb.

Infants especially need to have readily adjustable prostheses to adapt to their rapidly changing needs. Suspension can be a problem with infants since there is little firm tissue on the stump on which to base a system. Suspension sleeves constantly fall down when the child is crawling, so often times we used a cuff strap and or waist belt to attain adequate suspension on small infants. I am not in favor of joint and corset or supercondylar suspension in growing children unless there is no other alternative. This type of suspension has the effect of constricting the use and growth of the quadriceps muscles just above the knee as well as the natural muscle timing of the knee.

When is it the right time to put a prosthesis on a congenital infant amputee? My wife is a pediatric physical therapist and believes the earlier the better. Normal human locomotion requires that an infant spend time crawling on his or her hands and knees because this is one of the few times in childhood development that there is weight bearing on the hands. Children generally take a while to get used to wearing a prosthesis and it is critical that the parents are involved and supportive of the process. The sooner the child incorporates the prosthesis into his or her life, the better the chances for a successful outcome.

One of the techniques that we used to foster greater acceptance of the prosthesis was to always cover the leg with some type of cosmetic cover. We knew that we were going to adjust the prosthesis frequently so we tried to make the cover as accessible as possible. Admittedly, the strenuous activity level of the child often destroyed the covers but we felt it was worth it because of the acceptance factor. Another reason that soft covers are advisable is that when a child or toddler is playing with other children, he or she won't injure the other children with the leg. An exoskeletal leg or the aluminum parts of an endoskeletal leg are very hard, especially when they attain velocity by kicking or being thrown. Putting a soft, cosmetically appealing cover on a child's prosthesis might seem like an exercise in frustration but the benefits in acceptance are worth it.

Emotional Issues

Children born without limbs will realize that they are different than other children by the time they are 1 year old. When they receive a prosthesis, they begin to achieve more integration with other children. Mental adaptation to this process is generally pretty smooth in my experience, primarily based upon the attitude of the parents. If the parents are accepting and positive, the child will make the transition with minor complications. If the parents are laden with guilt or shame, the child will recognize this and take on some of those characteristics regarding the disability.

When a child loses a leg from trauma or disease, there can be a different set of circumstances. There is the psychological process of dealing with either the traumatic event that resulted in amputation or the illness that necessitated removal of the leg. Either way, in addition to the obvious difficulties that wearing a prosthesis entails there is the baggage of trauma or illness. Again, the deciding factor seems to be the parent's reaction to the event and how it affects them. In my experience there is no substitute for strong parental positive attitude. Encouragement to keep trying and praise when success is achieved can go a long way in giving children a positive self-image. In the United States and Europe, there are few social stigmas attached to amputation and plenty of role models that get regular media coverage.

In my practice, all of the children with which we worked did very well with their prostheses and led active lives with lots of friends. They seemed to have a zest for life that many others did not, even though being an amputee did have some minor limitations. They were rough on prostheses and tested the limits of systems as well as components with their activities. I was always glad to see a beat up leg come in the door because I knew that the child was out having a life, not being worried about what he or she could or couldn't do. Whenever children came into the lab it was like a shot in the arm for the entire staff. They enriched us all with their energy and determination, and we used them to motivate others who could only see the tragedy in their situation.

The real challenge in emotional issues was rarely with the children; it was with parents or siblings who had a tough time dealing with the loss. When child amputees have a sense of humor, they can use this to put loved ones at ease and most do this without even thinking about it. It is a technique that can be learned as well. If a child can tell a joke or poke fun at him- or herself, he or she has developed a powerful tool to aid in creating acceptance. Parents of child amputees need to be considerate of the limitations of the child without catering to them. For example, if the child has a blister on his or her stump and the leg is too painful to wear, then it is appropriate to go get him or her a drink from the refrigerator. On the other hand, if the parent waits on the child even when there is not a prosthetic problem, they are teaching the child poor habits in using other people. It is important for parents to have some rudimentary knowledge of prostheses and how they work in order to keep an eye on things in between prosthetic visits. Even if parents are not mechanically inclined, it is possible to learn how to diagnose minor skin problems or recognize when the height of the prosthesis is off.

It is my experience that children with below-knee amputations will function quite well in today's society, especially in the United States or Europe. Sports programs in the mainstream schools provide access for amputees and there are many programs specially designed for amputees that give them a wide choice of activities. Life as a below-knee amputee should not be that different from other children's lives, providing that the parental role models are positive and considerate.

CHAPTER 10

Legal Issues

Stories

Dylan

Dylan had just turned 18 years old 3 days before his accident. He was out riding his Harley Davidson motorcycle, looking cool and feeling like he owned the world. He had just been accepted to Arizona State University and offered a full athletic scholarship in football. He had been the star offensive tackle and defensive linebacker for his high school team, which had won the state title thanks to his prowess. He was 100 kg (220 lb) of pure muscle and could bench press over 180 kilos (400 lb) easily. Not only was he built like the proverbial freight train, he was good looking and quick-witted. The girls would not leave him alone and since it was the 1970s, he took full advantage of their offers.

He felt great on that spring day with the sun beaming down and his whole life to look forward to. "I am going to get out of this town and make something of myself," he thought as he slowly motored down one of the back streets of his neighborhood. In the small town where he was raised he was known as a wild man, but since his dad knew the local chief of police and sheriff he was given much more latitude than most other young people. Dylan rounded the corner and slowly motored in front of a house where a particularly attractive young lady lived. To show off, he decided to ride his bike up into her front yard. He knew that it would anger her father, but he truly didn't care. He figured that if it made her father mad, it would make her secretly happy.

As the big motorcycle drove onto the grass, Dylan could see that there was moisture on the newly mowed lawn. He decided to turn sharply and do a spin out with his back tire. The engine on the big bike roared as he gunned it to spin the tire and chew up part of the lawn. The grass was really wet, having just been watered and when his back tire spun, he temporarily lost control of the bike and it went down, pinning his right leg beneath it. He felt a sharp pain behind his knee as the bike came down on top of him. With his massive arm strength he lifted the heavy bike off of his leg and stood up. Immediately, he was jolted by the pain behind his knee and had to hop to get around to where he could right his motorcycle. He felt stupid enough spinning out in the front yard and didn't want to be there when the old man came out to see about the commotion. He mounted the bike and rode home with a screamer pain behind his knee that didn't seem to get any better.

When Dylan got home he laid down on the couch and put some ice behind his knee, but it didn't help the pain at all. Apparently, the foot peg of the bike had jammed right into the middle of the back of his knee. The skin wasn't broken but the swelling was getting bad and the pain was nearly unbearable. His mother came home from work and immediately took him to the emergency room where the doctor told him that he had a serious bruise, stating that ice was the best thing he could do for the injury. He was given some pain pills and sent home. The next day he couldn't put any weight on the leg and was in incredible pain. His mom called their local doctor who agreed to see him back at the emergency room in the hospital. They took an X-ray of the knee and nothing showed up to indicate a bone break, but due to the amount of pain that Dylan was in the doctor admitted him to the hospital. Over the next couple of days it became obvious that there was some type of serious infection going on in his leg because he started to run a very high fever. The pain never went away and they continued to administer morphine in increasing amounts to help him cope with the agony. The doctors that examined him could not figure out what was going on. Since there was no external penetration of the skin, they were baffled by the infection.

On the fifth day that he was in the hospital his aunt who was a surgical nurse came in to visit with him. He was very groggy because of the heavy medication but when she examined his leg and saw the skin color beginning to turn reddish purple she immediately called his mom. "Get him out of that hospital or they will kill him," she said to Dylan's mom. The family agreed that they had to get him to a hospital where he could receive better treatment, so they arranged to have him flown to another hospital in an emergency helicopter. Dylan died 3 times on the way to the hospital and was resuscitated each time by astute paramedics on the flight.

What had happened to Dylan that the doctors at his local hospital had failed to diagnose was that the foot peg of the motorcycle had severed the major artery that carries the blood to the foot. This effectively cut off circulation to the bottom of the leg, causing the infection to set in and become gangrenous. The gangrene began to move into the rest of the body and that's what caused him to go into cardiac arrest on the trip to the hospital. The doctors at the hospital immediately saw what was happening and put him on massive antibiotics. Within hours they determined that the leg was not salvageable because so much of the tissue had been destroyed by the gangrene. His right leg was removed the next day below the knee.

In the space of 5 days Dylan's life had gone from perfection to disaster. Arizona State didn't want a 1-legged football player and his family could not even afford to pay his hospital bills let alone send him to college. Through a family friend they retained a local lawyer to represent Dylan in a medical malpractice lawsuit. The attorney was not particularly experienced in medical malpractice but took the case anyway. Dylan and his family thought that they had a pretty open and shut case of malpractice that their attorney reinforced with exaggerated overconfidence. The lawsuit was for $1.5 million, a very large sum of money at that time. Although Dylan was very depressed about the loss of his leg, he figured that life would be bearable when he won the suit.

After 18 months the case came to trial. The defense hadn't made any settlement offers, which had made Dylan's attorney suspicious. The attorney made his case in front of a local jury made up of people from the small town where Dylan was from. He neglected to call any expert witnesses either for an alternative medical perspective or for a projection of future prosthetic costs. When it came time for the defense to make its case, they basically admitted to most of the errors but then called the 2 surgeons to the stand. The surgeons who had treated Dylan at the hospital were the only surgeons in the town. As a matter of fact, they were the only surgeons in the entire county, a point that was brought up by the defense. Their testimony was that if a punitive verdict was reached in this case that they would be forced to close their practices and move elsewhere. Faced with the threat of losing the only 2 surgeons for a 160 km (100 m) radius of town, the jury returned a verdict of not guilty.

Dylan got nothing but legal bills from the lawsuit. He was also strapped with $50,000 in unpaid hospital bills and the specter of bankruptcy was staring him in the face. Fortunately for him, he was made of tough stuff and decided that he would somehow overcome this situation. He had always been good with his hands and knew metalworking from helping his father who made a living as a sheet metal worker. Even though his prosthetic provider was mediocre at best, he obtained a job as a welder and over the next 8 years paid off all of the hospital bills.

Dylan's story is an example of the failure of the legal system to provide compensation to someone who was a victim of incompetent medical treatment. His determination was such that he overcame the adversity and went on to work as a volunteer fireman, raise a family, and eventually get into prosthetics. Losing his leg should not have ruined his opportunities for a college education or forced him into manual labor to pay for his poor medical treatment.

Gayle

It was not the kind of job that her father had necessarily approved of, a delivery person for Airborne Express. He did not think that driving a step-van and running in between deliveries was a very feminine occupation for his pretty, blue-eyed, blond daughter. Gayle thought it was the perfect job for her. She had always had a shapely body, but the running and carrying all day long had firmed her up more than any gym could have ever done plus the money was great. No one stood over her to make sure she did her work and this suited her just fine. She was on her own the minute she walked out of the warehouse and the responsibility she was given drove her to be her best.

It was a typical day with deliveries all over the county. She loved studying the maps and trying to figure out where some of the addresses were located. She had just pulled off of the road to study her detailed map. This was a back county road with very little traffic but to be on the safe side she pulled off of the road and onto the shoulder so her full concentration could be on the map.

Unbeknownst to Gayle there was a large semi tractor-trailer barreling down the road behind her. The driver was late to get the machine parts to the warehouse, which was another 5 km (3 miles) ahead, so he was pushing it a bit. He had just glanced over at his cassette tape storage box to pick out a new cassette and when he looked up he saw the cow standing right in the middle of the road looking up at him with uncaring eyes. Reacting on instinct, the driver turned the wheel of the semi sharply to the left, avoiding the cow but causing his left front tires to go into the shoulder. His attempt to overcorrect and brake at the same time caused the overloaded trailer to skid out of control. When he looked ahead, he saw the delivery van on the shoulder right in front of him and although he tried to steer away from it, the trailer slammed into the side of the parked van with the force of a locomotive.

Gayle had no time to even react. Her concentration on the map was broken as she heard the screeching of tires and spitting of gravel. The next thing she knew she was being tossed sideways, held into the van by her seat belt. The big van rolled over and she was suspended upside down for a second before the heavy trailer with all of the machine parts crushed into the overturned van. When all of the motion ceased Gayle took stock of her situation. The cab of the van was crushed all around her, her left leg was bent back behind her, and there was a stabbing pain coming from the injury there. She began to have a hard time seeing and realized that there was blood dripping into her eyes. She felt her forehead and discovered a large gash that was bleeding profusely onto her face. Her hands were free and the rest of her body seemed to be OK, but her left leg was pinned behind her and the cab was smashed all around her. Even through the white-hot pain in her leg and the growing headache, she realized that she was very lucky to be alive.

She heard someone calling in a cracked voice and asking if anyone was in there. She replied that she was alive but was injured and could someone please call an ambulance. The faraway voice kept apologizing to her over and over again, and she finally screamed for him to call an ambulance. Things got silent for a while. The period of silence seemed to last forever until she finally heard the approaching sound of sirens in the distance. She never thought that she would be glad to hear the sounds of sirens but she knew they represented her salvation. Gayle had no idea how much blood she was losing from her leg or if it was even cut since she couldn't see it but she began to feel sleepy. Soon she heard voices talking to her but she could feel that consciousness was slipping away. The next thing she remembers is the sensation of floating and the "whap whap whap" of helicopter blades. She thought she was either dead or on a flight to the hospital.

The paramedics and firefighters who arrived at the accident scene immediately began to cut the cab of the van away to extract Gayle from the wreckage. As they carefully pulled her out of the cab she was unconscious but still alive. The cut on her head was bleeding badly but what concerned them most was her left leg, which had been nearly severed by a piece of the van that had wedged it behind her. They got her in the helicopter and began administering fluids to try and keep her from going into deeper shock. She was in critical but stable condition when she reached the hospital.

Gayle was not married and it took a couple of hours before the authorities could reach her parents who lived several hours away. The emergency room surgeon saw no hope of saving her leg but needed the permission of either Gayle or her parents to perform the surgery. Since her condition was stable both the surgeon and her parents decided to wait until Gayle was awake and more lucid to obtain permission for the amputation. That evening Gayle regained consciousness and her parents and the surgeon explained what had occurred. Before she would agree to the amputation she demanded that she be able to see the injury. Her mother broke down and left the room sobbing. The surgeon lifted the sheet to reveal the mangled leg that was only attached by a piece of skin. Her father turned white but choked back the tears to see his baby girl injured in such a way. Gayle on the other hand stared at her leg for a long time exhibiting a surprising distant objectivity that surprised even herself afterward. She looked at the surgeon and told him in a steady voice that the leg had to come off and she was prepared to accept the situation.

The surgery went smoothly and Gayle's leg was removed 13 cm (5 in) below the knee and they were able to use good skin from the back of the calf to cover her stump.

The pain was pretty rough at first, and she had her thumb on the self-injection morphine distributor until it made her pass out. Each day got a little better and she consciously made the effort to go longer and longer in between pain medication until she was not using the morphine after the fourth day. A physical therapist came in every day to help her keep the rest of her body active and by day 3 she was able to stand up on crutches. A man came the same day and introduced himself as her prosthetist. He taught her how to wrap her residual limb and use a shrinker sock, which began to help her stump feel better after the initial discomfort.

Gayle was released from the hospital after 8 days and went into a rehabilitation center where she received physical therapy twice a day. The prosthetist came back to see how she was doing and informed her that as soon as the stitches were out he would make her a preparatory prosthesis. He left her with literature and videos that explained the process of her prosthetic rehabilitation, and she couldn't wait until the next week when the stitches would be removed. People from her work came to visit her as well as her friends, which cheered her up. They were all amazed at her attitude that was optimistic and full of humor. One day her father came for his daily visit and brought along a man dressed in a business suit. He introduced the man as an attorney and told Gayle that he thought it would be best to have someone looking into the legal issues of her accident. Gayle hadn't even thought about any of this. Her focus was on getting well and healing. She told him the story of her accident and agreed to meet with him when she got out of the rehabilitation hospital.

Gayle went home after 3 weeks in the rehab hospital with her preparatory prosthesis. She was able to use the leg with crutches since her stump was still very tender and the rest of her body was a bit shaky. She had lost 7 kg (15 lb), most of it muscle that she had worked so hard to develop. She was determined to learn to use a prosthesis and go back to work as before. When she talked to her boss from work, he told her that there would be some kind of position for her at work but he didn't think it would be best for her to return to delivery due to the physical requirements that the job entailed. This was a big disappointment for Gayle, but she was still determined to show her boss that she could do the job.

A week after she returned home, her father drove her to the office of the attorney that had come to visit her in the rehab hospital. He explained the legal process of how and why people seek redress for negligent damages. After hearing her account of the accident again, he said that he thought there was negligence on the part of the driver of the truck that hit her, as well as negligence on the part of the trucking company that employed him. She didn't quite understand the whole issue of negligence but since she felt she could trust this man, she agreed to have him pursue a lawsuit against the negligent parties. He also explained that the legal system also would look at her negligence in the cause of the accident. He then asked detailed questions about how far off of the road she had pulled and whether she had her emergency blinkers on. After an hour of questioning, he was satisfied that they had enough of a case to pursue then he explained how his firm gets paid. He said that all court costs or document acquisition would be totaled and paid for by the law firm up front. If the case is won or settled favorably those costs would be deducted from the judgment and then the law firm would be entitled to 20% of the balance. Gayle and her father agreed to the arrangement and went home.

Gayle had to go into the attorney's office several times over the next 3 months for conferences and depositions. The deposition was grueling with her lawyer asking her questions then another lawyer asking a lot of the same questions over and over again. The other lawyer seemed like a pretty nice man but it was apparent that he represented the defense because he kept asking about whether she had taken proper safety precautions when she pulled off of the road. After the deposition, her attorney explained to her that they would need to hire expert witnesses to testify as to her prosthetic needs for the rest of her life as well as someone who could address her loss of work capability. He said that this would cost money since good experts are expensive but that he felt that it would be worth it.

Gayle's attorney did his homework. He found a prosthetic expert witness who prepared a detailed needs analysis that projected her prosthetic costs for the rest of her life based upon her life expectancy. Then he researched and retained a life care planner who prepared a detailed analysis of Gayle's employment history as well as her projected loss of employment opportunity. He also retained a medical expert who addressed the pain and suffering that was associated with amputation and recovery. He took depositions of the driver of the truck, the men at the loading dock where he picked up the machine tools that he was on the way to deliver, as well as the driver's supervisors at the trucking company. This process went on for 6 months in the legal process called discovery and a trial date was set for 6 months after that.

Gayle's attorney advised her to go about her life as if there were no lawsuit for $1.8 million because there was no guarantee that she would receive anything from the litigation. She took his advice and returned to work with Airborne but had to sit at a desk all day checking orders for delivery. She didn't like the work and it only paid half of what she made as a delivery person. She had been fitted with her first permanent prosthesis after 4 months and her prosthetist said she was doing spectacular. She had regained some of her weight but not the hard body she had when she was delivering packages. This disappointed her and she was very nervous about getting back into the dating scene. She was still the pretty, blond, blue-eyed, woman that she had always been and even though she no longer had the hard body that she had before the accident most women would be envious of her build. The scar on her forehead healed nicely even though it required 15 stitches, and she found that if she wore her bangs down on her forehead no one could see it.

The day of Gayle's trial was approaching and her attorney had prepared her for the possibility that the other law firm would probably make a settlement offer prior to trial. Sure enough, a week before her case was due the defense made an offer of half a million dollars to Gayle's lawyer. They met to discuss the offer but her lawyer recommended that they reject the first offer and see if they would come back with a better counter. It took until the day before the trial but the defense finally made a counter offer of $1.2 million and after a discussion with Gayle and her father, they decided to accept it.

After the experts and the court costs were paid, there was $1,125,000 left of which the law firm received $225,000 as their 20%, leaving Gayle with $900,000. This money was supposed to compensate Gayle for the loss of her leg as well as any outstanding hospital bills. With the help of her father she consulted with a financial planner who recommended that they place a large portion of it in an investment portfolio. The investment would pay her a dividend that she could use to cover her prosthetic costs for the rest of her life based upon the needs analysis prepared by the expert. She kept a relatively small portion of her settlement to splurge on herself, buying a new car and some new clothes then taking a cruise with her best girlfriend. On the cruise she had a romantic affair with a handsome young man who gave her back the confidence she needed to reenter the dating world. Gayle eventually returned to her delivery job after a year and a half when her stump had matured and her prosthesis worked well. She had to prove to her boss that she could still perform up to their requirements but she exceeded all expectations.

This is an example of how the judicial system in this country is supposed to work. In an ideal scenario, the damaged plaintiff is able to recover sufficient funds to compensate him or her for his or her loss and provide for his or her needs. The critical factor is the competency of the plaintiff's attorney and the strength of the case. If the case is strong and the attorney is competent, then there is a good chance that a positive conclusion will be reached. It is still never wise to bank on a verdict that isn't in.

Projecting the Prosthetic Costs of an Amputee

When I lost my leg 30 years ago, I felt that I needed to bring a suit against the construction company that had been managing the site where my accident occurred. I knew a good attorney from Ohio and asked him to do some research to find a good attorney in Georgia who could take my case. He called my dad back and made a referral. After I got out of the hospital, we went to visit the attorney and he explained how the legal process worked and what we could expect. No one in my family had ever been in a lawsuit before so we had no idea of how to proceed or how to choose representation. My attorney and his assistant were very knowledgeable and we decided to trust their judgment. The fee for their service seemed a bit high. We didn't know that 50% was on the very high side of the attorney fee charges, but we were novices.

One of the first things that the attorney requested was a projection of the costs for prostheses for the rest of my life from my prosthetist. Grant, who was my prosthetist, admitted to me that he didn't know how to go about determining the costs but did the best that he could. The process that he went through was very disruptive to the rest of his business and he complained to me several times that he really felt inadequate to the task. My attorney also hired a psychologist from California who studied my diaries to develop a psychological profile of me. I was keeping a journal of my experiences since the accident at the request of my attorney so I mailed these off to this man I had never met. I recently read the psychological profile and besides the fact that I find it humorous, it bears little resemblance to my makeup. It was also the advice of my attorney to maintain my residence in Ohio so that my case would be tried in a federal court instead of a county court, which he said would give me a more sophisticated jury.

My attorney was always very guarded about my chances to recover the big dollars; the total suit was for $350,000, even in 1974 that was not a very significant amount. The best advice that he gave me was to forget the whole lawsuit thing and concentrate on my education. I did follow his advice and tried not to let the thought of having some money influence my decisions about my future. I had been in the hospital with 2 other amputees who had talked about nothing other than their lawsuits and the Corvettes that they were going to buy with their money. I was careful not to fall into that trap, so after my last 2 years of college I took the teaching job overseas and started teaching in Egypt. My activity level and traveling were not conducive to an image of the poor disabled amputee, but my attorney said that I shouldn't count on any kind of settlement. He explained that juries in the south did not look favorably on motorcycles or the people who rode them.

The case was finally due to come to trial after 3.5 years of waiting. I was living in Egypt teaching in the American school and having the time of my life traveling as well as experiencing the novelty of overseas life. One month prior to the trial date the defense made an offer to settle the case. My attorney recommended that we try to negotiate a settlement, and I gave my permission for him to exercise authority over the settlement decision. After a week of dickering, he finally accepted a total settlement of $50,000 of which he got half. I didn't have to leave my job and I got $25,000, which seemed like an awful lot of money at the time. Little did I know that that sum would-n't provide for 5 years worth of prosthetic costs let alone the rest of my life.

I became a prosthetist partially out of self-defense since I didn't have the resources to provide prostheses for myself. In the early 1980s I was asked to determine the life-time prosthetic costs for one of my clients. Like Grant, so many years before, I had no idea how to go about the task but I determined that I needed to develop a consistent system to form a projection. Based upon my experience with amputees and prosthet-ics, I came up with a systematic approach to projecting prosthetic needs that has been used as a model by numerous professionals since then. I have also adapted my system based on the cases that I have been involved in and the changes that have occurred in the field. I now have a consultant business that provides expert witness testimony all over the United States and I have even testified in other countries. I lecture and write articles on this systematic approach that is used by many other prosthetists when they are asked to provide a similar service.

In order to project the prosthetic needs of an amputee, I start with one basic prem-ise. My job is to project what it would cost to return the amputee to as close a style of life as he or she had prior to amputation considering the limitations of prosthetic tech-nology. It is not my job to determine whether my projection is what he or she deserves or will get, only to provide what is necessary to continue his or her life as close as pos-sible to his or her previous life. I make the same projection whether I am representing the plaintiff (injured party) or the defense.

If you or someone you know is involved in a lawsuit over the loss of a leg, then I have some advice. Be very careful in choosing an attorney. In my experience there is a wide range of competency levels in attorneys. It is wise to take the time to find one who will do his or her homework as well as someone that you can trust. Try not to become obsessed with the thought of future financial gain. If you have a good attor-ney that you can trust, let them do all of the worrying and you should get on with your life. If you receive a positive judgment, then that is great, but if you don't, then you should still have your life to fall back onto. Make sure you understand the process of the litigation and have a good idea of how long it is going to take. The experience is never fun and often causes the amputee to have to dredge up painful memories.

Product Liability

Prostheses break and amputees suffer. This is the major reason that amputees will want to seek redress against the prosthetist or a manufacturer of prosthetic compo-nents. I have always avoided getting involved as an expert witness in product liability since my consulting business depends upon the goodwill of prosthetists and manufac-turers across the country.

Amputees need to know that they do have some recourse if their prosthesis does not function properly or breaks during use. The first recourse for an honest person is always to contact the prosthetist who made the limb and see if he or she will repair or replace any damaged or broken parts. If there was an injury due to the lack of function of the prosthesis, then it should be made clear to the prosthetist and an opportunity provided for them to compensate for damages. Whenever 2 parties cannot work out a problem and it has to be negotiated by attorneys, the only people who will always benefit are the attorneys. Work things out if possible. If not, seek advice from an attorney you can trust.

Most prosthetists will have a period of time in which they guarantee their work and most are honorable people who will do whatever it takes to make it right for the amputee. Most manufacturers of prosthetic supplies and components have a warranty policy that allows for the replacement of defective parts or materials. It is wise to be aware of the various warranties that exist on your prosthesis, and all manufacturers provide cards that explain the limits of their liability. The best relationship is one that is clear about expectations from the beginning, so make sure that there is minimal ambiguity on how long the prosthesis is guaranteed.

If, in the worse case scenario, there is some type of defect in the prosthesis that causes bodily injury to the amputee, there may be no alternative to litigation. Choose an attorney who has experience with product liability cases and who is willing to do their homework. Manufacturers and large prosthetic firms have legal representation that have extensive experience in defending against such suits so the plaintiff needs to be sure of his or her case. Work things out if possible and if it is not possible, seek council with someone who will advocate in a straightforward and honorable way.

CHAPTER 11

More Amputee Stories

My Story

For those of you who just couldn't get enough of what happened to me, here is a brief summary of the rest of my life up to present. I had moved to New Hampshire by the mid-1980s and taken a position with a prosthetic company as chief of prosthetics. I was married to Jane and not only was a member of the U.S. Disabled Nordic Ski Team but was the vice president of the National Handicapped Sports Association. We had purchased a small 13-acre gentleman's farm near the border with Massachusetts and settled into a lifestyle that centered around my activities.

I was now in my thirties and was beginning to wonder if I would ever become a father. Jane was not too keen on having children and as the years passed, this became an increasingly touchy issue. I used every strategy that I could conjure up to avoid dealing with our problems. I was busy, I kept someone living with us all of the time to distract us from our issues so the inevitable occurred—Jane and I slowly drifted apart. I sought solace outside of our marriage, which went even further in destroying any remaining trust.

I had worked for 2.5 years at the facility in New England and had continual problems with the business manager of the place. He and I had very different philosophies of patient care that were not likely to rectify themselves, so in 1987 I left my job there and started a small private practice in conjunction with a sports medicine clinic. In 1988, I met a woman while ski racing that I fell in love with. She was my age and in a similar circumstance as myself. I saw her as my last chance at having a family so I forsook 8 years of marriage. Jane and I got a divorce. I moved out west to be near to her and as everyone who cared about me predicted, she dumped me after about 6 months.

I had started a private practice in Reno, Nevada where I knew one person in the whole state. Undaunted, I dove into my work since my love life was a disaster and I was able to survive long enough to establish my business. I gave up any idea of having a family. I was 36 years old, one-legged, heartbroken, and owner of a struggling business. Not much of a resumé for anyone seeking a mate. Maybe I am just too hard headed to give up but I began dating again. One afternoon I gave an in-service at the local hospital and during my talk, I was attracted to a very cute blond with a southern accent who asked some good questions. Later I got a friend of mine in the hospital to introduce me to her and a friendship developed. I never thought that Jill would later become my wife and the mother of my 2 boys.

I began to devote my time and energies to the business and no longer had the time to continually train for the ski team. I had also become burned out with the sport to some degree. Training took 10 to 12 hours a week and the race schedule meant that I would not have time to take care of my clients. I left the team in 1989 after having my best season racing in the able-bodied biathlon circuit. I actually placed 95th in the US out of 250 racers in my age group. On my 35th birthday I raced my only marathon, a 50-kilometer race where I finished in the middle of my age group. I liked ending on a high note so I quit racing and devoted my energies to developing my business.

I also felt that I could no longer maintain the commitment to the National Handicapped Sports Association and I resigned from the board. This organization that had given me so much in the way of confidence was changing and growing so I felt that after 10 years it was time to move on. I replaced my need to give back to my community with Rotary International, a business group that has chapters all over the world. I joined the local Rotary Club and enjoyed the camaraderie as well as the opportunity to serve my community. After having been involved with the nonprofit world for almost 10 years, I was not very keen on how donated money was being spent. I was very impressed with how the Rotary Club used its local chapters in developing places to disburse funds and manage projects. You knew that there was someone just like you making sure that the eye clinic in Bolivia was really getting built and that no one was skimming money from the project.

My business was taking off and I had hired a person who was also an amputee to help me out around the shop. I slowly developed a plan for my business that centered on hiring amputees to work for me as a means of demonstrating my products. This created an environment that made most amputees comfortable and was highly motivational to people who had just lost their limbs. After 2.5 years at a small somewhat rundown house in Reno, I had saved up enough money to be able to think about buying a place. I had been successful by not only providing quality prostheses and backing it up with excellent service, but I also had been conservative in my business approach. I had no experience or training in finance but I had the value of not spending what I didn't have so I saved money along the way and by 1992 I was ready to buy a building. I was looking for a place that I could live and work out of so that I would only have one payment a month. I found that place in Washoe Valley, a short distance south of Reno and about halfway to Carson City, the capital of Nevada.

The building had been the county home for runaway girls and was in a state of disrepair when I bought it. All of my friends thought that I was crazy to buy the place since it was so far out of town and in such bad condition. I knew that if I provided the best prosthetic service around that people would drive the 20 minutes to have me make them a prosthesis. I also had a significant percentage of my clients who came from out of town so it was important that I have room to house them as well as a scenic facility where they would feel comfortable. The building was large and perfectly suited to my needs with a comfortable house section and had a large two-story annex attached to it that became my prosthetic facility. It took me 3 months to renovate the place doing a majority of the work myself on weekends and afternoons. I had generous help from friends and my father to finally have the place ready for me to move into and begin seeing patients.

It was at this time that the business really took off. I hired one of my clients to work for me and added a secretary to help with the paperwork in addition to the part-time billing person. Jill moved in with me. The first Christmas we were in the house, I proposed to her and she accepted. Neither of us was totally sure of the whole marriage thing so we decided to have a long engagement and see how it would work.

Business really started to boom and I continued to add employees. I hired amputees whenever possible, usually people for whom I had made limbs. This created a staff that had natural understanding of the amputee and provided a positive role model to anyone visiting our shop. A typical scenario was that a new amputee would be sitting in the waiting room and he or she may overhear the conversations of the employees. He or she would hear the secretaries talking about the cute man they saw at the health club where they had worked out the night before, or the guys in the shop telling fish stories. The effect was almost magic. The new amputee would then realize that all of these people were amputees and that the stuff he or she was hearing was just like the stuff they would hear anywhere. This had the effect of inspiring through demonstration that life could return to normal and that the things they thought they had lost were still within reach.

Jill and I married in March of 1992 with our close friends in attendance. We got married in the oldest church in Nevada, but we had no music for the occasion. Our friends hummed "Here Comes the Bride" as Jill came down the aisle. Jill became pregnant shortly thereafter, surprising us both. I was so excited I couldn't believe it. I was finally going to be a father, the only thing I had ever known that I wanted to be. Our first son, Jeff, came into the world and fulfilled my deepest desire. He was a healthy, very happy baby who brought joy to all who came into contact with him.

Life was busy then. The pressures of being a father, husband, and small businessman were tremendous but it was what I wanted to be doing. Business continued to grow and I added employees to keep up. I was constantly renovating and adding to the shop and home. After 20 months our second son, John, was born, a healthy boy that was not so happy to be in this world. He cried all night and adding sleep deprivation to my mix of stress didn't help. One of my employees also had a son the same age as Jeff so I began to provide a nanny for their care during business hours. This was great to have the boys close by so that I could pop up to the house during work to see them.

After 2.5 years in the new building, I realized that I needed to have a home separate from my business in order for my family to survive intact. The stress of never being able to leave work was not making my relationship with Jill any better. She is a strong personality and needs a more private life then the current set-up could provide. The business was also beginning to consume me as I grew. My overhead was high due to the number of employees and the benefits that I provided. I still was making a good living but the minimum amount I had to make each month to meet expenses was beginning to get pretty big. I needed help but had no clue as to where to go.

I love to hike and would routinely walk the mountains behind my shop. We had dogs and I would be gone for hours, traipsing through the woods and admiring the views from the hills behind me. I had a favorite spot that I would stop at to drink the one beer I would pack with me. Beer is heavy so it is a special treat to drink one when hiking. One day while sitting on my favorite log overlooking the valley, I wondered who owned the land I was on and whether any of it was for sale. The next week at the Rotary Club I cornered a hungry looking realtor, Harvey, who agreed to help me find out if there was any property for sale in the area. We found out that there was 120 acres for sale behind where my shop was located but I couldn't afford the price for the whole parcel. He recommended that I form a real estate partnership to purchase and develop the land. I had never done anything like this before but with the help of Harvey, I took the plunge. Now in addition to being a small business owner, I was a real estate developer.

The boys were growing and business was steadily improving so in order to get away from it all we began to go to Mexico for our vacations. Cozumel, an island off of the Mexican coast in the Caribbean was our favorite spot and both Jill and I took up scuba diving to experience the greatest attraction of the island. Scuba diving is the perfect sport for the amputee since being under the water removes the pull of gravity that makes wearing a prosthesis so demanding. It is like being on another planet and being able to fly. I had to construct a scuba diving prosthesis, which I have described in a previous chapter, in order to be able to keep up with my wife and the other divers; but once I did it became easy. Boat diving was a piece of cake, someone put your tanks on while you sit on the edge of the boat then all you have to do is fall over backwards, a skill I had perfected in second grade. We went there for 5 years in a row, usually going with 2 other families with kids and renting a villa that had a cook and maid. It provided the perfect getaway.

Back home in the real world, business was rapidly growing beyond my skills to manage it. I had also entered into a partnership with a man whom I met in the Rotary Club named Dave. He made sensors for robotics and we had come up with an application of the technology in prosthetics. We developed a sensor that would "beep" if the amputee's stump got too deep into the socket. We began a company named Prosthetic Sensing Technologies and started to try to market our product to the industry. After several years of very frustrating attempts to break into the industry, we both realized that the technology was just not going to be a quick sell and no larger company was willing to pick it up. We dissolved the partnership and basically let the product die.

Dave and I, however, became close friends and he introduced me to TEC, an organization of CEOs that helps businesses develop as well as grow. Through TEC I became a real businessman who used the reports and balance sheets produced by my accountant to manage my business. I was able to get control of the money that was owed to me and develop a long-term plan to grow the business. One of the strategies I learned from a speaker at our group was that if I could have my business prepared for sale (a concept that I had never really entertained) I would be managing it in the most efficient manner. I worked nonstop for 6 months to learn the nuances of finance and organization that would give me a clean record of Specialty Prosthetics. During the time that I was cleaning up my numbers, a big prosthetic company approached me about selling my business. I had no intention of selling, but I thought it would be a good exercise to submit my books to the biggie and see what they thought my business was worth.

When they came back with an offer I was floored. This was six times earnings and even in 2000 when the value of businesses was often over-inflated, I had to seriously consider this offer. I crunched numbers for days trying to determine if I had a better exit strategy. I didn't and so I entered into negotiations to sell Specialty Prosthetics and merge my practice with their local facility. My employees were equally surprised when I informed them of my decision and many of them were downright upset at me. The transition to the new facility went alright but there were immediate signs that this was not going to be the situation that I had envisioned. After 6 months I could no longer work at the new company. I was not in charge and their way of treating amputees conflicted with my way. I left the company and decided to continue my consulting business as an expert witness. This was a very difficult decision and there were a great number of former employees and clients that were very disappointed with my actions.

My boys were 7 and 9 years old so Jill and I decided to take a year and move to Spain. My friend Miguel lives in Granada, which is a city deep in the heart of the Sierra Nevada Mountains in southern Spain. It is ancient and beautiful and we were able to rent a house in the oldest part of the city, Albaicin, only about a block from Miguel. The boys went to a Spanish school where only 2 other people spoke English so they had the challenge of their lives learning to cope. We lived there for 16 months while Jill studied Spanish and I drank a lot of the local wine while enjoying the café lifestyle. We met some great people and this was where I started writing this book.

We moved back to the United States in the summer and the boys returned to their old elementary school where they have reintegrated beautifully. Jill got a job working in her profession for the school district and I have labored on this book, a labor of love. It is now almost over and as I sit in my house that overlooks the valley below, I am almost sorry for it to end. I hope that by sharing my story you have seen some of yourself in my adventures and learned that the trick to survival is to never give up.

Miguel

When Miguel was 18 years old he was one of Spain's most famous young mountain climbers. He and a fellow climber decided to attempt to summit the north face of the Eiger in November, the latest month that had ever been attempted. The Eiger is a mountain in Switzerland that has an enormous vertical face over a kilometer and a half (1 mile) in all directions. To make it even more difficult it actually has a bit of an outward bulge at the top. This is one of the most dangerous climbs in the world and has claimed the lives of many excellent climbers. They were climbing in November in order to avoid the almost constant avalanche of rocks and boulders that shower down during the summer month; the only problem is the risk of storms that can hit the region that late in the year.

They had been climbing for 5 days and were nearing the top, expecting to summit that afternoon then enjoy the relatively easy walk to the train station on the nearby glacier. Miguel was leading the pitch and was roped to his partner with 120 feet of line. He dug his ice ax into a ledge of snow and began to haul himself up when the ledge began to give way. He quickly dug his other ax into the ledge of snow but the snow was rotten and it broke free. Down he fell, trying to dig his axes into anything he could find but nothing slowed down his descent. Fortunately, his partner pulled in the rope and was able to stop Miguel's fall but not before his feet slammed against a ledge, snapping both of his ankles. His partner slowly pulled him up to a tiny rock outcropping to survey the damage. Both of Miguel's ankles were broken and they didn't dare to remove the boots for fear of not being able to get them back on. They used their radio to call for help and Miguel's partner dug a cave from a snow-filled crevasse in the side of the mountain.

Unfortunately for them, the first major snow storm of the year hit. No rescue attempt could be made until the storm abated and they had already nearly used up all of their food. On the second day in the cave their stove refused to work and so they could not melt snow for water. Miguel's legs didn't hurt much anymore which he knew was a bad sign since severe frostbite doesn't hurt once the tissue is dead. On the fifth day they had both resigned themselves to the fact that they were probably going to freeze to death. Miguel got to spend many hours with God during the 5 days stuck in the snow cave and it has since given him a presence that surfaces under pressure. They hadn't given up but they also realized that with the storm still raging any attempt to rescue them was fruitless. The fifth day when they reported in on the radio they were told that the storm may take a break for a couple of hours and that if it did there would be a rescue attempt. God smiled upon them that day and a helicopter with a rescuer was able to extract them from the side of the Eiger in a dangerous rescue that was right out of the movies. Miguel would later relate that the most terrifying part of the entire ordeal was when he was dangling from a rope as the helicopter was descending to the hospital. He realized that he wasn't going to die and that he would now have to live with the loss of his feet.

He was taken to a local hospital where they had to amputate both feet, leaving stumps that were not quite a Syme's amputation and not quite a partial foot amputation. The skin from the bottom of his feet was dead so they used grafts to cover them, preserving the ankles and some of the forefoot bones. He spent months recovering in the hospital before he received prostheses from a Swiss prosthetist. He immediately was able to walk and get around on crutches much to the surprise of all of the people who worked with him. He returned to Spain where he lived with his parents for a while until he was independently mobile again. Miguel is not one to dwell for long on his misfortune. He maintained his self-confidence and actually returned to climbing again. He met a young American girl who was studying Spanish at the University and they started dating.

One day, 2 years after his accident, Miguel was back climbing in the Sierra Nevada Mountains near to Granada with a good friend named Pepe. His buddy was leading the pitch and Miguel was roped to him on a 40-meter (120-ft) line. They were traversing a sheer 160-meter (500-ft) drop that was covered with ice. Pepe decided to use a protruding boulder as an anchor to swing onto a ledge about 3 meters (10 ft) in front of him. He swung the rope over the boulder and pulled hard on the rope to test the boulder's stability. Feeling that everything was safe, he slowly moved beneath the boulder. Just as he got beneath it, the boulder came loose and it along with Pepe plunged down the face of the cliff. Pepe landed on a small protruding ledge and the boulder landed on top of him, then they both continued their descent to the rocks below. Miguel was strapped to Pepe and there was only one ice piton hammered into the cliff to arrest Pepe's fall. Miguel thought fast and pulled as much rope through the piton as he could before Pepe's full weight tested the piton's strength. If the piton let go, Miguel and Pepe would plunge to their deaths on the rocks below. As he felt the weight on the rope he let it out to arrest the descent and the piton held. Miguel looked down to see the slumped head and limp body of Pepe dangling below. With all of his strength, Miguel dragged Pepe back up to a nearby ledge and examined the damage to his friend. When the boulder had landed on Pepe, it had crushed his legs, severing one completely and smashing the other one flat. Most people would have panicked but not Miguel.

Miguel is not a big guy, at the time he was only 68 kilos (150 lb) and had two artificial legs. He put tourniquets on Pepe's legs and began the laborious process of getting him to medical attention. This was before the time of cell phones and they didn't have a radio so he had to put Pepe's dead weight body on his shoulders to haul him out. It took Miguel 11 hours to bring Pepe to safety but they made it and Pepe is alive today because of Miguel's efforts.

Miguel went on to marry the American girl and they have a daughter who is the same age as my oldest son. I met Miguel when he and his wife were in the United States teaching in a prep school in New Hampshire. I liked him the minute I met him and through my efforts we adopted him onto the U.S. Disabled Ski Team and he joined us for the 1986 race season. He ended up winning a silver medal in the 1988 Olympics and went on to win more medals for Spain than any other athlete. He then moved to bicycle racing where he won many more medals including Olympic gold and European championships. He raced for 8 more years until he broke his hip in a long bicycle race in Belgium. Unfortunately, family life and world class racing rarely mix well and his wife left to return to the United States with their daughter. Miguel is one of my best friends in the whole world and I cherish the time that we have spent together.

Art

The first time that I met Art I thought that this guy was close to death. He was in his 70s and was so skinny that a slight wind might blow him away. He had just lost his right leg due to peripheral vascular disease and was diagnosed with leukemia to boot. You still couldn't help but be impressed by the firm handshake, the twinkle in his eyes, and the large diamond earring in his right ear. We made a preparatory leg for Art and he returned to driving big rigs that moved trailers all over the west. This was his business and he wasn't about to let the loss of a leg get in the way. He told me that when his leg hurt he would use a cane to push in the clutch so he wouldn't have to miss a haul.

I always love to hear stories from my clients, so one day when I was working on Art's leg and we had some time to kill, I asked him to tell me a little about himself. He had grown up in Cleveland in a very rough part of town. His father was abusive and his mother had left when he was young so Art grew up as a tough street kid. His best buddy was the son of the local Mafia don and Art lived with them off and on throughout high school. After graduation the 2 buddies went to work for the Mafia doing errands and performing jobs for the organization. Their big chance came when they were asked to perform a "hit" on someone who owed money to the mob and they jumped at the chance to make a name for themselves.

After the hit, the police were very suspicious of the two and so they decided to hide out in Canada for a while. The year was 1941 and World War II was raging all over Europe and Asia. The heat from their hit was getting intense so in order to hide even deeper, they decided to join the Canadian Army under false identity where they figured they could remain anonymous. They were just finishing boot camp up in Alberta when one day they were called into the Commandant's office where a man in an American military uniform was sitting. The American officer knew all about them, their names, where they were from, and more importantly whom they had killed. He gave them a choice, extradition back to the United States to face trial for murder or they could join an elite commando squad that he was organizing. Since this was not much of a choice, the 2 men decided to become commandos.

They returned to the United States to a training school somewhere in the West. It was so secret that they didn't even know where it was. There they learned how to use explosives and the art of hand-to-hand combat. They learned to jump from airplanes and to swim undetected onto beaches as well as to leave no evidence of their presence. The United States had not entered the war yet but anyone in the know knew that it was only a matter of time. The only hint at what they were being trained for came when they were given a crash course in Chinese for 2 weeks. After 6 months of intensive training, their team of 8 men was flown to Singapore where they parachuted into China. They were met by Chinese soldiers and spent the next 6 months blowing up bridges and trains all over northern China. China had been at war with Japan for nearly 10 years by this time and the Japanese controlled most of the coastal cities and countryside. The Chinese armies under Chang Kai Shek had retreated to the interior of the country and avoided pitched battles with the superior Japanese army. Art and his buddy were working in the north where the Chinese Communists under the leadership of Mao Tse Tung were fighting the Japanese in a constant guerrilla war.

The United States entered the war in December of 1941 and when the Dolittle Raid occurred in the spring of 1942 some of the pilots had to ditch their planes in China. Art and his unit were some of the commandos who helped rescue these pilots and keep them out of the hands of the Japanese who executed any pilots they captured. They continued their espionage of the Japanese war effort through 1942 and were then taken out of China to enter a new theater of the war. Art and his unit had no dog tags, no identification of any type since they technically didn't exist. Whenever they came out of the fighting and returned to some form of civilization, they were generally a bit wild in the local bars. These were not men that even the toughest Marine wanted to mess with. Just the look in their eyes told you that they had no regard for life or death and that they were living for the moment. They couldn't obtain transport via regular military channels so they were always scrounging around to find discreet ways of moving to their next assignment.

Next, they found themselves in the Mediterranean where their assignment was to parachute into Yugoslavia and destroy radar bases there. British and American bombers were flying regular missions deep into Nazi-occupied Romania to bomb the Polesti oil fields in order to cripple the German war effort. The radar stations were the early warning for the German fighter interceptors that were taking a terrible toll of pilots and aircraft. Destroying the radar stations would make it much safer for the Allies to bomb the oil fields and shorten the war. During this operations Art had saved his buddy's life on 2 occasions while they were laying explosives and were caught by the guards. After the radar stations were blown up, Art's buddy swore that he would make it up to Art when they got back to the real world at the end of the war.

Art couldn't help but smile when he related the rest of his wartime adventures to me. They had to fight their way out of Yugoslavia and back into Italy where the closest Allied lines were located. They worked their way down to Naples where they were at last told that they could go back to the United States. They would receive honorable discharges but the details of their involvement in the war were to remain top-secret. They still had the problem of traveling with no identification and no orders. There were several occasions where they had to fight their way out of encounters with the military police to keep from being thrown into jail and their identities discovered. In Naples, they befriended a pilot in a bar who told them that he could fly them as far as Tunis, Tunisia where he was sure they could get a ship bound for the United States.

They made it to Tunis but were stuck there for several weeks trying to arrange transport via ship. Art says that he befriended a little monkey in the bar by the waterfront where they hung out all day. He really liked that monkey and took it with him everywhere he went. One very inebriated evening they were talking to a Brazilian man who claimed to be a boat captain and was headed to Miami where he was dropping off a shipment. He told them that they could crew for him as far as Miami and that Art could bring his monkey if he wished.

When Art and his buddy finally recovered from their massive hangover, they found themselves pressed into semicaptivity on a leaky tramp steamer that was not bound for Miami. It was on its way to Recife, Brazil and by the looks of the boat may not even make it there. They were tempted to take over the ship but they had no weapons and the rest of the crew treated them with a distanced respect. Three weeks later, they arrived in the shabby port of Recife and began their search for transport to the United States. Finally, after 2 more weeks of miserable life in the seedy port, they managed to secure berths on another tramp steamer that was headed for New Orleans. The monkey had disappeared in Recife. Art thought that one of the women he had been with had stolen it from him, but due to the abundance of rum he couldn't be sure.

Finally, they were on their way to the United States and home. Art and his buddy were still alive after all of those adventures even though they couldn't tell anyone about them. It was late 1944 and the war was drawing to an end. Some said it would be over by Christmas but for Art it was already over. German U-boats still prowled the Caribbean and as luck would have it one of them torpedoed the tramp steamer that Art and his buddy were on. Once again, Art saved his friend's life by hauling his unconscious body onto a life raft. They and 6 other men were on the raft with little food and water for 3 days before they were picked up by a fishing boat and taken to Cuba. It had been a long trip home but after a few days recovering in Cuba they arrived back in the United States.

After a 5-year absence, the 2 boys that had become old men returned to Cleveland to find that the Mafia don had died the month before. Art's best friend and comrade in arms was now the de-facto head of the Cleveland Mafia. He told Art that he could have anything that he wanted; all he had to do was ask. Art never hesitated. "I want out," he requested. Once you are in the Mafia, the only way out was to die, so this was a serious request. Honoring his promise, the Mafia don released Art from his blood obligation.

Art moved out West and started a trucking company specializing in hauling mobile homes and trailers. He had a reputation as a man not to be trifled with but that was honest and true to his word. He married and raised a family as well as ran his business even after his health started going. When I met him he looked like hell, but there was still that look in his eye that hinted at his past. He passed away several years ago and I have always been grateful that I had the privilege to know him.

Johnny One-Foot

There were still several more hours before dark as John made the decision to take a short cut on his way home. The road was not as good as the main highway. Some of it was not even gravel, but it shaved almost 60 miles off of the trip and it would get him to his next destination, Mt. Hood, an hour earlier. He had been up since 4:30 am which was early even for him and had spent the day climbing on Mt. Rainier. He hadn't summited the 4300 meter (14,000 foot) peak but had spent the bulk of the day at an altitude of over 2800 meters (9,000 feet) and his body could feel it. He had been out of the military where he had been a Green Beret medic for almost 2 years but had still managed to keep in top physical condition.

The setting sun and the winding gravel road mesmerized him and he succumbed to the seductive power of his fatigue. He never felt himself fall asleep or the car plunge off of the steep embankment that bordered the road. The first realization of danger was the rush of adrenaline that jolted him awake, as the car was in mid-air. He braced for the inevitable impact and the sickening crunch of steel buckling and branches cracking. When he came to it was almost dark. He was wedged into the floor of the car, his right ankle was on fire and he was bleeding from several cuts on his body. Having had extensive medical training he immediately attempted to diagnose what was wrong with his body. He couldn't move his right foot; it was wedged inside of a 64-centimeter (2 foot) piece of tree root that had punched through the windshield. He found his sleeping bag and fell into a fitful sleep as the gloom turned to dark, resigning himself to a night trapped in his car.

John was not one to panic. His situation wasn't so bad, he thought. The road was just above him, only a mere 50 meters (150 feet) up the embankment and other cars would certainly pass by and see the wreckage. When he didn't arrive at work someone would inform the authorities and a search party would find him in short order. He couldn't see much beyond the interior of the car but he could hear the rush of water not far away. His ankle was broken for sure. The pain was just too intense for anything else, he just didn't know how much it was bleeding or how much blood he had lost. There was little sleep for him that first night. He lay awake worrying that a bear might discover him and have him for a late night snack. He thought of Mary, his fiancé and childhood sweetheart, and how she must feel when he was reported missing.

The dawn finally arrived and with it he could finally see his true dilemma. His right foot and ankle were wedged beneath the dash of his car by a large tree root that had penetrated the windshield of the vehicle. His ankle might be broken as he could see a great deal of swelling. The ankle was swollen to the size of a cantaloupe but was not bleeding. He was stuck in a very awkward position that caused him to have to twist his torso in order to lie on his side. The twisting was already causing his back to ache in addition to the ankle. He was very thirsty but had nothing to drink in the car. He had planned to stop when he hit the highway and pick up some sodas.

Survival training served John well. He surveyed his situation and saw his pack in the back seat of the overturned car. He couldn't reach it with his hand but he found a broken tree branch and used it to pull his pack to him. Inside he didn't find any water, but he found an apple that he devoured with relish. "Best apple I've ever eaten," he thought to himself. This quenched his thirst somewhat but if he were down here long he would still need to get some water. He could hear water very close by and he twisted the other way to see the rushing stream no more than 3 meters (12 ft) away. How could he get at the water? It was too far away to reach. They say that necessity is the mother of invention, and this was one of those circumstances where it ended up meaning life or death. John took several articles of clothing from his pack and tied them together to form a rope of clothes. With the help of his stick, he used it like a fishing pole and was able to throw the end of the clothes rope into the stream and then wring it out in his mouth to get at the moisture. He could survive now and it would only be a matter of time before he was found.

Meanwhile, John had made himself as comfortable as possible. He wedged the pack beneath his leg so that gravity was not pulling downward on the swollen ankle. He squeezed a little more water into his mouth and drifted off into a pain-filled, uneasy sleep. He awakened with a startle at the sound of tires on gravel. He could hear a car coming down the gravel road above him. Finally, he would be saved. They had to see where his car went off of the side and all it would take would be a glance over the side of the embankment to see his overturned car. To his dismay, he heard the car come to the curve in the road but just keep going. His heart sank; they didn't see his tracks. Next time he would yell with all of his might to attract attention. He checked the car horn and the lights, but the battery must have become unattached in the crash because neither worked. He drifted off again and it wasn't until almost dusk that he heard the sound of another vehicle approaching. John is a big guy and has a booming voice but despite all of the yelling he could muster, the sound was drowned out by the rushing stream next to him. The car kept on going and John felt despair.

Night passed into the next day and each time a vehicle passed by he would fall a little deeper into depression realizing that he might actually die there. The ankle was now a dull throb that never abated and was superseded by gnawing hunger pangs that shot through his body at regular intervals. In addition his back was cramping from the twist that it was in all of the time. He dismantled the inside of the car to create tools that might be helpful to him. The crash had occurred on a Sunday night and he had been trapped for 5 days now but he felt sure that someone would find him. The weekend was coming and more cars would be on the road. He took the rear view mirror and would use it to signal to cars, surely one of them would see his signal.

By now a full-blown search was underway that used all of the modern techniques available at that time. Several times John thought that he heard airplanes going overhead but he could never be sure. His brother actually drove the road that John had crashed on but there wasn't a trace of where John's car had gone off so no one bothered to look over the embankment. Because the station wagon was upside down the car was similar in color to the surrounding rocks and boulders so it was not visible from the air. After 10 days the Highway Patrol called off the search and Mary, his fiancé, began to lose all hope of ever seeing John again.

He had awakened from a troubled sleep one morning to the sound of birds chirping outside the car and something inside of him had changed. All of the pains were still there but the hunger had abated somewhat. He thought clearly for the first time in days and he decided right then and there that there was only one person in the world who could get him out of this situation. It was he. He had to find a way out of there or he would die for sure. The infection or starvation would eventually kill him. He surveyed his situation anew. If he could only free his foot, he could climb up the embankment and flag a passing car. But how could he free his foot? He contemplated cutting it off but thought there must be a little more palatable solution. Still, the decision that it would be better to lose the foot than his life gave him a certain serenity that allowed him to move on.

The next day John located the tire iron that had been in the trunk. He pulled it to him with his trusty stick and began to sharpen it on one of the flat rocks nearby. If nothing else he would be able to hack off his foot with it. The tire iron just bounced off of the tree root when he jabbed at it. He needed leverage but there was nothing in the car with which to hit the tire iron. He used his suitcase to pull in a large stone that he used as a hammer. With the first strike he felt the iron bite into the root. Within a few hours, he had freed the foot and the pain of the blood returning to the foot could not mask his exuberation at being free. Even in his weakened state, he dragged himself up to the edge of the gravel road in 1 hour. His luck finally changed and he hadn't been waiting by the road for more than 30 minutes when a dump truck came around the bend. He flagged down the truck and was rescued.

He was taken to the hospital where they had to remove his foot and ankle midway down his calf. He had been trapped in the car for 16 days and had lost 12 kilos (25 lb). John was just happy to be alive and reunited with Mary. She never thought she would see him again, and their reunion was full of emotion.

John adapted to life as an amputee with ease. Nothing was as bad as what he had been through. He went on to participate in many competitive events, including Nordic skiing and triathlons. John became a vice president of several corporations that dealt with medical devices. He and Mary have 2 daughters who are grown. He even was on the "To Tell the Truth" show back in the 1970s as the guy who had survived 16 days trapped in a car. I met John while skiing and we have stayed friends ever since.

What is it about a person that causes them to not give up when others would have succumbed? I don't know exactly but I think that it has to do with faith, with that inner something that no one can quantify or catalogue. John has it and to meet him today, you would never know that this man had experienced such trauma. Life is sweet. Even the bad times have their place.

The Raft Trip Boys

Every year for the past 14 years I have had the dubious privilege of going white water rafting with a group of guys. These are the greatest guys I know. Most of them are Vietnam Vets who lost legs in the war but one is a motorcycle victim like myself. One is not even an official amputee but nearly got his arm blown off so he qualifies. We raft the rivers of California over a weekend in the spring when the water is flowing and the weather is pleasant. Or so it would seem.

We have rafted in the snow with the water temperature nearly freezing, in the rain, and the boiling sun. One year, we skipped rafting and went land sailing, a sport that takes place on the dried up lakebeds of Nevada called playas. After having to take one of the participants to the hospital for a broken collarbone, we opted once again for the relative safety of the water. The trip that actually resulted in the most injuries never even made it to the river. We met at one of the guy's houses to pack up but after multiple beers we opted to just hang out at his pool for the weekend. The resulting falls and near drowning at the pool were more severe than any injuries sustained on even our class V rivers. It just seems like every time we get together we have to celebrate our lives so much that we come close to losing them.

We have had some legitimate rafting adventures, however. We rafted the Tuolumne River in Central California 2 years in a row. This river comes out of the Sierra Nevada Mountains just north of Yosemite National Park and runs through a narrow gorge that has no access to it until you arrive at the take-out. This was a 2-day trip and we camped half way through. The second day started out macho enough with some class III rapids. We were feeling pretty competent since it was too early to have had anything to drink yet, and we were all strong despite our disabilities. We even had a guide who was in an oar boat with the 2 less experienced rafters. I was in the lead raft with

7 other men full of testosterone. As we cruised down the rapids we knew that there was a big class V coming up. We were so overconfident that we didn't even get out to scout the rapids and we just paddled on.

As we rounded a bend in the river, the roar of crashing water caused us all to stop our babbling and pay attention. Up ahead we could only see the water disappear in a haze of mist. We started paddling hard to get into the middle of the entry to the hole that was as big as a house. I am not exaggerating. This hole was enormous, so much so that as we entered it the 5-meter (16-ft) raft ended up almost vertical pointing down into the frothing center of the enormous abyss. I was in the front and was paddling for all I was worth because I did not want to end up in the water. We headed up the other side of the hole and all of us were paddling for all we were worth and just as we were about to crest the top of the hole I felt the raft shudder. I tried to dig my paddle into the water, but all I got was air since I was almost perpendicular to the water at that point. I fell over backward and was only stopped by running into the steersman at the back of the boat. Somehow the raft made it up over the far edge of the hole, and we were free of the sucking vortex. We pulled off into an eddy where we could rest and watch the guide oar boat attempt the hole.

Keep in mind that the oarsman on the other boat was our professional guide, so he was supposed to know more than we did. In the boat with him was Chris who weighs about 140 kilos (300 pounds) of mostly muscle and Herman who lost both legs in Vietnam and even with the legs only weighed about 70 kilos (150 pounds). As the guide hit the hole, the raft was not square as it entered. The high side of the raft had Herman and the low side down in the hole had Chris. We could see the guide try to correct by digging in with the high side oar but all he got was air. The next thing we saw was the raft disappearing into the enormous whirlpool and then Herman came shooting into the air. I kid you not; he flew out of the hole and landed at least 10-meters (30 ft) from the hole where we retrieved him. Then we saw the guide go floating by and we figured we would catch him further downstream. Next came Chris who was entangled by the ropes that we lashed our gear onto the raft with. He was holding onto the raft for dear life and it took 2 of us pulling with all of our might to get him onto the raft. As he flopped onto the bottom of the raft I looked up to see the front of our raft enter a class III hole that we also barely survived.

This was the last time we attempted the Tuolumne since we all did have jobs and families that depended on our surviving our outings. I do have to tell a Herman story though. I had the honor of getting to make prostheses for Herman on several occasions and there is a story of his previous prosthetist that I must relate. Herman had always identified heavily with his time in Vietnam; some would say that he never really came home. He is an extremely active guy who does everything for himself despite the fact that he has no legs. Therefore, it is critical for him to have prostheses that function and don't hurt. Apparently, he was having difficulties with getting a good fit from his previous prosthetist and in frustration he paid them a visit. Herman also has an unhealthy fascination with firearms and so in order to prove a point he sneaked into the back door of the prosthetic facility. He took out his 45-caliber handgun and held it to the router, a piece of equipment that is unique to the prosthetic profession. He held their router hostage until they reimbursed him for the bandages that he had used to treat his skin breakdown that he felt was their responsibility. Herman was not to be trifled with.

Like I said these are the greatest guys I know. I have gotten to share moments with each of them over the last 14 years and their candor has helped me on numerous occasions. We still get together every spring, but our thirst for danger now revolves around watching action sports instead of participating in them. This year we plan to go sailing, a seemingly innocent sport, but I am sure that by the end of the adventure there will be stories to tell.

CHAPTER 12

Resources for Amputees

Unlike when I lost my leg 30 years ago, today there are a multitude of organizations that provide help and support for amputees. They range from sports-oriented groups to gatherings of amputees that offer support for emotional adjustment. I am listing all of the organizations that I have been able to find through my research, but I am sure that it doesn't represent all of the groups that exist. The best place to find support is through the Internet. There are numerous sites that provide information on whatever you may have an interest in. Another source of information is your prosthetist; they are usually aware of and can contact a local amputee support group in your area.

Support Groups

The Amputee Coalition of America (ACA) is undoubtedly the best organization in the United States for information about amputees. Whether you need a referral for a support group or wish to purchase a publication, you will find help from these dedicated people.

Amputee Coalition of America
900 East Hill Avenue, Suite 285
Knoxville, TN 37915-2568
(888) 267-5669 or (865) 524-8772 (local)
Fax: (865) 525-7917
www.amputee-coalition.org

Email Listings for the ACA

ACA Membership	membership@amputee-coalition.org
ACA Marketplace	sales@amputee-coalition.org
Annual Conference	meeting@amputee-coalition.org
*in*Motion Magazine	inmotion@amputee-coalition.org
*in*Motion Editor	editor@amputee-coalition.org
*in*Motion Advertising	stracy@amputee-coalition.org
biofit Program	biofitinfo@amputee-coalition.org

Youth Activities Program	yapinfo@amputee-coalition.org
Parent ListServ	parentlistserv@amputee-coalition.org
Youth ListServ	youthlistserv@amputee-coalition.org

The ACA maintains chapters and affiliations with Amputee Support Groups in 39 states and 7 countries. They offer peer counseling as well as information about local services that are available for amputees. Many of the Support Groups are run by amputees and are not necessarily a substitute for legitimate counseling by trained professionals if that is what you require. However, they will provide the best, most honest feedback about life as an amputee and the resources available. These listings can be found at www.amputee-coalition.org/npn_group_list.html.

Other Resources for Amputees

American Amputee Foundation (AAF)
PO Box 250218
Little Rock, AR 72225
(501) 666-2523
Fax: (501) 666-8367
www.americanamputee.org
info@americanamputee.org

The AAF is a referral source for amputees that helps connect relevant organizations with those in need. It has contacts to prosthetic and orthotic providers as well as sports organizations. They also can provide peer counseling and assist with financial support.

Disabled Sports USA
451 Hungerford Drive, Suite 100
Rockville, MD 20850
(301) 217-0960
Fax: (301) 217-0968
www.dsusa.org

DSUSA is the organization in the United States that has representation on the U.S. Olympic committee that sanctions skiing competitions. They have chapters around the United States and sponsor competitive and recreational ski events.

National Amputee Golf Association
11 Walnut Hill Rd
Amherst, NH 03031-1228
(800) 633-6242
Fax: (603) 672-2987
www.nagagolf.org
info@nagagolf.org

The National Amputee Golf Association is an organization that provides golf opportunities for amputees. They sponsor tournaments and gatherings that I understand are a lot of fun. It also provides a forum for amputees to learn about adaptive prosthetic devices that allow full participation in the sport.

National Sports Center for the Disabled
PO Box 1290
Winter Park, CO 80482
(970) 726-1540
Fax: (970) 726-4112
www.nscd.org
info@nscd.org

This organization is the premier competitive program for selection to the Disabled U.S. Ski team. They provide programs geared toward the competitive racer. There are also recreational programs as well.

Wheelchair Sports, USA
1668 320th Way
Earlham, IA 50072
(515) 833-2450
www.wsusa.org
wsusa@aol.com

This organization provides opportunities for amputees who cannot participate in ambulatory activities and need to use a wheelchair. They sponsor various sports, especially wheelchair basketball on a national and international level.

American Academy of Orthotists and Prosthetists
526 King Street, Suite 201
Alexandria, VA 22314
(703) 836-0788
Fax: (703) 836-0737
www.oandp.org

This is the professional organization for orthotists and prosthetists. They provide literature and training for the industry and have information about new products and innovations.

American Orthotic & Prosthetic Association
American Board for Certification
National Commission on Orthotics and Prosthetics Education
330 Carlyle St. Suite 200
Alexandria, VA 22314
(571) 431-0876
Fax: (571) 431-0899
www.aopanet.org
academy@oandp.org

This triad of organizations is the certifying and industry supporting body for the prosthetics profession. They certify prosthetists and can tell you which practitioners have maintained their credentials as well as the requirements to become certified.

Orthotic and Prosthetic Assistance Fund
1666 K Street, Suite 440
Washington, DC 20006
(202) 223-8878
www.opfund.org
opaf@opfund.org

The Orthotic and Prosthetic Assistance Fund aims to enable individuals who are served by the orthotics and prosthetics community to enjoy the rewards of personal achievement, physical fitness, and social interaction. This organization was established to provide financial support for the Paralympics.

ActiveAmp.com
P.O. Box 9315
Wilmington, DE 19809
(302) 683-0997
www.ActiveAmp.com or www.Ampsoccer.org
rgh@activeamp.org

An amputee who was frustrated by the lack of available information about activities for amputees founded this organization. It is a clearinghouse for information with an emphasis on amputee soccer (played on crutches).

Amputee Resource Foundation of America, Inc
2324 Wildwood Trail, Suite F104
Minnetonka, MN 55305
(612) 812-7875
www.amputeeresource.org
info@amputeeresource.org

The Amputee Resource Foundation of America, Inc is an organization dedicated to providing outreach and information to the amputee community. It is the oldest information resource for amputees on the Internet.

Stumps R Us
2109 Skycrest Drive, #1
Walnut Creek, CA 94595
(925) 952-4408
www.stumps.org
DanSorkin@stumps.org

This amputee support group that was founded by amputee Dan Sorkin in the San Francisco Bay area. It uses humor and information to help amputees get back into life.

Limbless Association
Rehabilitation Centre
Roehampton Lane
London
SW15 5PR
20 8788 1777 Ext. 21
Fax: 20 8788 3444
www.limbless-association.org
enquiries@limbless-association.org

This British organization provides support and information for amputees. They publish a monthly newsletter that is full of interesting data for amputees.

Resources for Children
(courtesy of Mary Free Bed Hospital)

Parent/Peer Resources

Family Resource Center on Disabilities
20 E. Jackson Blvd., Room 300
Chicago, IL 60604
(312) 939-3513
TDD: (312) 939-3519
Fax: (312) 939-7297
www.Ameritech.net/users/frcdptiil/index.html
frcdptiil@ameritech.net

This organization is focused on organizing an effective parent advocacy group as well as assisting parents on how to move the bureaucracy.

National Peer Network
Attn: NPN
900 East Hill Avenue, Suite 285
Knoxville, TN 37915-2568
(888) 267- 5669 or (865) 524-8772
Fax: (865) 525-7917
www.amputee-coalition.org/npn_about.html

Like the Family Resource Center, this is a parent advocacy group that focuses on parental involvement through being assertive.

Other Children's Resources

Mary Free Bed Hospital
Center for Limb Differences
235 Wealthy Street SE
Grand Rapids, MI 49503
(800) 528-8989
www.mfbrc.com
info@maryfreebed.com

This is probably the single best source for information and programs for children with amputations. The resource and library center has full time staff that can provide contact information that is up to date and reliable.

Association of Children's Prosthetic-Orthotic Clinics
6300 N. River Road, Suite 727
Rosemont, IL 60018-4226
(847) 384-4226
Fax: (847) 823-0536
www.acpoc.org
king@aaos.org

This organization provides information and resources to assist in finding facilities that specialize in the care and treatment of child amputees.

Cancer Information Service of the National Cancer Institute
NCI Public Inquiries Office
6116 Executive Boulevard, MSC8332
Bethesda MD 20892-8322
(800) 422-6237
TTY: (800) 332-8615
www.nci.nih.gov

Candlelighters Childhood Cancer Foundation
National Office
PO Box 498
Kensington, MD 20895-0498
(800) 366-2223 or (301) 962-3520
Fax: (301) 962-3521
www.candlelighters.org
staff@candlelighters.org

Federation for Children With Special Needs
1135 Tremont Street, Suite 420
Boston, MA 02120
(617) 236-7210
Fax: (617) 572-2094
www.fcsn.org
fcsninfo@fcsn.org

National Information Center for Children and Youth With Disabilities
PO Box 1492
Washington, DC 20013
(800) 695-0285
Fax: (202) 884-8441
www.nichcy.org
nichcy@aed.org

Camps and Other Recreational Organizations
Wilderness Inquiry
808 14th Avenue SE
Minneapolis, MN 55414-1516
(800) 728-0791 or (612) 676-9400
Fax: (612) 676-9401
www.wildernessinquiry.org
info@wildernessinquiry.org

American Camping Association
5000 State Road 67 North
Martinsville, IN 46151
(765) 342-8456
Fax: (765) 342-2065
www.acacamps.org

Children's Oncology Camping Association International
(515) 243-6239
www.coca-intl.org/list.html

Easter Seals
230 West Monroe Street, Suite 1800
Chicago, IL 60606
(800) 221-6287 or (312) 726-6200
TTY: (312) 726-4258
Fax: (312) 726-1494
www.easter-seals.org

Other Internet Sites

Alberta Amputee Sport & Recreation Association
www.aasra.ab.ca

International Child Amputee Network
www.child-amputee.net

Amputee Coalition of America's National Limb Loss Information Center
www.amputee-coalition.org/nllic_about.html

Closing the Gap: Computer Technology in Special Education and Rehabilitation
www.closingthegap.com

Internet Resource for Special Children
www.irsc.org

LimbDifferences.org: An online resource for families and friends of children with limb differences
www.limbdifferences.org

OntheOtherHand.org: Information for families and children with hand differences
www.ontheotherhand.org

Reach. The Association for Children With Hand or Arm Deficiency
www.reach.org.uk

Superhands Network
www.superhands.us

Superkids (archive only site)
www.super-kids.org

Linda's one-armed web site, ADL tips with photos
www.toysrbob.com/onearm

Bibliography and Resource Books

Before beginning this project I bought and read all of the books listed below. I gained knowledge from every one of them and am in debt to all of the authors for their work. All of the information that I have written about has been printed before, somewhere in the below listed books and pamphlets. Most of them can be obtained through the library maintained by the Amputee Coalition of America, and I also used the library at Northwestern University's Prosthetic and Orthotic Center.

Adil JR. *Accessible Gardening for People With Physical Disabilities. A Guide to Methods, Tools, and Plants*. Bethesda, MD: Woodbine Press; 1994.

Barn Builders: A Peer Support Network of Farmers and Ranchers with Disabilities and Caregivers. West Lafayette, IN: Purdue University; 1999.

DiLillo J. *Soccer My Life, My Passion*. Lincoln, IL: Author; 2001.

Eugstrom B, Van de Ven C. *Therapy for Amputees*. Toronto, Canada: Churchill Livingstone; 1986.

Goldman J, Cagan A. *Up and Running: The Jami Goldman Story*. New York, NY: Pocket Books; 2001.

Kostuik JP, Gillesie R. *Amputation Surgery and Rehabilitation, The Toronto Experience*. New York, NY: Churchill Livingstone Press; 1981.

Lusardi MM, Nielsen C. *Orthotics and Prosthetics in Rehabilitation*. Boston, MA: Butterworth Heinemann Press; 2000.

Madruga L. *One Step at a Time: A Young Woman's Inspiring Struggle to Walk Again*. Lincoln, NE: 2000 Universe.com Inc.; 1979.

Marshall SC. *One Can Do It: A How to Guide for the Physically Handicapped*. Highland City, FL: Rainbow Books Inc; 1994.

Martin P. *One Man's Leg: A Memoir*. Pine Brook, NY: Greycore Press; 2002.

Maxfield G. *The Novel Approach to Sexuality and Disability*. Sparks, NV: Author; 1996.

May BJ. *Amputations and Prosthetics: A Case Study Approach*. Philadelphia, PA: F.A. Davis Company; 1996.

Mesch G, Ellis PM. *Physical Therapy Management of Lower Extremity Amputations*. Rockville, MD: Aspen Publishers, Inc; 1986.

Mooney RL. *The Handbook: Information for New Upper Extremity Amputees, Their Families and Friends*. Lomita, CA: Mutual Amputee Aid Foundation; 1995.

Ott K, Serlin K, Serlin D, Mihm S. *Artificial Parts, Practical Lives, Modern Histories of Prosthetics*. New York, NY: New York University Press; 2002.

Ratto LL. *Coping With a Physically Challenged Brother or Sister.* New York, NY: The Rosen Publishing Group; 1992.

Ratto LL. *Coping With Being Physically Challenged.* New York, NY: Rosen Publishing Group, Inc; 1991.

Rehabilitation Institute of Chicago. *Lower Extremity Amputation.* 2nd ed. Gaithersburg, MD: Aspen Publications; 1992.

Sabolich J, Sabolich S. *You're Not Alone.* Oklahoma City, OK: Authors; 2001.

Sanders GT. *Lower Limb Amputations: A Guide to Rehabilitation.* Philadelphia, PA: F.A. Davis Company; 1986.

Seymour R. *Prosthetics and Orthotics, Lower Limb and Spinal.* Syracuse, NY: Lippincott, Williams, and Wilkins; 2002.

Wallace CS. *Challenged by Amputation, Embracing a New Life.* Carmichael, CA: Inclusion Concepts Publishing House; 1995.

Wilson A B. *A Primer on Limb Prosthetics.* Springfield, IL: Charles C. Thomas, Publisher, LTD; 1998.

Winchell E. *Coping With Limb Loss: A Practical guide to Living with Amputation for You and Your Family/Sound Information from an Emotional Recovery Counselor Who Has Herself Experienced Amputation.* Garden City Park, NY: Avery Publishing Group; 1995.

Books and Pamphlets

Area Child Amputee Center at Mary Free Bed Hospital and Rehabilitation Center of Grand Rapids. *Adolescents With Limb Differences, A Handbook for Adolescents and their Families.* Grand Rapids, MI: Author; 1996-2002.

Area Child Amputee Center at Mary Free Bed Hospital and Rehabilitation Center of Grand Rapids. *Children With Hand Differences, A Guide for Families.* Grand Rapids, MI: Author; 1996-2002.

Area Child Amputee Center at Mary Free Bed Hospital and Rehabilitation Center of Grand Rapids. *Children With Limb Loss: A Handbook for Families (birth-5 years).* Grand Rapids, MI: Author; 1996-2002.

Area Child Amputee Center at Mary Free Bed Hospital and Rehabilitation Center of Grand Rapids. *Children With Limb Loss, A Handbook for Families (6-12 years).* Grand Rapids, MI: Author; 1996-2002.

Area Child Amputee Center at Mary Free Bed Hospital and Rehabilitation Center of Grand Rapids. *Children With Limb Loss, A Handbook for Teachers.* Grand Rapids, MI: Author; 1996-2002.

Broyles N. *For the New Amputee.* Chapel Hill, NC: Duke University Medical Center; 1991.

Kicken T, Edwards M, Miceli N. *Below-Knee Amputation. A Guide for Rehabilitation.* Chicago, IL: Rehabilitation Institute of Chicago; 2002.

Shurr DG. *Patient Care Booklet for Above Knee Amputees.* Washington, DC: American Academy of Orthotists and Prosthetists, Inc; 1998.

Swagman A, Novotny M. *Upper-Limb Prosthetic Options for Kids: Below Elbow.* Grand Rapids, MI: Area Child Amputee Center of Mary Free Bed Hospital and Rehabilitation Center of Grand Rapids; 1992.

United Amputee Services Association, Inc. *A Survivor's Guide For the Recent Amputee.* Winter Park, FL: Author; 1992.

Vellendahl JE. *Patient Care Booklet for Below-Knee Amputees.* Washington, DC: American Academy of Orthotists and Prosthetists, Inc; 1998.

Wilke HH. *Reflections on Managing Disability.* Nashville, TN: Amputee Coalition of America; 1984.

Wilke HH. *Using Everything You've Got.* Nashville, TN: Amputee Coalition of America; 1977.

Index